Lippincott's Pathophysiology Series

ENDOCRINE PATHOPHYSIOLOGY

William M. Kettyle, M.D.
Assistant Clinical Professor of Medicine
    Harvard Medical School
      and
    Harvard–MIT Division of Health Sciences and Technology
Associate Medical Director
    Medical Department
Massachusetts Institute of Technology
Cambridge, Massachusetts

Ronald A. Arky, M.D.
Charles S. Davidson Professor of Medicine
    Harvard Medical School
Master, Francis Weld Peabody Society
    Harvard Medical School
Boston, Massachusetts

D0713918

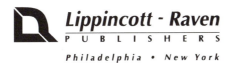

Lippincott - Raven
PUBLISHERS

Philadelphia • New York

Acquisitions Editor: Richard Winters
Developmental Editor: Delois Patterson
Manufacturing Manager: Kevin Watt
Supervising Editor: Liane Carita
Production Service: P. M. Gordon Associates, Inc.
Cover Illustrator: Patricia Gast
Medical Illustrator: Christopher Burke
Indexer: Katherine Pitcoff
Compositor: Maryland Composition
Printer: Courier/Kendallville

Printed in the United States of America

9 8 7 6 5 4 3 2 1

Library of Congress Cataloging-in-Publication Data

Kettyle, William M.
   Endocrine pathophysiology / William M. Kettyle, Ronald A. Arky.
      p.   cm.—(Lippincott's pathophysiology series)
   Includes bibliographical references and indexes.
   ISBN 0-397-51376-3
   1. Endocrine glands—Pathophysiology.   2. Endocrine glands—
Diseases.   I. Arky, Ronald A., 1929–   . II. Title. III. Series.
   [DNLM: 1. Endocrine Diseases—physiopathology.   2. Endocrine
System—physiopathology.   WK 140 K43e 1998]
RC649.K48   1998
616.4′07—dc21
DNLM/DLC
For Library of Congress   98-18408
                                                        CIP

Lippincott's Pathophysiology Series

ENDOCRINE PATHOPHYSIOLOGY

For our students, past, present, and future.

To Cindy, Elizabeth, and David

for their sustaining contributions of wisdom, humor, and love.

William M. Kettyle, M.D.

To Marie

Ronald A. Arky, M.D.

CONTENTS

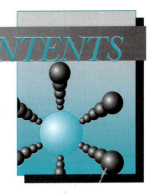

CONTENTS

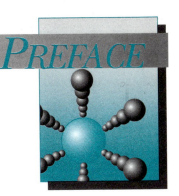

Problem solving is the essence of clinical medicine. Teaching effective clinical problem-solving skills traditionally has been left for clinical clerkships and house staff and fellowship training. Many medical schools, however, now add case-based teaching exercises, patterned on problem-based learning initiatives in other professional schools, to the preclinical curriculum to introduce and develop clinical reasoning skills earlier in the educational process. An additional benefit is that the introduction of clinical material often provides a more interesting and dynamic framework for the basic science curriculum. The New Pathway learning initiative at Harvard Medical School relies on the use of clinical cases discussed in small tutorial groups. These tutorials usually are coordinated with a lecture and a laboratory session on the topic.

This volume, *Endocrine Pathophysiology*, captures some of the dynamics of the problem-based learning process in a form that students can use on their own to supplement and reinforce classroom materials. Many of the cases included are patterned on problem-based learning materials that we have developed as part of The New Pathway. Some of the materials were prepared as part of the Endocrinology Curriculum of the Health Sciences and Technology Division, a joint program of medical education of Harvard University and the Massachusetts Institute of Technology.

Each chapter is designed to parallel some aspects of the case-based learning process and is organized as follows:

- Anatomy
- Chemistry
- Hormone action
- Regulation of function
- Overview of pathophysiology
- Clinically useful tests
- Clinical cases with discussion
- Key Points and Concepts
- Suggested Reading

As the cases unfold and evolve, the reader sees the dynamic aspects of both the disease process and the effects of treatment. Several cases are presented in each chapter in an effort to illustrate additional aspects of the pathophysiology of the gland system covered.

This volume is not a comprehensive reference for the endocrinologist. Rather, it provides a clinically driven tour of the field for medical students through practitioners whose aim is to master the basics of endocrinology in a manner that nurtures problem-solving skills through the case-based method.

ACKNOWLEDGMENTS

In addition to expressing our appreciation to our students for their encouragement and support, we would like to acknowledge the input and help of the following colleagues:

Maria Bachini, Christine Coughlin, and Kari Knutson provided administrative support.

Erin Yeh, M.D., and Ricardo Sanchez, M.D., provided some of the radiographic images.

Mark Laufgraben, M.D., and Howard Heller, M.D., reviewed parts of the manuscript.

At Lippincott–Raven, Richard Winters provided the stimulus to start this project and Delois Patterson and Diana Andrews shepherded the manuscript into a finished volume. Christopher Burke rendered our sketches into many of the illustrations.

Thank you.

Introduction: Problem-Based Learning

Problem solving is an integral part of clinical medicine. Renowned physicians gain their reputations through adroitly employing problem-solving skills in the diagnosis and treatment of their patients. Until recently, teaching the principles of problem solving to medical students was left until the clinical clerkships of the third and fourth years of the curriculum. Since the early 1980s, however, a number of medical schools have elected to introduce these concepts at the beginning of the student's course of study, and to challenge the first-year medical student with "real-life," patient-based problems to introduce the basic sciences. Medical educators have borrowed from the experiences of other professional schools, which regard the educational process as more than a series of lectures and laboratory exercises; rather, it is seen as an opportunity to develop the student's skills of inquiry, to foster the concept of teamwork both in the learning process and in the resolution of problems, and to enable the student to practice integrating these skills in the diagnosis and treatment of patients.

As long ago as 1899, the famous clinical educator William Osler recognized that the complexity of medicine was such that no faculty could teach, nor any student learn, everything. He urged that the major amounts of time allocated by the faculty for lectures and by the students for memorizing the lecture materials be curtailed and replaced with time for independent study, observation, and reasoning. He urged that medical educators focus on "how students learn" rather than "what the student should learn." The attraction to problem-based learning by an increasing number of medical educators in the past decade has been generated by the same concerns as Osler's.

The retention of new knowledge depends on its integration with existing knowledge and its organization and reorganization into long-term memory. Problem-centered learning should stimulate students to integrate, use, and reuse newly learned information in the context of a patient's problem. One major objective of the problem-based approach is to ensure that the medical student acquires a strong, comprehensive knowledge of the basic sciences and that through repetitive encounters he or she can retain, retrieve, enhance, and use that knowledge to resolve clinical problems. A second goal of patient-centered learning is to develop and nurture the clinical reasoning skills of the student—that is, to apply the scientific method in the approach to the patient. These skills include the ability to evaluate the patient's problem, decide what is wrong, and then make some decisions about the appropriate diagnostic tests and treatments the patient needs. These processes are analogous to the hypothesis–deduction approach of the bench researcher. Problem-centered learning is intended to activate the student intellectually and to connect the acquisition of new knowledge to active experiences of the student.

This text is designed for medical students who desire to apply the principles of problem-based learning in the acquisition of a background in the pathophysiology of the endocrine system. Vital to this process is a working understanding of the basic principles of anatomy, physiology, biochemistry, genetics, immunology, and pathology. In most instances, medical students will be in their second year of training and will already have been introduced to these fundamentals. The process of recall will be activated as the student notes cues that are implicit or explicit in the clinical problem used to exemplify specific pathophysiologic phenomena. This activated old knowledge is assimilated into the context of the new information imparted by the case and should stimulate the learner to analyze the issues and questions posed by the problem. From this analysis, the student formulates a "learning agenda." The learning agenda, in turn, is the impetus for seeking other sources, references, or consultants who will provide new knowledge. Knowledge acquired from these resources in the effort to resolve a clinical problem is then structured in the memory of the student in an organized fashion so as to be more accessible for future use.

Educators refer to the collation and analysis of new information from several sources coupled with prior knowledge as the *comparison phase* in the problem-solving process. In the world of clinical medicine, this is analogous to the differential diagnosis. Using both inductive and deductive reasoning, the learner limits the possibilities (the *inference phase* of the educational theorist) and arrives at the working diagnosis. Employing diagnostic studies or therapeutic trials, the clinician then assesses the approach that was used and applies the *evaluation phase* of the educator.

In the classroom, problem-based learning is commonly a small-group exercise facilitated by a tutor or member of the faculty. The problem consists of a set of phenomena or clinical events that are real and for which students attempt to define the mechanisms or abnormal physiologic principles that account for these phenomena. The learning agenda is compiled by the entire group of students, who then assign responsibilities for specific items of the agenda to individual students. This text is designed to individualize this learning process. To assist in the recall process, we have included a brief review of applicable anatomic, biochemical, and physiologic information before the presentation of the clinical problem. The individual student is expected to develop a learning agenda and to seek further references or consult other resources when that is deemed necessary. When appropriate, the text will assist the learner's analysis of the history, physical examination, laboratory, and other observations to develop a differential diagnosis.

OBJECTIVES OF PROBLEM-BASED LEARNING

- To stimulate the student to become an active learner as well as a life-long learner
- To develop the skills required for critical analysis of a problem
- To acquire the abilities needed to develop a personal learning agenda
- To become familiar with the multiple resources available for active learning and the abilities to use all of those resources
- To acquire the ability to collate new information with prior knowledge in a logical, systematic manner to resolve clinical problems
- To recognize the means of assessing the learning process of the individual and to evaluate its effectiveness

SUGGESTED READING

Bond D, Feletti G, eds. The Challenge of Problem Based Learning. London: Kogan Page.

Schmidt HG. Problem-based learning: rationale and description. J Med Educ 17: 11–16, 1983.

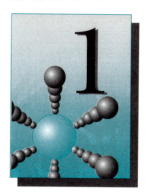

Introduction to Endocrinology

Endocrinology is the study of hormones, the glands that produce them, and the tissues that are affected by them. Hormones are chemical messengers that transmit information to cells and control a wide variety of physiologic functions. The endocrine system has many similarities to the nervous system, and these two control systems overlap and are integrated at many levels.

In the classic model of an endocrine system, a hormone produced by an endocrine gland is released into the circulation. Once released, the hormone is available to bind to a specific receptor on the target cell or tissue. The hormone then triggers a series of reactions that result in some change or modification of cellular function. An expanded view of endocrinology also takes into consideration the concept of chemical messengers that act locally on the cells that produce the substance (autocrine) and on neighboring cells (paracrine) (Table 1-1).

THE FUNCTIONS OF HORMONES

A large range of physiologic functions is controlled by endocrine systems. Table 1-2 outlines the principal functions of the endocrine system. A number of hormones act to stabilize acute challenges to the body's internal environment. Alterations in fluid balance, blood pressure, glucose availability, or electrolyte concentration trigger hormonal systems that respond rapidly—within minutes—and are vital to maintenance of the proper internal milieu. Hormones also control storage and utilization of energy by the body. Energy storage processes permit the organism to withstand sudden increases in the demand for energy and to survive periods when metabolic fuel is scarce.

The processes of growth and development also are controlled by endocrine systems. Hormones control the expression of the genetically programmed capacity of tissues to enlarge and mature. Growth hormone, sex steroid hormones, insulin, and thyroid hormone all are vital for normal growth and development.

TABLE 1-1. *HORMONE SYSTEMS*		
SYSTEM	**DESCRIPTION**	**EXAMPLES**
Endocrine	Hormone is released from a gland and circulates to a distant target tissue.	Thyroid hormone, cortisol, sex hormones, growth hormone.
Paracrine	Hormone acts on neighboring cells.	Pancreatic islet D cells influence the output of insulin from the B cell and glucagon from the A cell.
Autocrine	Hormone acts on the cell in which it is produced.	Insulin regulates its own production in the B cell of the pancreatic islets.

Hormones also are essential for reproduction. They regulate sexual development as well as the production and maturation of gametes. In addition, many aspects of male and female sexual behavior are under endocrine control. Interestingly, males and females have essentially the same hormones. Quantitative differences, differences in the secretory patterns and genetic programming, and differentiation of target cells account for sexual dimorphism.

Most hormones have multiple effects. One example is testosterone: among other effects, it plays a role in embryogenesis, in the growth and development of the male urogenital tract, in spermatogenesis, in hair growth, in the synthesis of red blood cells, in the development and maintenance of muscle, and in the enlargement of the prostate that occurs with normal aging. Although testosterone acts in very different ways, upon a variety of tissues, its diverse effects are modulated by a single molecular mechanism, a mechanism that is similar for each of the steroid hormones (see Mechanism of Action later in this chapter).

Most important homeostatic processes, especially those vital to survival, are controlled by multiple hormones. Examples of vital functions that are influenced by a complex series of hormonally mediated control mechanisms include the maintenance of electrolyte balance, blood pressure, and plasma glucose. Hormone systems, often working in an antagonistic or push–pull fashion, control vital functions in a way that allows for precise tuning of the controlled process and for

TABLE 1-2. *PRINCIPAL FUNCTIONS OF THE ENDOCRINE SYSTEM*	
FUNCTION	**EXAMPLES**
Maintenance of internal milieu and control of production, utilization, and storage of energy	Insulin, glucagon, cortisol, growth hormone, thyroid hormone, aldosterone, antidiuretic hormone
Growth and development	Growth hormone, sex hormones
Reproduction	Sex hormones

speedy adaptation to changes in the environment, availability of energy, or stressful events. Insulin lowers blood glucose, whereas glucagon sets in motion a number of processes that increase glucose availability. Cortisol, growth hormone, and catecholamines also are actively involved in the control of blood glucose. The input of several hormones, each of which in some way defends the concentration of glucose in the bloodstream, provides a redundancy of function—a safety net— that ensures maintenance of the internal environment.

In some processes hormones play a permissive role. They are not the driving or major controlling factor, but their presence is required for normal function. Thyroid hormone and cortisol, for example, are not the dominant controlling hormones in growth and development, but they are required for the process to be completed. Without thyroid hormone and cortisol, growth is retarded.

Feedback control of hormone production and secretion is a key aspect of endocrine function. Feedback loops have been identified for virtually all hormone systems. Although these loops usually are negative, with the end product of the system inhibiting its own production, there are instances of positive feedback in which the end product of the system stimulates further output, thereby magnifying the function of the system. The mechanisms of control in endocrine systems may involve cations (e.g., calcium controlling parathyroid hormone secretion), metabolic substrate (e.g., glucose controlling insulin and glucagon), tonicity or extracellular fluid volume (e.g., plasma osmolality controlling vasopressin [ADH] or effective blood volume controlling renin and aldosterone), or the hormonal product of a gland (e.g., T_3 controlling thyroid function). Complicated loops of feedback control with multiple input and modulation points have been described (Fig. 1-1). One of the most exten-

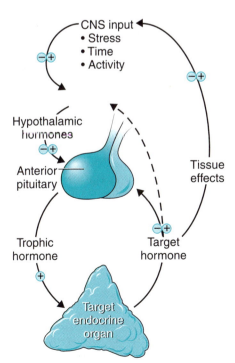

Figure 1-1. Feedback control. Hypothalamic–pituitary–target gland systems allow CNS input to control target gland function with additional modulation of axis function at several sites.

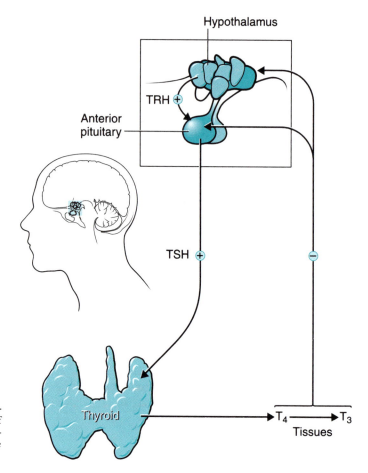

Figure 1-2. Control of thyroid function. T_3, the metabolically active form of thyroid hormone, controls its own production by negative feedback at both the pituitary and hypothalamic levels.

sively studied feedback mechanisms is the control of thyroid gland function (Fig. 1-2). T_3, the metabolically active form of thyroid hormone, exquisitely controls its own production (see Chapters 2 and 4).

Evaluation of clinical problems in endocrinology requires a thorough understanding of feedback loops and control systems. To understand the mechanism of thyroid hormone deficiency, the level of thyroid hormone (thyroxine [T_4]) must be correlated with the level of the hormone that controls the thyroid, thyroid-stimulating hormone (TSH). Concomitant assessment of the dynamics of the controlled parameter–controlling hormone pair is required to determine whether there is any endocrine pathology. Abnormalities in the relationship between the hormone and the controlled parameter are the basis for clinical endocrine disorders.

CHEMICAL STRUCTURE OF HORMONES

Virtually all hormones are variations of one of two chemical types. They conform to either the *peptide–amino acid* derivative model or the *steroid–cholesterol* derivative model. Among the *peptide–amino acid* group are those derived from single amino acids (catecholamines, serotonin, and dopamine), the dipeptides (thyroxine [T$_4$] and triiodothyronine [T$_3$]), the small peptide group (thyrotropin-releasing hormone [TRH]), the intermediate-sized peptide group (insulin and glucagon), and the complex polypeptide group (luteinizing hormone [LH] and thyroid-stimulating hormone [TSH]).

There are two subclasses of *steroid–cholesterol* hormones: those secreted by the adrenal cortex and gonads with an intact steroid nucleus (e.g., cortisol, aldosterone, estrogen, testosterone) and those in which the B ring of the steroid is broken (e.g., vitamin D and its metabolites).

HORMONE SYNTHESIS, STORAGE, AND SECRETION

Hormones are synthesized in the same fashion by which corresponding substances are produced in nonendocrine tissues. Endocrine glands do not possess unique enzymatic or synthetic capacities; in fact, many peptide hormones can be produced by cells in the central nervous system, the gastrointestinal tract, or the placenta. Although hormones are not produced exclusively by endocrine glands of the classical definition, these organs do possess the mechanisms to manufacture large quantities of the hormone, the capacity to process hormonal precursors, and the apparatus to secrete the product when appropriately signaled.

The steps involved in the synthesis of polypeptide hormones are analogous to those in the production of other proteins. Through the transcription process, information flows from the gene or genes encoded to produce the hormone. After posttranscriptional processing, messenger RNA (mRNA) carries the template from the nucleus to the protein synthetic machinery, located on ribosomes in the cytoplasm. The protein or polypeptide molecule is produced on the ribosomes, enters the endoplasmic reticulum, and, after a series of posttranslational events, migrates through the Golgi apparatus. The polypeptide then is transferred to a secretory granule, where it is stored until the appropriate signal is received to release the contents of the granule. Many polypeptide hormones initially are produced as large molecules that are progressively shortened to form the active hormone. This activation process often occurs in the storage granules before release of the hormone, but it also may occur after secretion of the hormone. An example is insulin, which starts out as a large precursor molecule, pre-proinsulin; then is cleaved to a smaller molecule, proinsulin; and then is cleaved yet again to the active hormone molecule, insulin, before release. Polypeptides present in secretory vesicles are released by exocytosis, fusion of the vesicle with the plasma membrane, and release of the granule contents into the extracellular space.

Steroid hormones also are synthesized in the organelles of the cytoplasm. The building block is cholesterol, which is modified through sequential, enzyme-controlled hydroxylations and cleavages of various carbon–carbon bonds to form the active products. The trophic hormones that stimulate steroid hormone synthesis—adrenocorticotrophic hormone (ACTH), follicle-stimulating hormone (FSH), and luteinizing hormone (LH)—act at the membrane of the adrenal cortical or gonadal cell. The presence of the trophic hormone activates adenylate cyclase, inducing an increase in cyclic adenosine monophosphate (cAMP), which, in turn, activates the enzymes that catalyze the production of steroid hormones. Steroid hormones usually are not stored in the cells that produce them and pass through the cell membrane, leaving the cell rapidly after synthesis.

Hormonal secretion may occur in different patterns or formats. Many glands secrete small amounts of hormone on a regular basis, a *basal rate*. Superimposed on this basal secretion rate are stimulation and suppression of hormone production and release. Hormone levels in the bloodstream usually are determined predominantly by the rate of secretion and not by the clearance or inactivation of the hormone. The rate of release of a hormone usually is determined by the rate of synthesis. Typically, only limited quantities of a hormone are stored. The pituitary and the endocrine pancreas usually have a small reserve of polypeptide hormones stored in storage granules, and more hormone is produced when stimulation occurs. Two important exceptions to the concept of limited storage and production on demand are the relatively large stores of thyroid hormone in the thyroid gland and vitamin D in fat, which provide protection against iodine deficiency and lack of exposure to sunlight, respectively.

Another important aspect of endocrine function is the phenomenon of disuse atrophy, the loss of function that follows long-term suppression of a gland. Like unused muscles, unstimulated endocrine glands develop functional and anatomic atrophy. The suppression of function that leads to atrophy may be the result of exogenous hormone or of autonomous, endogenous overproduction of hormone. Although in almost all cases recovery from the atrophy of prolonged suppression does occur, it may take several months and usually is associated with a period of relative hypofunction. This period of hypofunction provides the signal or stimulation that results in recovery of normal function.

TRANSPORT OF HORMONES

Once secreted, most water-soluble hormones—the hormones of the *peptide–amino acid* group—circulate in solution in plasma. Thyroid hormone and the less soluble steroid hormones are transported in the plasma by carrier proteins. Binding sites on the carrier protein hold hormone molecules in a dynamic equilibrium with a small amount of free or unbound hormone. In most cases it is only the free or unbound hormone that enters or interacts with the target cell. The transport protein acts as a reservoir that provides a ready source of hormone. As unbound hormone enters a cell, it is replaced by hormone newly released from the transport protein. A new equilibrium is established that eventually results in the secretion of more hormone, triggered by the feedback mechanism controlling the system. Albumin and transthyretin (formerly called pre-albumin) are general, nonspecific, transport proteins, whereas thyroxine-binding globulin (TBG), corticosteroid-binding globulin (CBG), and testosterone-estrogen–binding globulin (sex hormone–binding globulin [SHBG]) are specific transport proteins that have unique binding sites with high affinity for the hormone transported.

The clearance rate of a protein-bound hormone is related to the binding affinity of that hormone with the associated transport protein: the higher the affinity, the slower the rate of clearance. Hormones usually are cleared by hepatic metabolism or renal excretion of the free or unbound hormone molecule, or both. Most transport proteins have binding capacities that exceed the physiologic concentrations of the hormone that they bind. Thus, when hormones are overproduced or administered in pharmacologic amounts, enormous quantities of the hormone are potentially available.

Protein hormones typically have relatively short half-lives, ranging from a few minutes to about an hour. In addition to receptor binding, which takes the hormone out of circulation, enzyme systems rapidly inactivate protein hormones, resulting in the ability of protein hormones to transmit information in an agile, responsive fashion. Thyroid hormone and steroid hormones, largely as a result of their association with binding proteins, have longer half-lives. In addition, it is important to note that the effects of a hormone on the target tissue usually far outlast the presence of the hormone in the circulation. The thyroid hormone released in response to stimulation of the thyroid by TSH has an effect that lasts for days beyond the life of the triggering hormone, TSH.

Hormones are present in the circulation in very low concentrations. Levels of the steroid and thyroid hormones are measured in picomolar and micromolar amounts. Several adaptive mechanisms ensure that hormones have an impact on the target tissue or tissues, in spite of low concentration. Target tissues contain specific receptors that bind hormone avidly. In most cases, the principal target cells of a hormone contain a high concentration of receptors for that hormone. These receptors usually have a high affinity for the hormone and catch hormone molecules as they flow by in the circulation. Hormones can also be directed to a specific target by delivery within a limited circulation. Glucagon, for example, is released from the pancreas into the portal circulation, which results in relatively high concentrations of the hormone being presented to glucagon receptors in the liver. A third mechanism by which hormonal action is focused is direct diffusion of a hormone into adjacent cells, a paracrine effect. Testosterone produced by the Leydig cells of the testes is available in high concentration to promote spermatogenesis in the nearby seminiferous tubules. Local formation of a hormone from a circulating precursor or prohormone provides yet another means to magnify or focus the action of a hormone. Thyroxine (T_4), the precursor, is deiodinated to triiodothyronine (T_3), the active hormone, in several tissues, resulting in high levels of the active form of the hormone at sites of deiodination.

MECHANISM OF ACTION

It is misleading to say that any one hormone has a single target tissue. Most hormones affect many tissues either directly or indirectly, through interactions with other hormones.

The mechanism of action of most hormones of the *peptide–amino acid* group begins with binding to a receptor at the outer cell membrane. These receptors typically are transmembrane proteins that have an external ligand, or hormone-binding domain. A transmembrane portion of the receptor may span the membrane one or more times, anchoring the receptor molecule. The intracellular component of the receptor is the effector portion of the molecule and initiates transduction of the signal when the receptor is occupied. A number of intracellular signaling strategies have been identified, including activation of protein kinases, activation of G-protein complexes, and ion channel opening, among others. The signal transduction process may involve a second or intracellular messenger, such as cAMP. A wide variety of intracellular processes is controlled by these transmembrane receptor systems.

The principal site of action of the *steroid–cholesterol* hormones (steroid hormones, vitamin D) and thyroid hormone is in the nucleus of the cell. These hormones do not require specific carrier proteins to cross the plasma or nuclear membrane. High-affinity receptor molecules for each of these hormones are present in the nucleus. The C-terminal end of the protein receptor molecule is the hormone binding site. The central part of the receptor molecule is configured to bind to DNA. The presence of the hormone on the receptor results in a modification of gene transcription. The modification may involve inhibition or facilitation of gene transcription, but, in any case, the hormonal signal results in some change in protein production in the target cell.

HORMONAL BIORHYTHMS

Many hormones are secreted in a rhythmic fashion that results in marked variation in hormone concentration in the plasma (Fig. 1-3). Some hormonal levels fluctuate so widely during the day that the nadir or the peak values, if maintained, would produce adverse effects. For example, in healthy people, cortisol levels may range from 80 to 690 nmol/L (3 to 25 μg/dL) during the course of a day, but if the peak value were to be maintained throughout the day, the individual soon would develop the symptoms and signs of hypercortisolism. Similarly, if the nadir value were to persist throughout the day, signs and symptoms of hypocortisolism would become apparent. Pathological states may exist in which the level of a hormone appears to be "normal" yet is inappropriate for that time of the day or environment.

The rhythms of hormonal secretion vary widely in interval and pattern. Hormone levels may change over minutes to hours (e.g., the pulsatile secretion of LH and insulin), over the course of a day (e.g., the circadian fluxes in the ACTH–cortisol axis), over weeks (e.g., the menstrual cycle), or over longer periods (e.g., the seasonal variability in thyroxine production). In some cases these patterns of secretion are age-dependent, as exemplified by the sleep-associated

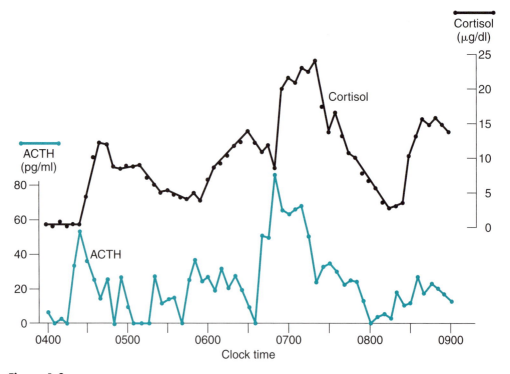

Figure 1-3. Diurnal hormonal rhythm. Between 4:30 a.m. and 6 a.m., ACTH is episodically secreted, resulting in a rise in cortisol levels that peaks at about 7 a.m.

surge of gonadotropic secretion during puberty, a pattern not seen in older adults or in young children. Hormonal rhythmicity may be neurogenic, related to environmental factors, or, in some cases, modulated by the involved hormones themselves.

ENDOCRINE PATHOLOGY

Most clinical endocrine disorders are the result of hyperfunction, hypofunction, or some anatomic abnormality of the gland or target tissue. In some cases—a pituitary tumor, for example—all three pathologic mechanisms may be present in the same patient. A pituitary adenoma is an anatomic abnormality that can overproduce a hormone, while at the same time the pressure of the adenoma on adjacent normal tissue also may result in hypofunction of other cells in the anterior pituitary.

Syndromes of endocrine hypofunction may result from a variety of mechanisms. Autoimmune destruction of glandular tissue is one of the most common causes of endocrine hypofunction. Insulin-dependent diabetes mellitus, primary hypothyroidism, primary adrenal insufficiency, and primary hypogonadism are all associated with autoantibodies and other destructive processes that characterize autoimmune syndromes. Other processes such as granulomatous diseases (e.g., sarcoidosis), infectious agents (e.g., tuberculosis), neoplastic disease (e.g., metastatic carcinoma of the lung), or infarction (e.g., after postpartum hemorrhage) may destroy or partially disrupt endocrine organs, causing subnormal hormone production and a hypofunctional clinical syndrome. Destruction by chemotherapeutic agents, radiation, and surgical removal are other causes of hormone deficiency states. Even this extensive list of causes, however, cannot explain some deficiency syndromes.

A gene mutation that alters the structure of a hormone usually affects its function and results in a hypofunctional clinical state. At times target tissues may not respond to a hormone, and a "hormone-resistant" state is present. Syndromes of resistance exist for a number of hormones and involve abnormalities in the cell surface and intracellular receptors, defective metabolism of the hormone within the cell, or other defects in signal transduction that are vital for the action of the hormone. Resistance to hormone function may be hereditary and genetically determined (e.g., pseudohypoparathyroidism) or acquired (e.g., insulin resistance of obesity) or both (e.g., type 2 diabetes). Most resistance states are diagnosed by the presence of excessive quantities of the hormone in the blood because, in most feedback systems, the failure of hormone action leads to increased hormone production. Because of this compensatory mechanism, many resistant states go unrecognized until the compensatory mechanisms fail.

The mechanisms for hyperfunctional endocrine states also are variable and, in some instances, difficult to define. Circulating substances may simulate a hormone by binding to its receptor, initiating the intracellular sequence of events that the true hormone would effect and producing a hyperfunctional state. For example, the overactivity of the thyroid seen in Graves' disease results from thyroid-stimulating immunoglobulins that occupy thyroid-stimulating hormone (TSH) receptors on the surface of thyroid cells and produce a hyperfunctional state. Endocrine or nonendocrine tumors that overproduce hormones or hormone-like substances also may induce a clinical picture of a hyperfunctional state. In these instances normal homeostatic controls are either absent or abnormally reset. Thus, when the level of parathyroid hormone (PTH) is elevated in the face of a high serum calcium concentration, parathyroid function is abnormal because the level of parathyroid hormone is not appropriately suppressed by the high calcium concentration. Hyperplasia or neoplasia of one or more of the parathyroid glands must be suspected. Hormone excess states also may be the result of exogenous sources or of inappropriate release of preformed hormone, as in thyroiditis. Viral infection or autoimmune inflammation of the thyroid may result in the inappropriate release of stored thyroid hormone and a transient syndrome of thyroid hormone excess.

EVALUATION OF ENDOCRINE DISORDERS

Abnormalities of endocrine function usually are suggested in the clinical presentation of the patient. Characteristic patterns of symptoms and physical findings often point to the presence of too much or too little hormone or to some anatomic abnormality related to endocrine function. Definitive diagnosis, however, requires a careful correlation of the patient's history and physical findings with laboratory data. Single hormone levels occasionally are diagnostic but can at times be misleading. Paired hormonal values (e.g., cortisol and ACTH; T_4 and TSH) or a similar matching of hormone and controlled parameter (e.g., calcium and PTH) often leads to the appropriate diagnosis (Fig. 1-4). In some circumstances, testing that stimulates or suppresses the endocrine system in question is necessary to provide a clear diagnosis. Syndromes of hormonal deficiency may require a stimulation test, whereas syndromes of hormonal excess may require a suppression test. Other testing strategies include evaluation of hormonal secretion or of a controlled parameter over time. A 24-hour urine collection with measurement of a hormone or its metabolite may give valuable information about hormone secretion over a 24-hour period and provide more information than can be obtained from a single blood level or series of blood levels. Similarly, the percentage of hemoglobin that is glycosylated can give an indication of the average

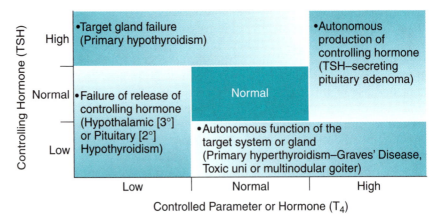

Figure 1-4. Relation between controlling hormone and controlled parameter. Analysis of paired hormone values, target gland hormone, and controlling hormone or parameter provides valuable diagnostic information. Thyroid axis abnormalities are presented in parentheses.

glucose levels during the preceding 3-month period and can be very helpful in assessing diabetic control.

After a hormonal imbalance or abnormality is found, further information can be generated with imaging studies. Nuclear scans, ultrasound studies, X-rays, computed tomographic (CT) scans, and magnetic resonance imaging (MRI) studies all can provide valuable information but must be interpreted in light of the clinical and laboratory findings. Incidental, nonfunctional anatomic variations and abnormalities may not represent significant pathology and can be misleading.

TREATMENT OF ENDOCRINE ABNORMALITIES

Syndromes of hormonal deficiency usually are treated with replacement of the missing hormone. Some hormonal replacement regimens are relatively simple. When thyroid function is deficient, synthetic or animal-derived thyroid hormone can be taken orally, once a day, with excellent restoration of normal function. Insulin replacement is more complex, for several reasons. Because insulin is a protein hormone, the oral route of administration is not effective. Insulin, like other ingested proteins, is digested, and although the amino acids may be nutritious, the structure and function of the hormone are lost. Injection of insulin into subcutaneous tissues avoids the digestive process and allows insulin to enter the circulation. The short half-life of insulin and other protein hormones, however, presents additional obstacles. Frequent injections and the use of preparations of insulin that are released more slowly are ways in which insulin can be replaced in a manner that mimics normal physiology. In addition, although the dose of thyroid hormone may vary from patient to patient, the daily dose usually is the same over long periods of time. Careful control of diabetes with insulin, however, requires frequent testing of the blood glucose concentration and adjustment of each dose of insulin based on glucose level, meal plans, and anticipated activity.

In some cases of hypofunction, only the end product of an axis needs to be replaced, whereas in others the function of nearly the entire axis must be replaced. When anterior pituitary failure is caused by hypothalamic failure, replacement of adrenal cortical and thyroid function can be done easily with oral preparations of the target gland hormones, cortisol and thyroid hormone. Replacement of hormones for reproductive function can be done in several ways, depending on the needs of the patient and the nature of the lesion. End-organ gonadal steroid replacement is relatively easy and provides many aspects of normal sexual development and function. Gonadal development and fertility, however, require replacement of pituitary gonadotropins or hypothalamic releasing factors, a much more complicated project. If a child has hypothalamic or pituitary failure, growth hormone can be replaced with human growth hormone produced by recombinant technology to help the child achieve normal stature, but frequent injections of this protein hormone are required.

Syndromes of hormonal excess usually require one or more of four basic modes of therapy. *Inhibition of hormone synthesis and secretion* may control some hyperfunctional syndromes. Antithyroid drugs, for example, inhibit the production of thyroid hormone and lead to significant clinical improvement. They do not, however, cure the underlying condition. Other strategies include using *medications that block or inhibit the effectiveness of a hormone.* Spironolactone, for example, can be used to correct some of the effects of excess aldosterone. *Destruction of the overactive gland by surgery or radiation* is another therapeutic possibility for some conditions of hyperfunction. In some cases, one condition is traded for another—overfunction becomes underfunction. Because in many cases underfunction is more easily treated, this approach may be appropriate. In still other cases, *removal or destruction of the abnormal portion of a gland* may allow normal function to return. After removal of an adrenal adenoma, for example, normal adrenal cortical function usually returns after a number of months.

KEY POINTS AND CONCEPTS

- Hormones control a large range of physiologic functions:
    - Maintenance of internal milieu, including energy storage and utilization.
    - Growth and development.
    - Reproduction.
- Most hormones have multiple effects.
- Most vital physiologic functions are influenced by multiple hormones.
- Most hormones are one of two chemical types:
    - *Peptide–amino acid* molecules are water soluble and have relatively short half-lives.
    - *Steroid–cholesterol* derived molecules have longer half-lives and are, in some cases, transported in the circulation by carrier proteins.
- Mechanisms of hormone action:
    - *Peptide–amino acid* hormones usually work at the cell surface, binding to receptors that signal changes in cytoplasmic reactions and processes that result in the effect of the hormone.
    - *Steroid–cholesterol* derived hormones and thyroid hormone have their principal effect at the cell nucleus, where they alter transcription of DNA; this alteration results in changes in protein synthesis that bring about the hormonal effect.
- Hormone synthesis and release are tightly controlled and usually are subject to both stimulation and suppression.
- Prolonged suppression of gland function may result in significant anatomic and functional atrophy.
- Syndromes of hormonal deficiency:
    - Often are the result of autoimmune or other destructive processes.
    - May require a stimulation test for definitive diagnosis.
    - Usually are treated with replacement of the missing hormone.
- Syndromes of hormonal excess:
    - Often are the result of an abnormal stimulating factor or a defect in the normal control or set-point of secretion.
    - May require a suppression test for definitive diagnosis.
    - Usually are treated with medications that inhibit hormone synthesis or block hormone effect, surgery, or radiation therapy.

SUGGESTED READING

Cheatham B, Kahn CR. Insulin action and the insulin signaling network. Endocrine Reviews 16:117–142, 1995.

Guillemin R. Peptides in the brain: the new endocrinology of the neuron. Science 202:390–402, 1978 (Nobel Lecture).

Schally AV. Aspects of hypothalamic regulation of the pituitary gland: its implications for the control of reproductive processes. Science 202:18–28, 1978 (Nobel Lecture).

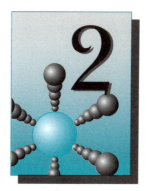

Neuroendocrinology and the Anterior Pituitary

Although the hypothalamus and the pituitary are anatomically separate and of different embryologic origin, they function as an integrated unit. For most of the 20th century, the anterior pituitary, also referred to as the adenohypophysis, was thought of as the "master gland." At least seven hormones affecting multiple target glands and tissues are produced and released by the anterior pituitary. Since the 1960s, further understanding of the anatomy and physiology of the hypothalamus and anterior pituitary has clearly demonstrated that the anterior pituitary is not the master gland at all, but a target gland. Hormones made by and secreted from the neurons of the hypothalamus stimulate or inhibit the release of the hormones of the anterior pituitary. In many instances the anterior pituitary appears to modulate and amplify the signals originating from hypothalamic centers. The neurohypophyseal unit controls a wide variety of functions—thyroid, adrenal, reproductive, and growth and development. The posterior pituitary, although closely related anatomically and functionally, is discussed separately in Chapter 3, and thyroid, reproductive, and adrenal function are discussed in the chapters covering these separate target gland systems. An overview of the anatomy of the hypothalamus and pituitary is shown in Figure 2-1.

HYPOTHALAMUS

Many of the neurons of the hypothalamus are capable of secreting chemical messengers or hormones. Although these molecules may have local effects in the hypothalamus, the major function of these transmitting agents is either to stimulate or to inhibit the release of hormones from the anterior pituitary.

The hormones of the hypothalamus fall into two categories—releasing and release-inhibiting, depending on whether their action leads to the release or the inhibition of the release of the designated pituitary hormone. All of the known hormones of the hypothalamus are polypeptides, with the exception of dopamine,

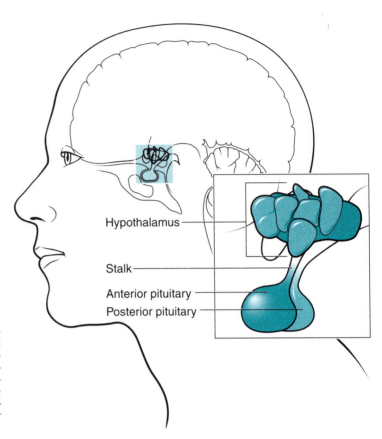

Figure 2-1. The anatomy of the hypothalamus and pituitary. A lateral view of the head at the midline reveals the hypothalamus and the anterior and posterior pituitary. The pituitary is housed in a recess of the sphenoid bone called the sella turcica. The stalk connects the posterior pituitary to the hypothalamus.

which is a modified tyrosine molecule. The hypothalamic peptides are synthesized as larger prohormone molecules with leader sequences that facilitate their transfer to the endoplasmic reticulum for further processing before release. Prohormone synthesis occurs in the cell bodies of the hypothalamic neurons. The prohormone is cleaved to form the active hormone in granules that travel down the axons of the synthesizing neurons. Release occurs in pulses into the perivascular space of a fenestrated capillary system, which leads to the delivery of the releasing or release-inhibiting hormone to the anterior pituitary below. The hormones of the hypothalamus and anterior pituitary are listed in Table 2-1.

The hypothalamus and the pituitary are located outside the blood–brain barrier, enabling them to sense and to respond to circulating levels of hormones and other blood constituents. In addition, the hormone products of the hypothalamus and pituitary can easily enter the circulatory system.

The chemistry and function of the hormones of the hypothalamus are listed in Table 2-2. These hormones are carried to the anterior pituitary by a vascular portal system. This portal system is very much like the portal system that brings nutrients, drugs, and other molecules from the absorptive surfaces of the gastrointestinal tract to the liver for first-pass hepatic processing. Capillaries in the hypothalamus lead to a plexus of veins that proceeds down the pituitary stalk. The venous system branches into another capillary bed to provide a relatively high concentration of the hypothalamic hormones to the cells of the anterior pituitary. Most of the hypothalamic hor-

TABLE 2-1. *HORMONES OF THE HYPOTHALAMUS AND ANTERIOR PITUITARY*

HORMONE	ABBREVIATION	OTHER NAMES
Thyrotropin-releasing hormone	TRH	
Corticotropin-releasing hormone	CRH	
Growth hormone–releasing hormone	GHRH	
Gonadotropin-releasing hormone	GnRH	LHRH
Somatostatin	SS	
Dopamine	DA	PIF, Prolactin release inhibitory factor
Arginine vasopressin	AVP	ADH, antidiuretic hormone
Thyroid-stimulating hormone	TSH	Thyrotropin
Adrenocorticotrophic hormone	ACTH	
Prolactin	PRL	
Growth hormone	GH	Somatotrophic hormone
Follicle-stimulating hormone	FSH	
Luteinizing hormone	LH	

TABLE 2-2. *THE CHEMISTRY AND FUNCTION OF THE HORMONES OF THE HYPOTHALAMUS*

HORMONE	CHEMISTRY	TARGET—ANTERIOR PITUITARY HORMONE
Stimulators		
TRH	Tripeptide	TSH Prolactin*
CRH	Polypeptide	ACTH
GHRH	Polypeptide	Growth hormone
GnRH	Polypeptide	LH, FSH
ADH	Polypeptide	ACTH*
Suppressors		
SS	Polypeptide	Growth hormone
DA	Modified amino acid	Prolactin

* Uncertain physiologic significance.
ACTH, adrenocorticotrophic hormone; ADH, antidiuretic hormone; CRH, corticotropin–releasing hormone; DA, dopamine; FSH, follicle-stimulating hormone; GHRH, growth hormone–releasing hormone; GnRH, gonadotropin-releasing hormone; LH, luteinizing hormone; SS, somatostatin; TRH, thyrotropin-releasing hormone; TSH, thyroid-stimulating hormone.

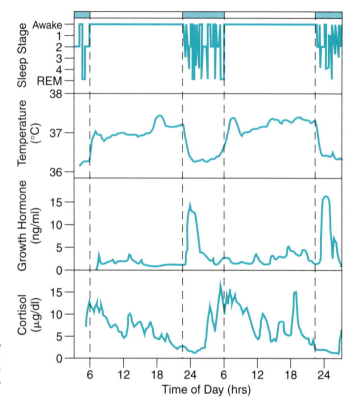

Figure 2-2. Circadian rhythm of pituitary hormone secretion. Growth hormone (GH) and ACTH, as well as other hormones, are secreted episodically in a pattern that is influenced by activity, sleep, and light.

mones are found in very low concentration in the peripheral circulation. Although the significance is unclear, a number of the releasing hormones of the hypothalamus also are found in other tissues, such as the brain, pancreas, and gastrointestinal tract.

The nuclei of the hypothalamus have multiple connections with the midbrain above. One of these centers, the supraoptic nucleus, also known as the suprachiasmatic nucleus, serves as an intrinsic pulse generator that provides an internal clock that appears to coordinate the rhythm of hormonal secretion. Light input from the optic system provides a mechanism for the effect ambient light has on certain aspects of hormonal secretion. Other brain centers provide information about sleep and other activities. Figure 2-2 correlates sleep stage with body temperature and the levels of growth hormone and cortisol.

ANTERIOR PITUITARY

The anterior pituitary, or hypophysis, is embryologically derived from Rathke's pouch. The cells of the future anterior pituitary migrate to their final location just under the hypothalamus. The posterior pituitary (see Chapter 3) is really an extension of the hypothalamus and is entirely of neural origin. The anterior and posterior pituitaries are housed in a well-protected recess of the sphenoid bone called the sella turcica (see Fig. 2-1). The pituitary stalk, which provides a connection between the hypothalamus above and the pituitary below, travels through a membrane referred to as the diaphragma sella. This membrane, which separates the pituitary fossa from the hypothalamus above, is an infolding of the meninges. Although it is not covered with meninges, the pituitary is bathed in cerebrospinal fluid (CSF), and the hormones of the anterior pituitary can be found in the cerebrospinal fluid. The stalk itself is largely made up of the axons of the cells of the posterior pituitary. These axons grouped together provide a structure for the portal venous plexus, which delivers hypothalamic hormones to the anterior pituitary. The contents of the sella turcica, the anterior and posterior pituitary, are surrounded by bone except at the superior aspect where the stalk and portal system enter the sella.

Just above the sella and beneath the hypothalamus is the optic chiasm. In the optic chiasm, nerve fibers from the nasal portion of the retina of each eye cross over to form the optic tracts. Pressure from a pituitary mass expanding within the bony confines of the sella turcica can cause dysfunction of the chiasm and result in altered peripheral vision, with a decrease in visual acuity in the fields of view served by the nasal retinae.

The six hormones of the anterior pituitary are secreted by five different cell types in the anterior pituitary (Table 2-3). Each of these five cell types appears to be derived from a common progenitor cell. The hormones of the anterior pituitary are all peptides. LH, FSH, and TSH are glycoproteins with two peptide chains, alpha and beta. The alpha subunit of each of these hormones is identical. Relatively small differences in the beta subunit sequence account for the marked differences in hormonal function. Both of the gonadotropins, LH and FSH, are secreted by the same cell line, the gonadotrophs (see Chapter 9).

Growth hormone, prolactin, and adrenocorticotrophic hormone (ACTH) are all single-stranded protein hormones. Although several of the hormones of the anterior pituitary may have local effects, the principal function of each appears to be on a specific target organ or tissue. Because of their rapid metabolism, all of the hormones of the hypothalamus and anterior pituitary have relatively short

TABLE 2-3. *THE HORMONES OF THE ANTERIOR PITUITARY*

HORMONE	CHEMISTRY	CELL OF ORIGIN	EFFECT
TSH	Glycoprotein	Thyrotroph	Stimulates growth and function of the thyroid gland
ACTH	Protein	Corticotroph	Stimulates growth and function of the adrenal cortex
PRL	Protein	Lactotroph	Prepares the breast for lactation, suppresses menstrual function
GH	Protein	Somatotrophs	Stimulates growth and development, multiple metabolic effects
FSH	Glycoprotein	Gonadotroph	Stimulates gonadal function
LH	Glycoprotein	Gonadotroph	Stimulates gonadal function

ACTH, adrenocorticotrophic hormone; FSH, follicle-stimulating hormone; GH, growth hormone; LH, luteinizing hormone; PRL, prolactin; TSH, thyroid-stimulating hormone.

plasma half-lives, usually less than 60 minutes. The kinetics of the effects on the target tissues, however, can be very variable and usually are much longer.

HORMONES THAT AFFECT THYROID GLAND FUNCTION: THE HYPOTHALAMIC–PITUITARY–THYROID AXIS

The function of the thyroid gland (see Chapter 4) is controlled by the hypothalamic–pituitary unit. TSH, which stimulates the synthesis and release of thyroid hormone from the thyroid gland, is released by the anterior pituitary in response to TRH. Feedback control of the hypothalamic–pituitary–thyroid axis is dramatically mediated by thyroid hormone modulation of TSH responsiveness to TRH (Fig. 2-3). The concentration of T_3, the principally active form of thyroid hormone, within the thyrotroph cells of the anterior pituitary controls the synthesis and release of TSH.

High levels of T_3, whether derived from the thyroid gland directly or from the monodeiodination of T_4 of any source, result in complete shutdown of TSH secretion. Low levels of thyroid hormone, resulting from thyroid gland disease or the effects of excessive antithyroid drug therapy, result in elevated TSH levels and a marked increase in the responsiveness of the thyrotroph to TRH. The effect of

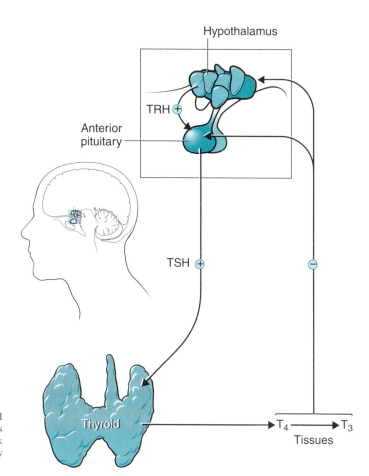

Figure 2-3. Control of thyroid gland function. Thyroid hormone controls its own production with negative feedback at both the hypothalamic and pituitary levels.

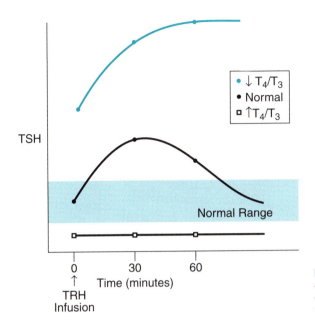

Figure 2-4. Modulation of TSH secretion. The level of circulating thyroid hormone modifies the secretion of TSH in response to the hypothalamic-releasing factor, TRH.

thyroid hormone on TSH secretion in response to TRH stimulation is shown in Figure 2-4. In addition to the modulating effects of thyroid hormone at the pituitary level, T_3 also has an inhibitory effect on TRH release from the hypothalamus.

Both the common alpha subunit and the specific beta subunit of the TSH molecule are synthesized by the thyrotroph. The subunits combine on the smooth endoplasmic reticulum to form the active TSH molecule. An inhibitory response element that binds T_3 inhibits gene transcription of both the alpha and beta subunits of TSH. TSH secretion is exquisitely controlled by the end product of the axis, T_3.

Although the physiologic significance is unclear, TRH also simulates prolactin secretion. The extrahypothalamic production of TRH seen in the cerebral cortex, spinal cord, pancreatic islets, and gastrointestinal tract is of unknown significance.

HORMONES THAT AFFECT ADRENAL CORTICAL FUNCTION: THE HYPOTHALAMIC–PITUITARY–ADRENAL AXIS

When released into the portal system, hypothalamic CRH stimulates the release of ACTH by the corticotrophs of the anterior pituitary. ACTH, in turn, stimulates the adrenal cortex to secrete cortisol (see Chapter 5). CRH is synthesized as a preprohormone in cells of the paraventricular nuclei of the hypothalamus. Release of CRH, with the resultant increase in ACTH and eventual increase in cortisol secretion, occurs in response to an intrinsic diurnal rhythm. In addition, the release of CRH and the cascade that follows can be stimulated by stress—both physical and emotional—by a mechanism that overrides the diurnal rhythm (Fig. 2-5). Cytokines, released as part of an inflammatory response, also can activate the

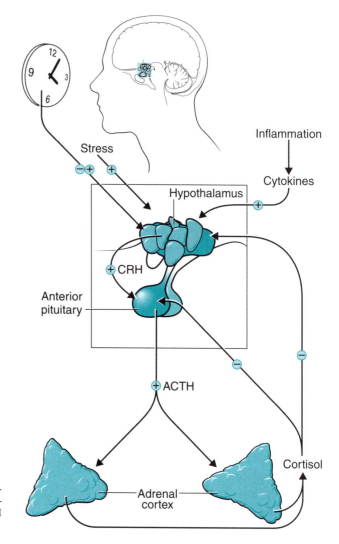

Figure 2-5. Control of adrenal cortical function. In addition to negative feedback by cortisol, multiple additional inputs control ACTH and cortisol secretion.

axis. Cortisol, the end product of the axis, inhibits the release of both CRH and ACTH.

ACTH is synthesized and secreted by the corticotrophs of the anterior pituitary in response to stimulation by CRH and also by AVP via the V_1 receptor (see Chapter 3). When engaged, the CRH receptor on the pituitary corticotroph cell activates a protein kinase system that results in the synthesis of the precursor molecule for ACTH. The physiologic significance of AVP stimulation of ACTH secretion is unclear and probably is not important in normal daily life. Severe stress, especially volume depletion or hemorrhage, leads to increased AVP production, which may further enhance the release of ACTH. The resulting increase in cortisol secretion could aid in the correction of the volume depletion that stimulated the AVP response.

Pro-opiomelanocortin (POMC), the precursor molecule for ACTH, is produced by the corticotrophs. This 268-amino-acid protein undergoes significant posttranscriptional processing that results in production of the active 39-amino-acid ACTH molecule and beta-lipoprotein, an 89-amino-acid molecule of uncertain significance. In some settings, this same precursor molecule can be split into melanocyte-stimulating hormone (MSH) and beta-endorphin. The synthesis of POMC and the eventual release of ACTH are inhibited by cortisol, which negatively regulates POMC gene transcription. As with other protein hormones, the plasma half-life of ACTH is very short, measured in minutes. Although it may have effects on other tissues, the principal effect of ACTH is to stimulate adrenal cortical production of cortisol and, when levels are high, the production of aldosterone as well.

GROWTH HORMONE AND ITS CONTROLLING HORMONES

Growth hormone (GH) is a 191-amino-acid peptide hormone that plays a critical role in growth and development from birth to young adulthood. In addition to stimulating the growth of bone and some soft tissues, GH has multiple metabolic effects. Although prenatal growth and development do not depend on GH, the effect of GH on growth and development is seen dramatically in children with syndromes of excess or deficiency. Excess GH before puberty and before epiphyseal closure results in gigantism, the growth of a giant. After puberty, when epiphyseal growth plates have closed and bones can no longer elongate, excess GH results in acromegaly, a syndrome marked by widening of bones, thickening of soft tissues, and multiple metabolic changes. Many of the metabolic effects of GH can be categorized as counteracting the effects of insulin. In other areas, the effects of GH are similar to those of insulin.

In children, deficiency or ineffectiveness of growth hormone results in short stature. The role of growth hormone in fully grown adults is uncertain. A clear deficiency syndrome for postpubertal adults has not been definitely established.

Growth hormone synthesis and release are under the control of both a stimulating hormone, growth hormone–releasing hormone (GHRH) and a release-inhibiting hormone, somatostatin (SS) (Fig. 2-6). Both the stimulating and suppressing hormones act via a protein kinase system, which controls the transcription of the GH gene. In addition, transcription and eventual release of GH are inhibited by one of its metabolic products, insulin-like growth factor-1 (IGF-1).

GH secretion is pulsatile and is highest in the first few hours after falling asleep. Exercise, stress—both physical and emotional—and the ingestion of certain foods stimulate GH secretion. Once secreted into the circulation, GH is available to bind to GH receptors in the liver and other tissues. In the liver, GH stimulates the production of IGF-1, also known as somatomedin C. This protein is released into the circulation and causes differentiation and clonal expansion of chondrocytes, especially those in epiphyseal growth plates. In other tissues, an insulin-like effect is seen with increased glucose and amino acid uptake. IGF-1 appears, in addition, to provide negative feedback on the secretion of growth hormone.

PROLACTIN

Prolactin (PRL) is a protein hormone that is similar chemically to GH. It is composed of 199 amino acids with three intramolecular disulfide bonds. Although the physiologic function of prolactin in males is unclear, in the female, prolactin plays a role in pubertal breast development and prepares the breast for postpar-

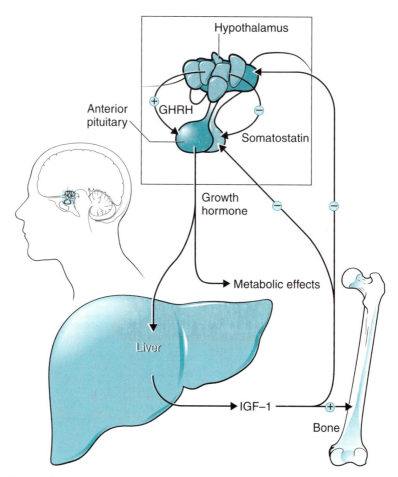

Figure 2-6. Control of growth hormone secretion. Hypothalamic stimulatory and inhibiting hormones regulate GH secretion. GH regulates growth via stimulation of the production of IGF-1 by the liver. In addition, GH has multiple metabolic effects.

tum lactation. Prolactin alone does not stimulate milk production; a developed breast and estrogen also must be present.

Unlike other hormones of the anterior pituitary, PRL is under tonic inhibition by its principal controlling hormone, dopamine (DA). When dopamine is present on the cell surface receptor of the lactotroph cells, PRL secretion is inhibited. When dopamine levels are lowered (for example, by suckling) via a spinal afferent pathway, prolactin secretion increases (Fig. 2-7). Any disruption in DA production, secretion, or delivery through the portal system may result in elevation of PRL levels.

Estrogen promotes the production of PRL via an estrogen response element on the PRL gene. The high levels seen in pregnancy and the low levels seen in children, males, and postmenopausal females are mediated by this estrogen response element that controls prolactin synthesis.

Although the physiologic significance is unclear, TRH and vasoactive intestinal polypeptide (VIP) also stimulate prolactin production. Prolactin affects men-

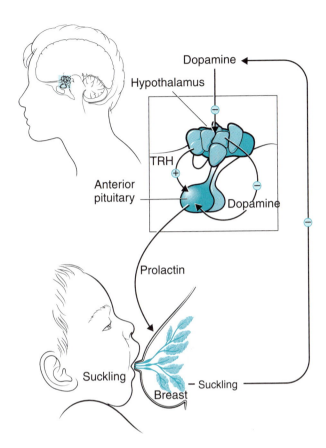

Figure 2-7. Control of prolactin secretion. Prolactin, unlike the other hormones of the anterior pituitary, is actively secreted unless inhibited by dopamine, the release-inhibiting factor for prolactin. Suckling inhibits the release of dopamine, resulting in an increase in release of prolactin.

strual function by inhibiting ovulation and shortening the luteal phase of the menstrual cycle. Elevated levels lead, in some women, to oligo- or amenorrhea.

GONADOTROPINS AND THEIR CONTROLLING HORMONES

The gonadotropins, LH and FSH, are named for their effects on the female gonad, the ovary. FSH leads to ovarian follicle stimulation and production of estrogen. In the male, this hormone stimulates sperm production. LH stimulates gonadal testosterone production in males, whereas it induces ovarian changes that result in ovulation and the production of progesterone in females. Like TSH, LH and FSH are glycoprotein hormones. They all share the same alpha subunit. The beta subunit of each is slightly, but importantly, different and accounts for the functional differences.

GnRH is the hypothalamic-releasing hormone for both LH and FSH. For a number of years it was called LHRH because the magnitude of LH response to an administered dose is much greater than the FSH response. GnRH is a 10-amino-acid polypeptide that is synthesized in the lamina terminalis of the hypothalamus. It, like many of the other polypeptide releasing hormones, is synthesized as part of a larger preprohormone precursor molecule (see Chapter 9). Figure 2-8 depicts the feedback loops involved in the function of the gonadal axis.

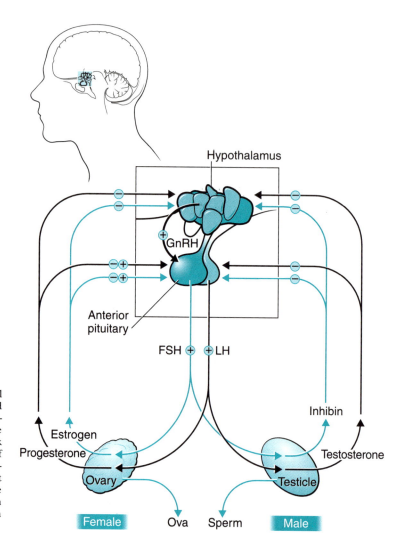

Figure 2-8. Control of gonadal function. The release of LH and FSH begins at puberty and continues through adulthood. In the male, classic negative feedback loops control the production of testosterone and sperm. In the female, a more complex system that involves both positive and negative feedback loops controls ovarian function until menopause, when ovarian function ceases.

DISORDERS OF THE HYPOTHALAMUS AND ANTERIOR PITUITARY

Anatomic and functional abnormalities of the hypothalamus are relatively rare. Developmental abnormalities can result in the improper development of some nuclei. Anatomic abnormalities, whether developmental or acquired as a result of tumors, surgery, radiation, or trauma, can impair the delivery of release-stimulating or release-inhibiting hormones to the anterior pituitary. Although the pituitary fossa rarely can be the site of metastatic disease, benign tumors of the various cell lines of the anterior pituitary are the most common cause of pituitary malfunction. If a pituitary tumor is capable of hormonal secretion, the hormone often is secreted without the usual controlling factors. This may result in a clinical syndrome that reflects the effect of the overproduced hormone.

The hormone most commonly produced by an adenoma or tumor of the pituitary is prolactin. Excessive production of growth hormone is the next most common condition. Overproduction of TSH, LH, or FSH is very rare. Overproduction of the alpha subunit of these hormones often is present, but a clinical constellation of symptoms is lacking. Although there are no clinical syndromes related to alpha subunit excess, the level of alpha subunit may serve as a marker to monitor the success of therapy.

Because the anterior pituitary is housed in a confined space, underactivity of the anterior pituitary is a frequent concomitant of a pituitary tumor. Pituitary tumors almost always are benign, but they may result in compressive damage to normal pituitary tissue and in the disconnection of unaffected pituitary cells from the portal system that delivers hypothalamic-releasing hormones. An enlarging adenoma may, if it grows slowly, result in erosion of the sphenoid bone and enlargement of the sella. Autoimmune inflammation, granulomatous infiltration, and other destructive processes are other causes of pituitary hypofunction.

CLINICALLY USEFUL TESTS OF HYPOTHALAMIC AND PITUITARY FUNCTION AND ANATOMY

SERUM HORMONE LEVELS

It is not currently possible to measure levels of the hypothalamic-releasing hormones in the peripheral circulation, and it is not anatomically feasible to measure hormone levels in the hypothalamic portal vein. All of the hormones of the anterior pituitary, however, can be measured in the peripheral circulation (Table 2-4). In special circumstances, it is possible to measure levels of the pituitary hormones in the venous effluent of the anterior pituitary by placing cathaters in the petrosal sinuses.

Occasionally, a random sample of a pituitary hormone level—especially if markedly elevated—provides important diagnostic information. Paired samples—measuring the stimulating hormone and the target gland hormone on the same sample—may provide valuable information. Examples of such pairs include TSH and T_4, FSH and estradiol, LH and testosterone, and ACTH and cortisol. In many cases, however, stimulation or suppression testing is necessary for thorough evaluation of pituitary function because randomly obtained levels of these short-half-life, episodically secreted protein hormones may overlap with levels seen in syndromes of hormone deficiency and excess.

When a syndrome of glandular insufficiency is suspected, stimulation testing often is required to provide definitive diagnostic information. Testing strategies are based on an understanding of the physiologic control mechanisms combined with some empiric observations. Because many of the hormones of the anterior pituitary are stress-responding hormones, creating a stressful situation, such as insulin-induced hypoglycemia, can be a very helpful testing strategy.

In cases of possible hormone excess, suppression testing often is necessary. Dexamethasone, a potent glucocorticoid (cortisol-like hormone) normally suppresses ACTH secretion and can be used to demonstrate suppressibility of ACTH and cortisol secretion (see Chapter 5). Although rarely necessary in the era of ultrasensitive TSH testing, a T_3 suppression test can be helpful in diagnosing thyroid hyperfunction.

TABLE 2-4.   *FACTORS INVOLVED IN THE ASSESSMENT OF ANTERIOR PITUITARY HORMONE LEVELS*

HORMONE	NORMAL LEVEL	CONDITIONS/NOTES	STIMULATION TEST	SUPPRESSION TEST
ACTH	<80 pg/mL at 8 a.m.	Plasma levels vary widely, affected by time of day and level of stress.	Insulin-induced hypoglycemia; CRH infusion	Dexamethasone
GH	2–6 ng/mL	Should be drawn fasting; levels affected by stress, activity, time of day.	Insulin-induced hypoglycemia; exercise; L-dopa	Glucose tolerance test
LH	3–35 mU/mL*	Levels vary widely depending on age, sex, and phase of menstrual cycle.	GnRH	—
FSH	5–20 mU/mL*	Levels vary widely depending on age, sex, and phase of menstrual cycle.	GnRH	—
TSH	0.3–5.0 mU/mL	Levels may need to be interpreted in light of clinical symptoms and T_4 level.	TRH	T_3 suppression
Prolactin	5–25 ng/mL	Levels are lower in males, children, and postmenopausal women.	TRH	—

* Levels of gonadotropins are <5 mU/mL in prepubertal children, vary during the menstrual cycle, and rise significantly at menopause in females (see Appendix of Normal Values).
ACTH, adrenocorticotrophic hormone; CRH, corticotropin-releasing hormone; FSH, follicle-stimulating hormone; GH, growth hormone; GnRH, gonadotropin-releasing hormone; LH, luteinizing hormone; TRH, thyrotropin-releasing hormone; TSH, thyroid-stimulating hormone.

ANATOMIC STUDIES

Imaging Studies

Magnetic resonance imaging (MRI) with gadolinium provides excellent views of the pituitary and hypothalamus. Figure 2-9 shows MR images of a normal pituitary. CT scanning with coronal views also can provide good visualization of the pituitary and hypothalamus. Although an abnormality occasionally can be seen on plain X-ray films of the skull, such studies usually are not very helpful clinically.

Formal Visual Fields

A careful history and physical examination may reveal evidence of visual field abnormalities. A pituitary tumor that extends above the sella turcica and compresses the optic chiasm can result in tunnel vision, a loss of peripheral acuity.

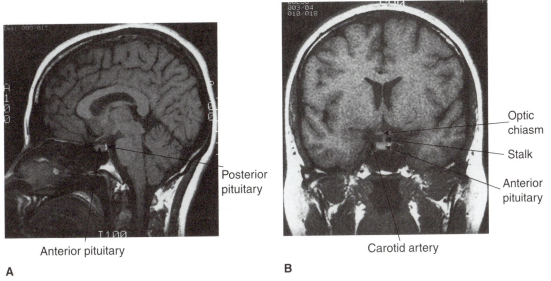

Posterior
pituitary

Optic
chiasm

Stalk

Anterior
pituitary

Anterior pituitary

Carotid artery

A

B

Figure 2-9. Normal MRI of the brain and pituitary. (**A**) Lateral view. Arrows label the anterior and posterior pituitary. The bright white signal is characteristic of the lipid-rich posterior pituitary. (**B**) Coronal view. Arrows label the anterior pituitary, the stalk, and the optic chiasm.

Formal testing of visual fields, similar to those done to monitor glaucoma, can provide vital information for the evaluation and long-term management of patients with pituitary disease.

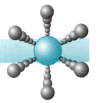

CASE PRESENTATION: CASE 1

A 14-year-old girl presents with short stature and delayed puberty.

Alice Atherton is 14 years old but looks more like a 10-year-old. She is 4 inches shorter than her 12-year-old sister, and, although her sister's menstrual periods started recently, Alice has not yet had a menstrual period. She has not had any appreciable axillary or pubic hair growth, nor has any breast development of significance occurred. She has always been the shortest child in her class. Her growth chart is shown in Figure 2-10.

Alice's general energy level has been normal, although she tires easily during athletic activities. Her performance in school is adequate, but not as good as it was a few years ago. Her past medical history is unremarkable. She is on no medications. A detailed review of symptoms reveals some headaches relieved by aspirin; occasional difficulty seeing the blackboard in school; some cold intolerance over this past winter; and increasing problems with constipation.

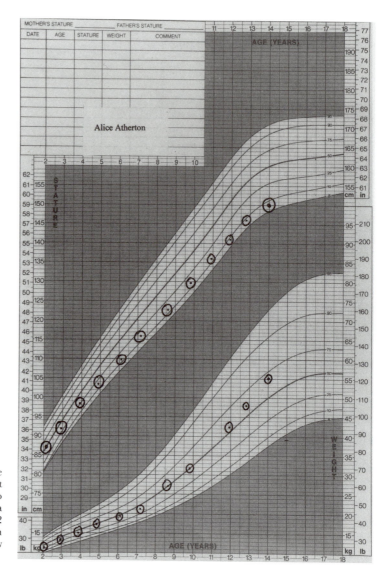

Figure 2-10. Growth chart: Alice Atherton. Although Alice's weight progressed steadily within the 25th to 75th percentile, her height crossed a number of percentile lines. At age 2 she was at the 50th percentile in height, but by age 14 she was below the 10th percentile.

Physical Examination

A young female who appears to be about 10 years of age

Vital Signs:	Blood pressure 100/58; pulse 58, regular
HEENT:	Full visual fields by confrontation, normal optic fundi
Chest:	Normal, very little breast development
Heart:	Normal
Abdomen:	Normal
Hair:	Essentially no axillary or pubic hair
Genitals:	External genitalia appear to be those of a normal 10-year-old female; vaginal exam shows very little estrogen effect

Laboratory Studies

Test	Alice Atherton	Normal Range
T_4	3.0 μg/dL	5–12 μg/dL
T_3RU (Resin Uptake)	23%	25%–35%
TSH	0.2 mU/L	0.3–5.0 mU/L
8 a.m. cortisol	6.8 μg/dL	15–25 μg/dL
LH	0.3 mU/mL	<5 mU/mL (prepubertal)
FSH	0.2 mU/mL	*Female:* Prepubertal: <5 mU/mL; Pre- or postovulatory: 5–20 mU/mL; Ovulatory surge: 12–40 mU/mL; Postmenopausal: >30 mU/mL
Growth hormone, fasting	0.1 ng/mL	2–6 ng/mL
Prolactin	34 ng/mL	5–25 ng/mL

Although the lack of sexual development led to Alice's clinical evaluation, there are other clues to a major problem of growth and development. Review of her growth chart reveals that she has crossed a number of percentile lines. She started near the 50th percentile and is now below the 10th percentile. Typical growth patterns for a patient with constitutional short stature and a normal child are shown in Figure 2-11. Alice's physical examination is remarkable for the disparity between her chronologic age and her physical appearance. She has not yet gone through puberty with the attendant secondary sexual development and the usual pubertal growth spurt.

Laboratory studies provide some clues to the cause of her problem. Levels of both thyroid hormone, T_4, and its stimulating hormone, TSH, are low, suggesting possible central or hypothalamic/pituitary hypofunction. The 8 a.m. cortisol level also is lower than expected. An ACTH level was not reported. If it had been elevated, end-organ adrenal dysfunction would be a possibility, and further evaluation should be directed toward end-organ adrenal failure. A low ACTH value might suggest hypothalamic or pituitary failure, but it would not provide definitive diagnostic information because ACTH levels may normally be quite low.

The low LH and FSH levels are appropriate for a prepubescent child and are consistent with Alice's apparent age of about 10, but are inappropriate for her chronologic age. The fasting growth hormone level also is low. Although none of these abnormalities is striking, one possible lesion that would explain all these findings is hypofunction of either the anterior pituitary or the hypothalamic–pituitary unit.

The elevated prolactin level, a value much higher than would be expected for a non-estrogenized, prepubescent girl, suggests either autono-

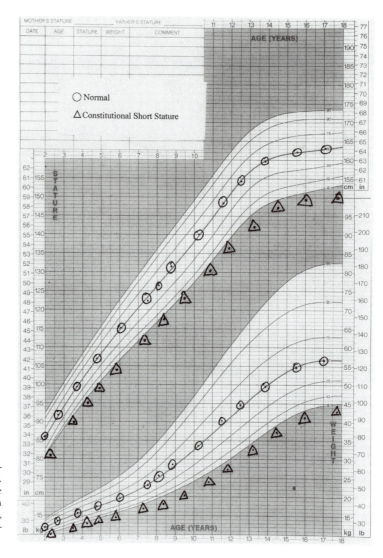

Figure 2-11. Growth charts—normal and constitutional short stature. The normal child follows a percentile line relatively closely. The child with constitutional short stature, similarly, does not deviate much from the percentile line.

mous overproduction of prolactin or, perhaps, disconnection of the lactotrophs of the anterior pituitary from the delivery of dopamine, the hypothalamic release–inhibiting hormone for prolactin. A disruption in delivery of dopamine or an expanding pituitary mass could explain the findings—both the clinical presentation and the laboratory results.

Additional Studies

Formal visual fields:	Normal
Pelvic ultrasound:	Normal uterus and ovaries for a 10-year-old
Skull X-ray:	Calcified suprasellar mass
Brain MRI:	Partially cystic, calcified suprasellar mass (Fig. 2-12)

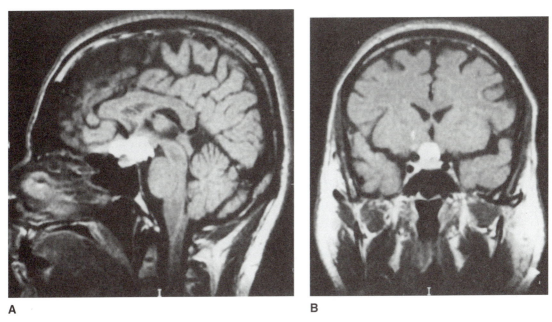

A   B

Figure 2-12. Brain MRI: Alice Atherton. (**A**) Lateral view. A large mass is present in the sella turcica and extends into the suprasellar area. (**B**) Coronal view. Significant suprasellar extension is clearly visible.

The pelvic ultrasound suggests that her primary sexual development has been normal. If evidence of hypothalamic/pituitary dysfunction were not present, other explanations for her lack of development would need to be considered, including Turner's syndrome (XO). The calcified suprasellar mass provides a possible mechanism for a disruption of the delivery of hypothalamic factors to the anterior pituitary. The location and appearance of this mass and the resultant endocrine abnormalities are diagnostic of a craniopharyngioma. Slow-growing rests of Rathke's pouch tissue migrate embryologically beyond the anterior part of the sella turcica and into the hypothalamus. In this location, they expand and can interfere with delivery of releasing and release-inhibiting factors to the anterior pituitary.

Shortly after her evaluation was completed, Alice underwent a transsphenoidal decompression of the suprasellar mass. The sphenoid sinus, located immediately below the sella, is separated from the pituitary fossa by a thin layer of bone. Relatively easy access to the sphenoid sinus can be obtained through the roof of the mouth.

Through this approach, a probe was placed into the mass and several milliliters of thick black fluid were removed, decompressing the suprasellar mass. Surgical removal of the cystic mass is extremely difficult and can result in significant damage to adjacent structures.

Following the decompression procedure, radiation therapy was started in an effort to destroy the epithelial cells that line the cystic mass. Destroying these cells should prevent further growth and enlargement of the cyst. At the time of surgery and during the radiation therapy, Ms. Atherton received replacement steroids to "cover" the stress of the surgery and radiation. It was assumed that she would not respond to the stresses of surgery and radiation with the normal increase in cortisol production that would occur if her hypothalamic–pituitary axis were functionally intact.

The radiation therapy was complicated by the development of hydrocephalus. The lateral ventricles became dilated because of radiation-induced edema, which resulted in aqueductal stenosis. In spite of this complication, Alice tolerated the treatments well. By 6 months following radiation therapy, she had tapered off the exogenous steroids completely and had grown almost 2 inches. In addition, she was beginning to show evidence of puberty. Two years after the surgery and radiation, Alice has grown an additional 3 inches, catching up to her younger sister. She now has normal breast development and is menstruating regularly. Her laboratory values, including her prolactin level, have returned to normal.

Her cold intolerance, constipation, and grade-point average have all improved. She feels well on no medications and will return for a follow-up MRI in about 6 months.

The resolution of all the aspects of Alice Atherton's presenting clinical situation without need for continuing hormonal replacement illustrates the importance of the appropriate portal connection between the hypothalamus and anterior pituitary. Successful treatment allowed delivery of the hypothalamic factors to the anterior pituitary.

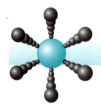

CASE PRESENTATION: CASE 2

Galactorrhea and amenorrhea in a 34-year-old woman.

For the first 8 years of their relationship, Janice and Arnold Dowd had been most concerned about contraception. They wanted to have children eventually, but graduate school, work, lifestyle, and financial pressures led them to plan to have children in their mid-30s. They are both now 34 and in good health. Nine months ago Janice stopped the oral contraceptives she had taken since she was 20 years old. She had one menstrual period shortly after stopping the pill and had one or two episodes of vaginal spotting a few months ago. The couple has intercourse without any form of contraception about three or four times a week and, so far, Janice has not become pregnant.

Janice has never been pregnant (para 0). Her menstrual periods started at about age 11, and after a few years of irregularity she had regular periods from age 16 until 20, when she started oral contraceptives. Her past medical history is unremarkable, and she takes no drugs or medications. Her weight has been stable, usually about 5 pounds heavier than she would like to be. She belongs to the local gym but gets there only once or twice a week for an aerobics class.

Physical Examination
   Healthy-appearing, well-nourished female

Vital signs:	**Blood pressure 110/68; pulse 78**
Height:	**5′4″**
Weight:	**132 lb**
HEENT:	**Normal**
Chest:	**Clear**
Heart:	**Normal**
Abdomen:	**Normal**
Breasts:	**No masses, but galactorrhea is present with a milking maneuver**
Pelvic:	**Normal external genitalia, normal vagina, normal cervix, and normal bimanual examination**

Laboratory Studies

Test	Janice Dowd	Normal Range
CBC (complete blood count)	Normal	Normal
Chemistry profile[a]	Normal	Normal
T_4	6.8 μg/dL	5–12 μg/dL
TSH	0.8 mU/L	0.3–5.0 mU/L
Prolactin	94.5 ng/mL	5–25 ng/mL
FSH	6.8 mU/mL	*Female:* Prepubertal: <5 mU/mL Pre- or postovulatory: 5–20 mU/mL Ovulatory surge: 12–40 mU/mL Postmenopausal: >30 mU/mL
HCG—beta subunit	Negative	Negative, not pregnant Positive, pregnant

[a] Includes tests of glucose, liver function, kidney function, and calcium.

Arnold Dowd's past history, physical examination, and semen analysis are all normal.

It may take several months for menses to resume after discontinuation of oral contraceptives. After 3 or 4 months of amenorrhea, however, further evaluation is indicated. Pregnancy, although unlikely based on the information available, should be ruled out. The negative beta subunit of HCG (see Chapter 9) indicates that it is highly unlikely for Janice to be pregnant. The presence of galactorrhea, milk production not related to a recent pregnancy or nursing, is an important physical finding that suggests hyperprolactinemia. Laboratory studies confirm the presence of hyperprolactinemia. Although not always linked, the combination of galactorrhea and amenorrhea is a common presenting clinical finding in patients with prolactin excess. Many medications—both legitimate and illicit–can raise the prolactin level. Drugs of the phenothiazine class, which deplete dopamine, are especially powerful elevators of prolactin levels. Drug-induced depletion of dopamine leads to a decrease in the inhibition of prolactin synthesis, and this results in hyperprolactinemia. Because Janice Dowd was not taking any medications or drugs, another explanation must be present.

After reviewing the data, an MRI of her brain was ordered. The MRI reveals a 4-mm right-sided adenoma of the pituitary (Fig. 2-13). The study is otherwise normal.

The gynecologist reviews the information with Janice and her husband and explains that a prolactinoma is present. A small group of prolactin-secreting cells is functioning excessively, and the resulting elevation of the prolactin level is causing galactorrhea and amenorrhea. The gynecologist recommends treatment with bromocriptine, a dopamine-agonist drug that suppresses the secretion of prolactin. Successful treatment, she explains, will lower the prolactin level and probably also shrink the adenoma. Lowering the prolactin level should stop the galactorrhea; allow regular, ovulatory menstrual cycles to return; and perhaps allow a pregnancy to occur.

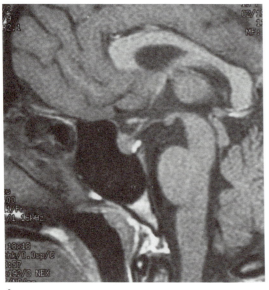
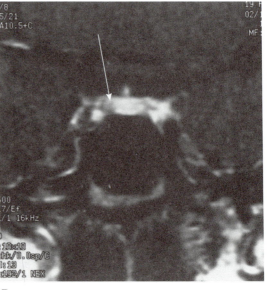

A   B

Figure 2-13. Brain MRI: Janice Dowd. (**A**) Lateral view. No significant abnormality is seen. (**B**) Coronal view. The arrow points to a hypodense area that is consistent with a 4-mm pituitary adenoma.

Bromocriptine is used to lower prolactin levels and to reduce the size of responsive pituitary adenomas. The fall in prolactin levels and, in some cases, the lessening of a mass effect within the sella usually allow ovulatory cycles to return.

After taking bromocriptine nightly for 2 months, Janice had had two periods and the galactorrhea was no longer present. Her prolactin fell to 23 ng/mL. The only side effects Janice had from the medication were some mild headaches and a stuffy nose.

The gynecologist explained that the normal pituitary expands about half again in size during a normal pregnancy and that much of this enlargement is in the lactotroph population of the anterior pituitary. Prolactin levels rise significantly during a normal pregnancy, probably because of the effect that estrogen in high doses has on prolactin synthesis and release.

The gynecologist feels that it is now reasonable for Janice to try to get pregnant and recommends that she stop the bromocriptine as soon as she thinks she might be pregnant.

Bromocriptine can have a remarkable effect in controlling the problems of elevated prolactin levels. If a large adenoma (greater than 1 cm) had been present, surgical removal or a prolonged course of bromocriptine before pregnancy might have been suggested. Because both prolactin-secreting adenomas and normal lactotrophs increase in size during pregnancy, it is possible for this enlargement in a closed space to threaten pituitary function and, in some cases, even threaten vision with chiasmal compression from suprasellar extension of the enlarging adenoma.

Two months later, Janice has missed a period, her pregnancy test is positive, and she has stopped the bromocriptine. The pregnancy continues normally and, after 39 weeks of gestation, Janice and Arnold's lifestyle changes dramatically with the addition of a healthy 8-pound girl to their family.

Postpartum, Janice breast-feeds her daughter for about 8 weeks but then weans the baby in preparation for her return to work. At 9 months postpartum, her menses still have not returned and she has some persistent breast milk. Her prolactin level is high, at 42 ng/mL. Janice is not yet ready for another pregnancy, but she learns from her gynecologist that she should not depend on her hyperprolactinemia alone for contraception and that oral contraceptives may enhance the growth of prolactinomas. Janice restarts bromocriptine, and the Dowds use condoms or a diaphragm for contraception. On bromocriptine, her menses return and the galactorrhea stops. At some point in the next year or 2, when the Dowds are ready for another pregnancy, Janice will have another MRI to check the status of the adenoma.

Estrogen, whether endogenously produced or exogenously provided (e.g., oral contraceptives, menopausal hormonal replacement therapy), activates the estrogen response element of the prolactin gene and leads to significant increases in prolactin synthesis and secretion. Oral contraceptives probably do not cause prolactinomas but may fuel their development and expression and usually are avoided in women with prolactinomas. Recent studies, however, suggest that some women with prolactinomas can tolerate oral contraceptives well without progression of their hyperprolactinemic problems.

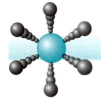

CASE PRESENTATION: CASE 3

Enlarging hat, glove, and shoe size in a 39-year-old woman with premature menopause and a gradual change in facial appearance.

Gladys Miller had worked for nearly 20 years as a nursing assistant in the newborn nursery of a major teaching hospital. During that time, not one of her coworkers mentioned the changes that had been occurring in Ms. Miller's appearance. A medical student starting his pediatrics rotation casually mentioned to Ms. Miller that he thought she probably had a pituitary tumor that was affecting her appearance and wondered if she were under treatment.

Ms. Miller was embarrassed, frightened, and concerned. Indeed, her face had changed. Her features were coarser, her lower jaw protruded, and her teeth had separated. These changes were most apparent when her present appearance was compared to her high school yearbook picture and to her 5-year-old hospital ID badge photo. Her hat, glove, and shoe size also had increased. Her fingers had enlarged to such a degree that it was hard for her to fasten the little snaps and tie the ties on the shirts the newborns wore in the nursery. In the hospital, it was easy to find rubber gloves and surgical scrub hats that were large enough for her, but shoes were a real problem. Her shoe size had gone from 7A to 8 DDD.

Eight years ago, at age 31, Ms. Miller's menstrual periods stopped suddenly. Although she had some vaginal dryness, the loss of menstrual periods did not alarm or concern her.

Her past medical history was unremarkable, and other than very oily skin and nocturia, 2 or 3 times per night, her review of systems failed to disclose any other problems.

Physical examination revealed a large woman with coarse facial features, a prominent jaw, and large, broad hands and feet.

Vital signs:	Blood pressure 160/100; pulse 88
HEENT:	Unremarkable except for prognathism; visual fields were intact to confrontation
Chest:	Clear
Heart:	Normal
Breasts:	Normal, no galactorrhea
Abdomen:	Normal
Pelvic:	Vaginal atrophy, healthy cervix, normal bimanual examination
Neuro:	Normal
Extremities:	Enlarged, widened hands and feet; fingers are impressively widened, with significant soft tissue thickening

Laboratory Studies

Test	Gladys Miller	Normal
Glucose, fasting	222 mg/dL	70–110 mg/dL, fasting
Growth hormone, fasting	78 ng/mL	2–6 ng/mL
FSH	4.2 mU/mL	*Female:* Prepubertal: <5 mU/mL Pre- or postovulatory: 5–20 mU/mL Ovulatory surge: 12–40 mU/mL Postmenopausal: >30 mU/mL
TSH	2.1 mU/mL	0.3–5.0 mU/mL
T_4	6.8 μg/100 mL	4.5–12.0 μg/100 mL
Prolactin	55 ng/mL	5–25 ng/mL
Cortisol, 8 a.m.	18 μg/dL	5–25 μg/dL
IGF-1	758 ng/mL	Adult female: 140–400 ng/mL

MRI: Large intrasellar mass with erosion and widening of the sella, some suprasellar bulging, but no chiasmal comprise is noted (Fig. 2-14)

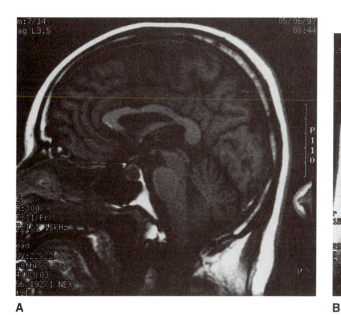
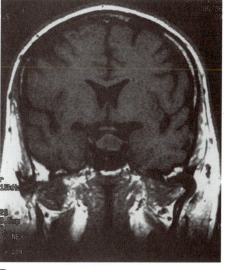

A   **B**

Figure 2-14. Brain MRI: Gladys Miller. (**A**) Lateral view. A sellar mass is present, pushing the roof of the sella turcica convexly upward. (**B**) Coronal view. The mass also is seen in this view. The optic chiasm is not compromised.

The changes that have occurred in Ms. Miller's appearance and health status went unnoticed for a long time by her friends, colleagues, and even herself. Ms. Miller has acromegaly. Although almost always benign pathologically, the effect of this slowly growing growth hormone–secreting adenoma can be devastating.

Because her epiphyses are closed, significant linear growth of her long bones is not possible. Chondrocyte stimulation, however, is intense because of the high levels of GH and the resulting elevation in IGF-1. This postpubertal stimulation of bone formation results in widening of bones, which is especially apparent in the skull and bones of the distal extremities or acral skeleton, hence the name acromegaly.

The growth of many tissues in addition to bone is stimulated by the excess growth hormone and IGF-1 levels. The skin thickens, and dermal appendages hypertrophy and hyperfunction, resulting in increased skin oil production. Cardiomegaly and renal hypertrophy, both functional and anatomic, occur commonly in acromegaly. Hypertension is seen often, and congestive heart failure often is the terminal event for patients with uncontrolled acromegaly. The bony changes result in alteration in weight-bearing forces that lead to significant osteoarthritis, especially in the knee.

Glucose intolerance is seen in many patients with acromegaly. The contra-insulin effects of growth hormone result in an increased need for insulin. In patients with a preexisting decrease in insulin secretory ability or resistance to the effects of insulin, diabetes mellitus may become manifest, as in Ms. Miller's case. Her nocturia most likely is the result of the osmotic diuresis that can be induced when glucose is present in urine (see Chapter 7).

The enlarging sellar mass has had a significant effect on other functions of the anterior pituitary. Her prolactin is elevated. Some growth hormone–secreting adenomas also secrete prolactin. In addition, the adenoma may have led to a disconnection of the lactotrophs in the pituitary fossa from the inhibitory effects of dopamine delivered by the portal system. Galactorrhea, however, may not occur because milk production requires the presence of both prolactin and estrogen. Ms. Miller's estrogen deficiency, as manifested by her amenorrhea and vaginal dryness and atrophy, is occurring in the face of a low FSH level. This indicates that her amenorrhea and estrogen deficiency are the result of hypothalamic/pituitary failure. Loss of gonadotropin function is a common and often an early concomitant of an enlarging intrasellar mass. The distribution of gonadotrophs in the anterior pituitary makes them especially susceptible to the effects of an expanding pituitary mass.

TSH and ACTH function often are relatively well preserved. The data available with regard to Ms. Miller do not, however, indicate what functional reserve is present in the hypothalamic–pituitary–adrenal axis, and further testing of the stress responsiveness of this axis with insulin-induced hypoglycemia might be indicated.

Gladys Miller was referred by her primary physician to an endocrinologist, who confirmed the diagnosis of acromegaly and ordered some additional studies.

Formal visual fields: Normal

Glucose Tolerance Test

Time	Gladys Miller: Glucose	Normal Glucose	Gladys Miller: GH	Normal GH
Fasting	197 mg/dL	70–110 mg/dL	94 ng/mL	2–6 ng/mL
½ hr	298 mg/dL	<200 mg/dL	102 ng/mL	<2 ng/mL
1 hr	337 mg/dL	<200 mg/dL	96 ng/mL	<2 ng/mL
2 hrs	288 mg/dL	<140 mg/dL	93 ng/mL	<2 ng/mL
3 hrs	227 mg/dL	<140 mg/dL	99 ng/mL	<2 ng/mL

Insulin Tolerance Test

Time	Glucose	Cortisol	Normal Cortisol
0	187 mg/dL	16 µg/dL	15–25 µg/dL at 8 a.m.
30 min	38 mg/dL	27 µg/dL	
60 min	62 mg/dL	42 µg/dL	A rise of cortisol to more than 18 µg/dL
90 min	156 mg/dL	21 µg/dL	after adequate hypoglycemia (glucose
120 min	170 mg/dL	20 µg/dL	<40 mg/dL)

These studies confirm the autonomous, nonsuppressible secretion of GH and demonstrate some preservation of ACTH and cortisol secretion in response to stress. Further testing of the TSH–thyroid axis and the pituitary gonadal axis is not necessary.

After an explanation of the diagnosis, several treatment options were discussed with Ms. Miller. The goals of treatment focus on lowering the growth hormone level to normal or below, managing the bulk of the adenoma, and replacing the pituitary function that has been lost. Surgery and radiation therapy can be used, individually or in tandem, to reduce the size of the adenoma and to control excess hormone production.

Although dopamine usually is a secretogogue for growth hormone in normal somatotroph cells, some patients with acromegaly respond to dopaminergic agonists (e.g., bromocriptine) with a reduction in both the size of the adenoma and the secretion of growth hormone. Somatostatin analogues also have been used with some success in managing patients with acromegaly. Transsphenoidal surgical removal of all or at least a large part of the adenoma usually is the treatment of choice. Surgery usually is effective both in controlling the mass effects of the adenoma and in reducing the systemic effects of the excessive growth hormone. Preservation of pituitary function and even restoration of previously lost function can be seen following surgical debulking of a growth hormone–secreting adenoma. Radiation therapy can be given as primary treatment but more commonly is used following surgery to destroy or prevent the proliferation of adenoma tissue that remains after surgery. All of the cell types of the anterior pituitary are susceptible to the effects of radiation therapy, and, although the more rapidly dividing adenoma cells are more severely affected, panhypopituitarism is a common long-term complication of radiation therapy.

Successful treatment of acromegaly requires reducing growth hormone levels into the normal range, or even below normal. Marked lowering of the growth hormone level may result in some slight improvement, but significant improvement requires low levels of growth hormone, usually less than 3 ng/mL. Diabetes mellitus and hypertension, if present, usually improve once the growth hormone level is under control. Soft tissue changes also may return toward normal, and the coarsening of features and puffiness of the hands and feet may decrease. The bony changes persist, however, in spite of good control of growth hormone levels.

Hormonal replacement therapy often is required to deal with the effects of the adenoma and its treatment. Thyroid hormone and adrenal corticosteroid replacement are required in many cases. Often, gonadal axis replacement therapy is also necessary and should be carefully tailored to the patient's needs.

Ms. Miller elected to have surgery. The transsphenoidal procedure successfully removed a large adenoma. During and immediately after the surgery she was "covered" with stress doses of exogenous glucocorticoids (see Chapter 5). Postoperatively, growth hormone levels fell to the normal range, and her glucose intolerance and hypertension markedly improved. Thyroid function tests have remained normal, and a repeat insulin tolerance test performed postoperatively and several months after exogenous glucocorticoids had been stopped showed a normal stress-responding reserve in the hypothalamic–pituitary–adrenal cortical axis.

Her menstrual periods did not return. Because she did not want to become pregnant, birth control pills offered an easy way to replenish her estrogen levels and protect her endometrium and her bones. Some of the coarsening of her facial features has abated, and her fingers are much more nimble.

Perhaps the medical student could have exercised his diagnostic expertise in a more sensitive and appropriate manner when he spoke to Ms. Miller about his observations. His comments did, however, lead to the discovery of an important clinical problem with a relatively good outcome. The changes of acromegaly usually develop very slowly and often go unappreciated, as in Ms. Miller's case, until the disease has progressed significantly. Whenever clinical findings suggest possible pituitary dysfunction, growth hormone excess must be considered.

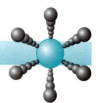

CASE PRESENTATION: CASE 4

A 65-year-old woman presents with a significant visual field defect.

After he replaced and repainted her left front fender for the third time, the auto body shop manager asked Mrs. Williams if her vision was okay. It wasn't an easy question to ask; both he and Mrs. Williams were embarrassed. Mrs. Williams said she didn't think she had a problem, but she had to admit to herself that something was not right with her vision. Her 65th birthday was in a few days, and it was time to renew her driver's license. She knew she would have an eye test then.

Although she could see virtually none of the letters on the left side of the viewer, the clerk sent her on to have her photo taken for her new license. The clerk did suggest that she see her eye doctor. Her eye examination showed no cataracts, the thing she feared the most, but it did show a significant problem with her fields of vision.

Mrs. Williams's past medical history was remarkable for mild hypertension, for which she was treated with a diuretic. She had had a hysterectomy at age 38 because of excessive bleeding caused by uterine fibroids. She specifically denied hot flashes; change in hat, glove, or shoe size; polyuria; cold intolerance; or constipation.

Her physical examination showed a blood pressure of 154/94, with a pulse of 80.

HEENT exam revealed a clear-cut left visual field abnormality. The remainder of her general physical examination was normal.

Visual fields (see Fig. 2-15)

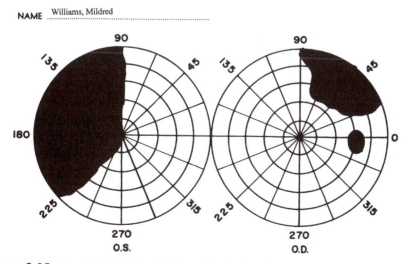

Figure 2-15. Visual fields: Mildred Williams. The darkened areas represent significant loss of visual acuity. A large upper, outer quadrant defect is seen on the left. A smaller defect is present in the right field of vision, just above the physiologic blind spot.

Laboratory Studies

Test	Mildred Williams	Normal Range
T$_4$	7 μg/dL	5–12 μg/dL
TSH	0.4 mU/L	0.3–5.0 mU/L
FSH	3 mU/mL	*Female* Prepubertal: <5 mU/mL Pre- or postovulatory: 5–20 mU/mL Ovulatory surge: 12–40 mU/mL Postmenopausal: >30 mU/mL
Prolactin	18 ng/mL	5–25 ng/mL

Insulin Tolerance Test

Time	Glucose	Cortisol	Normal Cortisol
0 min	88 mg/dL	11 μg/dL	15–25 μg/dL at 8 a.m.
30 min	22 mg/dL	14 μg/dL	A rise of cortisol to more than 18 μg/dL
60 min	198 mg/dL	16 μg/dL	after adequate hypoglycemia (glucose
90 min	134 mg/dL	13 μg/dL	<40 mg/dL)

MRI: **Large pituitary adenoma with significant suprasellar extension (see Fig. 2-16)**

Visual field abnormalities can be the presenting complaint for pituitary tumors. The gradual development of pituitary enlargement and malfunction may go undetected for long periods of time by patients and by their physicians. The lack of menstrual function or decline in sexual activity and interest may be seen as a normal concomitant of aging, therefore not leading to medical evaluation. Occasionally, illnesses such as the flu or gastroenteritis can precipitate a major crisis that leads to the appreciation of pituitary pathology. Prompt detection of the inability of the hypothalamic–pituitary unit to respond to the stress of the illness and treatment with glucocorticoids in stress doses can be lifesaving in such patients.

Although Mrs. Williams had some doubts about her vision, her denial was challenged by her auto mechanic and the licensing bureau. A visit to her eye doctor led to the discovery of the pituitary tumor and eventual therapy.

Because of the size of the tumor and the compromise of her vision, Mrs. Williams was offered transsphenoidal surgery as the best approach for her problem. She agreed to the surgery, and preoperatively she was "covered" with stress doses of a glucocorticoid. She tolerated the procedure well and postoperatively had significant improvement in her vision.

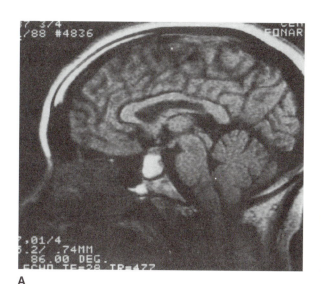

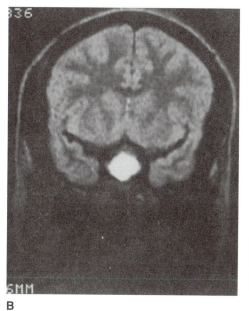

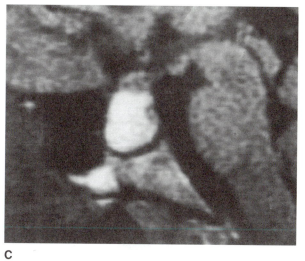

Figure 2-16. Brain MRI: Mildred Williams. (**A**) Lateral view. A large intrasellar mass with significant suprasellar extension is seen. (**B**) Coronal view. The mass compresses the optic chiasm. (**C**) Magnified lateral view.

Visual fields (Fig. 2-17)

The entire tumor could not be safely removed at the time of surgery. To further decrease the mass of tissue and to decrease the likelihood of regrowth, radiation therapy was begun. Her stress-dose steroids were tapered to physiologic levels. She started taking gradually increasing doses of thyroid hormone until her T$_4$ value was in the middle of the normal range. She elected not to have any estrogen replacement now but will consider it for the future. She selected the gold-plated version of the bracelet that provides medical information at the time of an emergency.

Mrs. Williams now drives more confidently and with less property damage. Her energy level and cold intolerance have improved significantly. The medications she has to take are not expensive, and the schedule of dosing is relatively easy to follow. She understands that she needs to increase her hydrocortisone dose at times of significant stress (see Chapter 5).

Mrs. Williams' visual fields did not return entirely to normal and probably will not return to normal. Fibers that were compromised but not destroyed recovered from the pressure effect of the pituitary lesion, with resultant improvement in her vision. Replacement of cortisol and thyroid hormone account for her improved energy and tolerance for the cold. A bracelet or similar system of identification is a vital part of the care of patients with pituitary lesions. When they are unconscious or otherwise unable to provide an accurate history, the information available via such a system should lead to prompt and potentially lifesaving administration of glucocorticoids in stress-level doses.

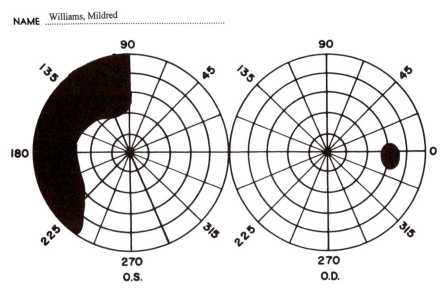

NAME Williams, Mildred

O.S.

O.D.

Figure 2-17. Postoperative visual fields: Mildred Williams. Significant improvement in peripheral vision has occurred on the left, and complete resolution is seen in the right field of view.

KEY POINTS AND CONCEPTS

- The hypothalamus and anterior pituitary function as an integrated unit.
- Feedback loops and CNS input control the secretion of the hormones of the hypothalamus and anterior pituitary.
- Normal function of the anterior pituitary depends on the delivery of hypothalamic releasing factors and release-inhibiting factors.
- All hormones of the anterior pituitary, except prolactin, require stimulation by a hypothalamic releasing factor for secretion. Prolactin is under tonic inhibition by hypothalamic dopamine.
- Syndromes of pituitary hormone excess may be the result of disconnection of the anterior pituitary from the hypothalamus (e.g., prolactin), or to autonomously functioning, hormone-producing tumors of the anterior pituitary.
- Syndromes of pituitary hormone deficiency may be the result of failure of delivery of hypothalamic releasing factors or to local factors within the sella turcica, including tumors, infiltration, and inflammation.
- Visual field compromise may be seen when pituitary tumors extend above the sella turcica and compress the optic chiasm.
- Syndromes of pituitary hormone excess may be treated with suppressing medications, surgery, or radiation.
- Syndromes of pituitary hormone deficiency usually are corrected with end-organ or target organ hormone replacement.

SUGGESTED READING

Elster AD. Modern imaging of the pituitary. Radiology 187:1–14, 1993.

Levy A, Lightman SL. The pathogenesis of pituitary tumors. Clin Endocrinol (Oxf) 38:559–570, 1993.

Melmed S. Acromegaly. N Engl J Med 332:966–977, 1990.

Serri O. Progress in the management of hyperprolactinemia. N Engl J Med 331:942–944, 1994.

Vance ML. Hypopituitarism. N Engl J Med 330:1651–1662, 1994.

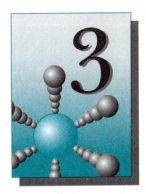

Posterior Pituitary

The neurons whose endings make up the posterior pituitary represent the quintessential neuroendocrine organ. These cells are part of the central nervous system; they also clearly function as hormone-secreting glands. Appreciation of this combination of neural and endocrine function led to the development of the concept of neuroendocrinology.

The posterior pituitary, or neurohypophysis, is merely one end of a neuro-secretory organ. It is the storage site and release point for the polypeptide hormones vasopressin (also referred to as antidiuretic hormone [ADH]) and oxytocin. The name *vasopressin* is derived from the fact that this molecule is a potent vasoconstrictor. In addition, this same molecule opens water channels in the renal collecting duct that result in the reabsorption of water and the elaboration of concentrated urine—hence the additional name, antidiuretic hormone. Secreted in response to increased osmolality or decreased effective blood volume, vasopressin allows the reabsorption of water by the kidney. This conservation of water tends to protect the osmolality and effective blood volume. Oxytocin, the other hormone of the posterior pituitary, stimulates uterine contraction and plays a role in parturition.

ANATOMY

The cell bodies of the neurons of the posterior pituitary are located in the supraoptic and paraventricular nuclei of the hypothalamus. The pituitary stalk is made up of a bundle of axons—the neurohypophyseal tract—that connects the cell bodies in the hypothalamus with their nerve endings in the posterior aspect of the sella turcica (Fig. 3-1). The neurohypophysis develops as an outpouching of the floor of the third ventricle of the brain and descends to its location in the pituitary fossa. The inferior hypophyseal artery, a branch of the internal carotid, provides a rich arterial supply. Venous drainage is into the cavernous sinus.

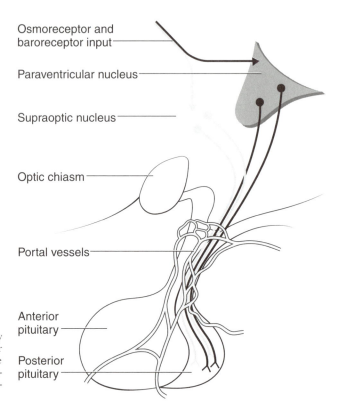

Osmoreceptor and
baroreceptor input

Paraventricular nucleus

Supraoptic nucleus

Optic chiasm

Portal vessels

Anterior
pituitary

Posterior
pituitary

Figure 3-1. Anatomy of the posterior pituitary and hypothalamus—lateral view. The posterior pituitary is made up largely of axons and nerve endings of neurons whose cell bodies are located in the supraoptic and paraventricular nuclei of the hypothalamus.

THE HORMONES OF THE POSTERIOR PITUITARY

CHEMISTRY

Vasopressin and Oxytocin

Each of the hormones of the posterior pituitary—vasopressin (ADH) and oxytocin—is an octapeptide with a five amino acid ring and a side chain containing three amino acids. These molecules differ from one another by only two amino acid residues (Fig. 3-2). Both ADH and oxytocin are synthesized as part of larger prohormone molecules in separate cells in the supraoptic and paraventricular nuclei of the hypothalamus. Once synthesized, each of the prohormones is packaged in intracellular storage granules. The storage granules travel down the axons from the hypothalamic nuclei at a rate of about 1 to 3 mm per hour. In these granules, the prohormone molecules are enzymatically split into the active hormone molecules and proteins called neurophysins. In the case of vasopressin, a glycopeptide also is part of the prohormone precursor molecule.

Binding between ADH and oxytocin and their respective neurophysins is highly specific, but weak. Depolarization of the neuron results in release by exocytosis of the active hormones together with the other contents of the storage granules. Fusion of the storage granules with the cell membrane of the axon allows the granule contents to spill into the extracellular space. Neurophysin is found in a 1 : 1 molar ratio with ADH in the hypothalamus and posterior pituitary, but in

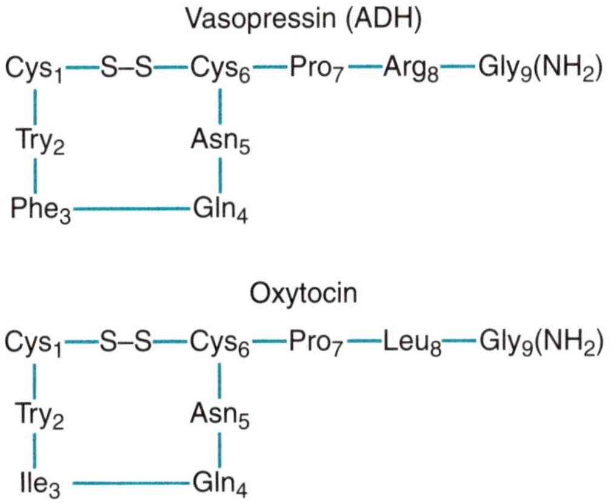

Vasopressin (ADH)

Cys$_1$—S–S—Cys$_6$—Pro$_7$—Arg$_8$—Gly$_9$(NH$_2$)

Try$_2$ Asn$_5$

Phe$_3$—————Gln$_4$

Oxytocin

Cys$_1$—S–S—Cys$_6$—Pro$_7$—Leu$_8$—Gly$_9$(NH$_2$)

Try$_2$ Asn$_5$

Ile$_3$ —————Gln$_4$

Figure 3-2. Vasopressin (ADH) and oxytocin molecules.

the circulation much more neurophysin is found, probably because of the very short half-life of ADH. Secretion of ADH occurs noncontinuously or in ''spurts'' in response to depolarization of the neuron. In addition to release of hormone in the posterior pituitary, some ADH and oxytocin are released in the area of the portal capillaries of the median eminence from axons that terminate before reaching the posterior pituitary.

Following secretion, ADH and oxytocin circulate as free polypeptides with short (1 to 10 minutes) half-lives. Degradation occurs in the kidney and liver.

CONTROL OF SECRETION

Osmoregulation

Via centers in the anterior hypothalamus, secretion of ADH is stimulated by rising serum osmolality and inhibited by falling osmolality. The osmoreceptors are not the supraoptic and paraventricular nuclei themselves, but they probably are nearby. Hypertonic NaCl or sucrose does stimulate ADH release, but hypertonic urea and glucose do not. The ability of osmotic particles to cross the osmoreceptor membrane may account for these differences. Because the osmolality of plasma is determined by the concentration of a number of different solutes—including urea and glucose—the total plasma osmolality alone is not always clearly related to the ADH level.

The osmoreceptor appears to have a threshold of about 280 mOsm/kg. Below this level, little or no ADH is secreted in states of normal blood volume. Maximal ADH levels occur with osmolalities of about 295 mOsm/kg (Fig. 3-3).

Baroregulation

Changes in blood volume and blood pressure also may lead to secretion of ADH. Receptors in the chest, left atrium, aortic arch, and carotid sinuses sense changes in blood volume and blood pressure. Via the vagus and glossopharyngeal nerves, impulses from these receptors eventually reach the supraoptic and paraventricular nuclei. Decreases in blood volume of 5% to 10% result in marked increases in ADH to levels that have important vasopressor as well as antidiuretic effects. Decreases in mean arterial blood pressure of 5% or more also can result

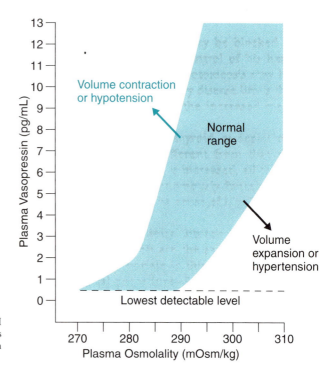

Figure 3-3. Relationship between plasma ADH and plasma osmolality. Volume contraction shifts the curve to the left, whereas volume expansion shifts the curve to the right.

in some increase in ADH secretion. This factor may mediate the rise in ADH seen during sleep.

The interaction between the baro- and osmoreceptor systems has long been of interest. Under ordinary conditions, when changes in volume are modest, the osmoreceptor system is the major regulator of ADH secretion. Figure 3-3 illustrates the relationship between ADH levels and osmolality. In states of volume depletion, the osmo- and baroreceptor systems appear to operate in an integrated fashion. Volume depletion lowers the osmotic threshold, shifting the curve of ADH level versus osmolality to the left, whereas volume expansion shifts the curve to the right. In certain situations of severe volume depletion, either effective or real, baroreceptor stimulation of ADH secretion occurs in spite of significant hypo-osmolality. In these situations, volume is conserved at the expense of tonicity.

Pain, severe stress, hypoxia, hypercapnia, and nausea also stimulate ADH release. The mechanism for these effects is unclear. Centrally, acetylcholine and alpha-adrenergic stimuli result in ADH release, whereas beta-adrenergic stimulation inhibits ADH release.

Effects of ADH

When ADH is present in the bloodstream, reabsorption of water from the distal convoluted tubule and collecting duct of the nephron occurs. This process results in the preservation of water and the elaboration of concentrated urine. The reabsorbed water is not excreted and remains in the individual's body, lessening the rise in plasma osmolality and helping to maintain both blood volume and total body water volume. This reabsorption of water completes the feedback loop and tends to decrease the secretion of ADH. The renal effect of ADH occurs at relatively low concentrations of the hormone. At higher concentrations, ADH has vasoconstrictive effects that result in increased blood pressure.

Two separate mechanisms of hormone action have been elucidated for ADH. The vasoactive effects are mediated by the V_1 receptor, which is located on vascular smooth muscle cells. The signaling initiated by ADH at the V_1 receptor occurs through activation of phospholipase C, which results in the generation of inositol trisphosphate and diacylglycerol. Diacylglycerol activates protein kinase C, and inositol trisphosphate mobilizes intracellular calcium. These events lead to smooth muscle contraction.

The renal effects are mediated by the V_2 cell surface receptor. Binding of the hormone to this receptor results in activation of adenylate cyclase, with resultant generation of cyclic adenosine monophosphate (cAMP) and activation of protein kinase A. This signaling results in the fusion of water channels with the cell membrane, allowing the movement of water out of the tubular lumen. Movement of water through the membranes of the distal convoluted tubules and collecting ducts results in the elaboration of concentrated urine and the conservation of water. The corticomedullary osmotic gradient developed by the countercurrent system and the cortical diluting segment of the nephron makes possible excretion of urine that is either very dilute (50 mOsm/kg) or highly concentrated (1200 mOsm/kg). In the absence of ADH there is no opportunity for the reabsorption of water, and a large volume of very dilute urine is excreted. When ADH is present, water is reabsorbed into the renal medulla and papilla, with the conservation of water and the elaboration of a small volume of concentrated urine.

OXYTOCIN

In women, oxytocin is secreted in response to nipple stimulation and in response to stimulation of stretch receptors in the vagina. The surge of oxytocin seen in the final stages of labor and the increase that occurs with sexual intercourse probably are mediated by vaginal receptors.

Although relatively normal labor and delivery are possible without centrally produced oxytocin, the hormone probably does play a role in normal parturition. Exogenous oxytocin often is used to induce labor or to stimulate uterine contraction. Oxytocin has been found to be produced by the uterus itself, suggesting a possible paracrine effect on the uterus. Oxytocin also is found in other tissues, including the spinal cord, where it may function as a neurotransmitter.

PATHOPHYSIOLOGY OF ADH

Both autoimmune-induced inflammation and anatomic disruption of the neurohypophyseal unit can lead to deficiencies of both ADH and oxytocin. ADH deficiency results in diabetes insipidus—the inappropriate formation of large amounts of dilute urine. With severe deficiency, water loss can be extensive, and it may be difficult for the patient to keep up with water intake to match the losses.

Diabetes insipidus also can be caused by a lack of renal responsiveness to ADH, in which case it is referred to as nephrogenic diabetes insipidus. Nephrogenic diabetes insipidus can be the result of a congenital, hereditary inability to respond to ADH or can be seen in certain conditions that lead to renal unre-

TABLE 3-1. *MEDICATIONS THAT AFFECT ADH*

LEVEL OF EFFECT	ENHANCE ADH	INHIBIT ADH
Hypothalamus—secretion	Amitriptyline	Ethanol
	Carbamazepine	Narcotic antagonists
	Chlorpropamide	Phenytoin
	Clofibrate	Vinblastine
	Morphine	
	Nicotine	
	Phenothiazines	
	Vincristine	
Renal—target organ function	Chlorpropamide	Acetohexamide
	Cyclophosphamide	Demeclocycline
		Lithium
		Propoxyphene
	Prostaglandin inhibitors	Tolazamide

ADH, antidiuretic hormone.

sponsiveness to ADH—hypercalcemia, hypokalemia, and some medications (e.g., lithium). The effects of various medications on ADH secretion and effectiveness are shown in Table 3-1.

Excess levels of ADH can be seen with CNS irritation, and in some cases excess ADH is produced by a malignancy, usually of the lung or upper respiratory tract. The resultant increase in water reabsorption limits renal free water excretion and can result in significant plasma hyponatremia and hypo-osmolality. In addition, a number of drugs increase ADH secretion, and still others potentiate the effects of ADH. These medications can be useful for some patients with partial, central ADH deficiency.

CLINICALLY USEFUL TESTS OF POSTERIOR PITUITARY FUNCTION AND ANATOMY

Serum Sodium Concentration. The concentration of sodium and its attendant anions, largely chloride, accounts for most of the total serum osmolality. Although extremes of sodium balance, excess, and deficiency, eventually may be reflected in abnormalities of serum sodium concentration, the concentration of sodium in the serum is essentially a function of the water balance state of the individual. Elevations of sodium concentration are seen in states of total body water deprivation. A serum sodium concentration lower than normal is seen with water overload or intoxication.

Urine Sodium Concentration. In the face of normal renal, adrenal cortical, and thyroid function, the concentration of sodium in the urine is helpful in evaluating effective volume status. In states of volume overload, urinary sodium excretion and concentration are increased. Volume depletion, on the other hand, results in a decrease in urinary sodium concentration and excretion. The test is readily available and does not require a timed collection of urine.

Plasma Osmolality. Plasma osmolality may be approximated by doubling the serum sodium concentration. A more accurate value can be obtained by adding the contributions of glucose (glucose concentration in mg/dL divided by 18) and urea (urea concentration in mg/dL divided by 2.8). In some situations, however, additional osmolar particles that are not measured in the usually available blood chemistry values may be present. In such cases, measurement of the total serum osmolality by freezing point depression techniques can be very helpful.

Urine Osmolality. Urine osmolality can be used to assess renal function and to evaluate abnormalities of water balance. The urine osmolality may be hyper- or hypotonic compared to serum osmolality. Inability to dilute or concentrate urine can be seen in renal dysfunction of various etiologies and in disorders of ADH secretion or function.

Urine Specific Gravity. In the absence of glucose or other chemicals that alter the specific gravity measurement, the specific gravity of urine is a rough approximation of the urine osmolality. A value of 1.010 is essentially iso-osmotic with normal serum.

Vasopressin Level. ADH levels are available in some clinical laboratories. These tests are expensive, and the sample must be handled very carefully. Elevated values are seen in nephrogenic diabetes insipidus and in states of inappropriate antidiuretic hormone excess. Low values are seen in states of water intoxication and central diabetes insipidus.

Dynamic Testing: Water Deprivation Testing. The differential diagnosis of polyuric states often requires a water deprivation test. Because both excess water intake (1° polydipsia) and central ADH deficiency are associated with a low level of ADH, additional dynamic testing is necessary to distinguish between these diagnostic possibilities. Lack of response to exogenous ADH after several hours of water deprivation is diagnostic of nephrogenic diabetes insipidus (Fig. 3-4).

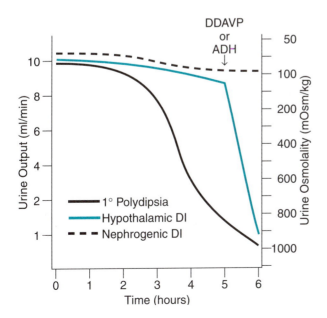

Figure 3-4. Water deprivation testing. A person with normal renal and posterior pituitary function decreases urine output and increases urine osmolality in response to water deprivation. When posterior pituitary failure (i.e., hypothalamic diabetes insipidus [DI]) is present, only a small decline in urine output occurs, but a marked decline in urine output and a rise in urine osmolality occur in response to ADH or its analogue, DDAVP. No response to either water deprivation or exogenous ADH is seen in nephrogenic diabetes insipidus.

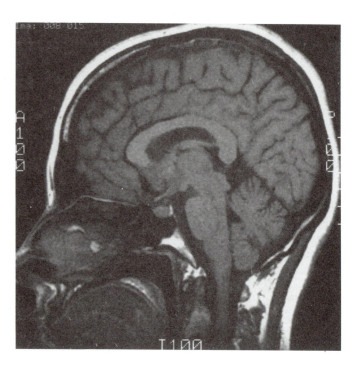

Figure 3-5. Normal MRI of the brain—
lateral view. The bright white signal is characteristic of the posterior pituitary.

Anatomic Testing: MRI. MR imaging of the hypothalamus and pituitary
can be useful in evaluating patients with apparent abnormalities of the hypothalamic–pituitary unit. The posterior pituitary typically is seen as a bright white signal
on the T1-weighted images of an MRI study (Fig. 3-5).

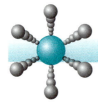

CASE PRESENTATION: CASE 1

Polyuria and polydipsia in a 24-year-old woman

Myra Wilson was about 24 years old when she began having to plan her
life and activities around the availability of water faucets and restrooms.
Over a 2- or 3-year period she had developed a persistent, unquenchable
thirst. Ice water was her preferred beverage, but even that didn't satisfy her
thirst completely. She drank several liters of water a day and urinated very
frequently, about every hour. She could not sleep for more than 2 hours
without having to get up to urinate and drink more water. In a classroom or
a movie theater she always sat close to the door, so she could exit quickly
and get to a restroom and water supply promptly.

Myra's past medical history was unremarkable. She had never had surgery and could not recall any significant trauma. She knows of no allergies.
She takes oral contraceptives, but no other medications, and denies any rec-
reational drug use. She does not smoke and uses very little alcohol. A detailed review of systems was unremarkable. Her menstrual periods are regular.

Physical examination revealed a healthy-appearing woman with a half-empty bottle of spring water in her hand. Her blood pressure was 106/66, and her pulse was 88. HEENT exam revealed a dry mouth. Her visual fields were full. Her chest was clear, and her cardiac and abdominal examinations were unremarkable. There was no edema.

Laboratory Studies

Test	Myra Wilson	Normal
CBC (complete blood count)	Normal	Normal
Serum sodium	145 mEq/L	135–145 mEq/L
Serum potassium	4.2 mEq/L	3.5–5.0 mEq/L
Serum osmolality	294 mOsm/kg	285–295 mOsm/kg
Urine osmolality	75 mOsm/kg	50–1200 mOsm/kg, depending on volume status
Urinalysis:		
Color	Yellow, clear	Yellow, clear
Specific gravity	1.001	1.001–1.020
Protein	Negative	Negative
Blood	Negative	Negative
Glucose	Negative	Negative
Ketones	Negative	Negative
Nitrite	Negative	Negative
Leukocytes	Negative	Negative

The lack of glucose in the urine sample indicates that Ms. Wilson's polyuric state is not caused by diabetes mellitus. If glucose-induced osmotic diuresis were the problem, the urine glucose would be strongly positive. The urine specific gravity and osmolality are both very low. These are the characteristics of renal tubular fluid as it leaves the ascending limb of the loop of Henle and enters the collecting duct system.

Although the production of large amounts of dilute urine can be physiologic—i.e., in response to the ingestion of large amounts of water—it also can result from deficiency of ADH or inability to respond to the hormone. Ms. Wilson's serum sodium and plasma osmolality are at the upper end of the normal range, but not frankly elevated. Lower values might be expected with water intoxication and higher values with ADH deficiency or ineffectiveness, but it is very difficult to separate the diagnostic possibilities based on random serum and plasma data. The differential diagnosis of polyuric states must, therefore, include all three possibilities:

Primary polydipsia. Although properly placed CNS lesions result in polydipsia in animals, clinically this disorder usually is a component of a psychotic state; it also may result from the use of antipsychotic drugs.

Central (hypothalamic) diabetes insipidus (DI). When less than 12% to 20% of the secretory capacity of the neurohypophyseal unit is functioning, central DI may result. Although some ADH may be present, the ADH reserve is not adequate to conserve water appropriately. This rare condition may be idiopathic, autoimmune, posttraumatic (surgical or nonsurgical), or the result of some local process—e.g., tumor, meningitis, or infiltrative disease.

Nephrogenic diabetes insipidus. Lack of renal responsiveness to ADH may be seen as a hereditary (usually sex-linked, expressed only in males) condition or it may be acquired because of an alteration in renal function that results in decreased ability to concentrate urine (e.g., lithium therapy, hypokalemia, hypercalcemia, sickle cell anemia, or pyelonephritis).

Ms. Wilson's 24-hour urine collection was measured at 8.9 liters, an impressively large volume.

An outpatient water deprivation test was scheduled shortly after her initial visit. Ms. Wilson was instructed to come to the medical center at 8 a.m. after a light breakfast. On arrival she was weighed, her vital signs were taken, both lying down and standing, and urine and blood samples were taken. After the test started, she could chew gum and suck on hard candy but could not eat or drink anything. Every hour she was asked to pass a urine sample; in addition, every 2 hours her vital signs and weight were measured:

Time	Urine Volume (mL)	Urine Specific Gravity	Urine Osmolality (mOsm/kg)	Additional Data
8:00 a.m.	450	1.001	57	Weight 143 lbs 110/70, P 78 supine 108/68, P 82 standing
9:00 a.m.	425	1.001	59	—
10:00 a.m.	420	1.001	69	Weight 141.8 lbs 108/68, P 88 supine 104/60, P 98 standing Very thirsty, uncomfortable
11:00 a.m.	400	1.003	70	—
Noon	375	1.003	78	Weight 141 lbs 90/54, P 100 supine 88/54, P 112 standing Very uncomfortable, dizzy on standing. *Given 5 units of aqueous vasopressin subcutaneously at noon.*
1:00 p.m.	25	1.015	958	
2:00 p.m.	Unable to void	—	—	Much more comfortable: Weight 141 lbs 90/52, P 100 supine 90/60, P 110 standing

The separation of polyuric states can be made by water deprivation testing (see Fig. 3-4). Unlike other hormone systems, ADH secretion systems do not appear to atrophy after prolonged suppression or to hypertrophy after prolonged stimulation. Water deprivation should, therefore, result initially in an osmotic and later in a a volume stimulus to ADH secretion. With urine osmolality as an end point, a patient with primary polydipsia usually shows a significant increase in urine osmolality in the face of water restriction. If there is little or no response after several hours of water deprivation, aqueous ADH or an analogue of ADH, DDAVP (discussed later in this chapter), can be given. Patients with central DI show improved concentration of their urine, whereas patients with nephrogenic DI show little or no response to either water deprivation or to exogenous ADH. The response to exogenous ADH can help determine whether a patient has with a mild form of central DI or primary polydipsia. The polyuric state itself—in central DI or in primary polydipsia—can reduce renal concentrating ability. This occurs by "washout" of the corticomedullary osmotic gradient. Because several hours of water deprivation is sufficient to cause enough ADH release for maximal antidiuretic effect, any response to exogenous ADH after significant water deprivation suggests a deficiency of ADH.

Ms. Wilson clearly was unable to respond normally to water deprivation, which eliminates primary polydipsia as the cause of her polyuric state. The slight rise in urine osmolality and fall in urine output that were seen during the test probably are caused by non–ADH-mediated renal responses to volume depletion. The prompt and impressive response to ADH indicates that renal responsiveness to ADH is present and that she does not have nephrogenic diabetes insipidus. Although an ADH level could be measured, it would be helpful only in excluding nephrogenic DI. Low values are seen in both central DI and primary polydipsia. An elevated value is seen in nephrogenic DI.

An MRI of the brain was normal. The sella and its contents appeared normal.

After completing the water deprivation test, Ms. Wilson started using DDAVP nasal spray. It seemed like a miracle. For the first time in 3 years her thirst was quenched, and for the first time in a long while she slept uninterrupted for 7 hours. Occasionally polyuria and thirst would return suddenly when the effects of the medication wore off. Luckily, her water balance came under control again within minutes of taking another dose of the DDAVP.

The cause of Ms. Wilson's central diabetes insipidus is unclear, but it does not appear to be caused by a mass lesion or destruction of structure in the hypothalamus or pituitary. Autoimmune destruction of the neurohypophysis is the probable cause.

Vasopressin replacement by various preparations and routes has been used to treat central diabetes insipidus. DDAVP—a modified arginine vasopressin molecule—can be administered as a nasal spray, a subcutaneous injection, or an oral form. Modifications of the natural hormone molecule, shown in Figure 3-6, result in a longer half-life and in very little vasoconstricting activity. DDAVP, although expensive, is the treatment of choice for central DI.

DDAVP

$$O=C\text{-}CH_2\text{-}CH_2 \text{—} S\text{–}S \text{—} Cys_6 \text{—} Pro_7 \text{—} D\text{-}Arg_8 \text{—} Gly_9(NH_2)$$

$$Try_2 \qquad Asn_5$$

$$Phe_3 \text{———————} Gln_4$$

Figure 3-6. DDAVP molecule.

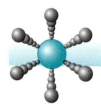

CASE PRESENTATION: CASE 2

Wide fluctuations in water balance following pituitary surgery in a 58-year-old man

Several weeks of tunnel vision led Charles McHenry to see his eye doctor for an evaluation. Visual field testing confirmed the presence of a bitemporal hemianopsia and led to an MRI, which showed a large sellar mass with suprasellar extension impinging on the optic chiasm. Endocrine evaluation showed evidence of gonadal hypofunction with a low testosterone and a low LH. The prolactin level was mildly elevated, at 44 ng/mL. Thyroid function tests were within the normal range, and an insulin tolerance test showed adequate adrenal axis reserve.

Because of the compromise of his vision, surgical decompression of the optic chiasm was recommended. The transsphenoidal surgery went well with the removal of a large, benign adenoma and decompression of the chiasm. Mr. McHenry was "covered" with stress-dose corticosteroids to correct possible adrenal axis hypofunction that might occur during the surgery and in the postoperative period.

Four hours after the surgery was completed the nurses in the surgical intensive care unit noted a significant decrease in hourly urine output, down to 10 mL per hour. He was receiving 5% dextrose in water intravenously at a rate of 200 mL/hour.

Laboratory Studies

Test	Charles McHenry	Normal
Serum sodium	123 mEq/L	135–145 mEq/L
BUN	6 mg/dL	8–22 mg/dL
Urinary sodium concentration	82 mEq/L	Volume depleted: <25 mEq/L Volume overloaded: >70 mEq/L

The low serum sodium, the low BUN, and the low urine output in the face of continued fluid intake indicate that a disorder of fluid balance is present. Mr. McHenry is unable to appropriately excrete the extra body water that he is accumulating. When adrenal cortical and thyroid function are normal, hyponatremia paired with an elevation of urinary sodium concentration points to an excess of ADH.

A syndrome of water intoxication or apparent "inappropriate" secretion of ADH (SIADH) is seen in several conditions. The term *inappropriate* refers to the fact that the secretion of ADH is continuing in the face of significant hypo-osmolality—a condition that ordinarily would shut off ADH secretion. In some instances, decreased volume—effective (e.g., severe congestive heart failure, liver failure) or real (e.g., diuretic therapy or large fluid loss, hemorrhage)—clearly is the stimulus for ADH release. SIADH also is seen in pneumonia and other inflammatory conditions of the lung and when tumors produce excessive amounts of ADH. In still other instances, the excess ADH is of central origin and is related to CNS pathology or surgery in the hypothalamic or pituitary area. Agents that potentiate ADH effect (especially chlorpropamide), including some of those listed in Table 3-1, also may produce a syndrome of ADH excess that is inappropriate for osmolality (see Table 3-1).

When increased ADH levels are combined with normal fluid intake, the extracellular fluid space expands with water and body solutes become diluted, with a resulting lower plasma osmolality and sodium concentration. The urine excreted in such situations often is more concentrated than the plasma, but in all cases it is relatively more concentrated than it would have been if more appropriate, lower levels of ADH were present. The relative volume expansion increases the glomerular filtration rate (GFR), decreases proximal renal tubular fluid reabsorption, and decreases renin-angiotensin stimulation of aldosterone secretion. Each of these factors tends to increase urinary sodium excretion. Edema is not present because total body sodium is not increased and the extra water is distributed evenly throughout the body. Mr. McHenry's apparent excess ADH is clearly related to his surgery earlier in the day. Trauma and mechanical irritation of the neurohypophyseal unit resulted in the release, inappropriate for both tonicity and volume status, of preformed ADH.

Ten hours after his intravenous fluid rate was decreased to the lowest volume possible, about 10 mL/h, Charles McHenry's sodium concentration rose to 128 mEq/L. He was alert and quite pleased with the improvement in his vision. He began to take fluids orally but was limited to 500 mL per day.

Thirty-six hours after the operation, Mr. McHenry's urine output increased markedly and he became very thirsty. His urine output was now 600 mL/hr, and the following laboratory studies were obtained:

Test	Charles McHenry	Normal
Serum sodium	158 mEq/L	135–145 mEq/L
BUN	28 mg/dL	8–22 mg/dL
Urinary sodium concentration	22 mEq/L	Volume depleted: <25 mEq/L Volume overloaded: >70 mEq/L

Now Mr. McHenry has evidence of volume depletion and free water deficiency. The hyponatremia of ADH excess has been replaced with hypernatremia. Hypernatremia is occurring in the face of an inappropriate diuresis of relatively dilute urine. These findings are consistent with a deficiency of ADH. Water deprivation testing is not necessary in this clinical setting to establish a diagnosis of ADH deficiency. The trauma of surgery in the area of the pituitary that earlier resulted in the release of preformed ADH has now led to a deficiency of ADH. Because of the short half-life of ADH, the effects of the traumatically released excess ADH wear off quickly and usually are replaced by a period of relative ADH deficiency. Fortunately, a return to normal fluid balance and ADH dynamics usually is seen by 2 to 3 weeks postoperatively. Neurons of the neurohypophyseal unit that were bruised by the surgery or trauma usually recover enough function to maintain normal fluid balance.

Three months after surgery Mr. McHenry is feeling quite well. His visual fields are even fuller than they were immediately postoperatively and are almost back to normal. Gonadal function has returned to normal, and postoperative testing shows maintenance of normal thyroid function and normal stress responsiveness of the hypothalamic–pituitary–adrenal axis. His serum sodium and thirst are now normal.

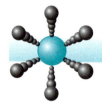

CASE PRESENTATION: CASE 3

Hyponatremia in a 65-year-old man with a lung mass

Donald Granger was very pleased that he was able to stop smoking last year. He is now 65 years old, and he had been smoking since he was 15. Although his cough had seemed to improve with discontinuation of cigarettes, it was now clearly worse and productive of small amounts of grayish sputum. He is on no medications, knows of no allergies, and uses moderate amounts of alcohol.

A detailed review of systems was unremarkable.

Physical examination showed a thin, tired-appearing man.

Vital signs:	**Blood pressure 140/84; pulse 88**
HEENT:	**Unremarkable for age**
Chest:	**Decreased air movement, no evidence of consolidation or wheezing**
Heart:	**Normal but distant heart sounds**
Abdomen:	**Normal**
Neurologic examination:	**Normal**
Chest X-ray:	**Left perihilar lung mass, 4 cm in diameter (Fig. 3-7)**

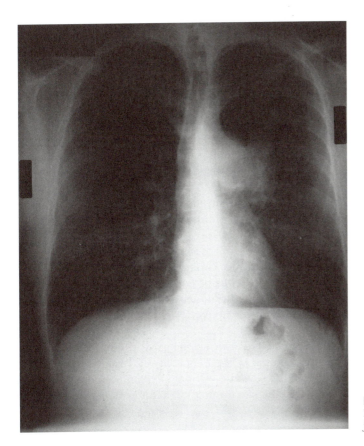

Figure 3-7. Posteroanterior chest X-ray: Donald Granger. A large hilar mass is seen just above the heart.

Laboratory Studies

Test	Donald Granger	Normal
Serum sodium	123 mEq/L	135–145 mEq/L
BUN	10 mg/dL	8–22 mg/dL
Urine osmolality	295 mOsm/kg	50–1200 mOsm/kg
Urine sodium	78 mEq/L	Volume depleted: <25 mEq/L Volume overloaded: >70 mEq/L
TSH	1.0 mU/L	0.3–5.0 mU/L
Cortisol, 8 a.m.	19 μg/dL	5–25 μg/dL

Hyponatremia in the face of normal renal, adrenal, and thyroid function suggests either significant volume depletion or inappropriate ADH levels. In the presence of volume depletion, the urinary sodium concentration should be relatively low, usually less than 25 mEq/L. The renal excretion of sodium is dependent on the glomerular filtration rate (GFR), proximal tubular sodium reabsorption, and distal, aldosterone-mediated sodium exchange. In the face of volume depletion, all three of these factors work to conserve sodium and decrease sodium excretion. The decrease in GFR results in the delivery of less sodium to the proximal tubule. Volume depletion increases proximal tubular sodium reabsorption; thus, even less sodium is delivered distally in the nephron. The stimulation of the renin-angiotensin system that occurs with volume depletion leads to aldosterone secretion. Aldosterone promotes further sodium reabsorption in exchange for potassium and hydrogen ions in the distal nephron. The net effect of these three factors, each of which is triggered by volume depletion, is the excretion of urine that has a very low sodium concentration.

Although Mr. Granger's urine osmolality is nearly iso-osmotic with normal serum, it is more concentrated than his serum and is therefore inappropriately concentrated for his hyponatremic, hypo-osmolal, volume-overloaded state. These findings all point to either an elevated level of ADH or an increased renal responsiveness to ADH.

The water restriction regimen Mr. Granger was told to follow was not easy. He was used to drinking three cups of coffee in the morning, a can of cola with lunch, another can in the afternoon, and at least two cups of tea after dinner. He now has to limit his intake to about three cups of fluid a day.

The chest mass was evaluated with bronchoscopy. Transbronchial biopsy revealed small cell carcinoma of the lung. Chest CT scanning indicated that it was not resectable. Next week he will begin chemotherapy. He plans to ask if there is anything else he can do that might allow him at least a little more fluid intake each day.

The treatment of SIADH involves looking for treatable causes and, if possible, correcting them. In Mr. Granger's case, the lung tumor is producing and secreting large amounts of ADH in an unregulated fashion. Water restriction often is helpful in returning plasma solute concentration toward normal. In severe cases, hypertonic saline may transiently improve severe hypo-osmolality. The sodium that is added is quickly excreted in the urine and has only a transient effect on the serum sodium concentration. Drugs that may cause renal unresponsiveness to ADH or nephrogenic diabetes insipidus—e.g., lithium and demethylchlortetracycline (see Table 3-1)—have been used with some success in patients with SIADH. Successful treatment of the tumor may also result in more normal ADH levels and increased ability to excrete free water.

After starting demethylchlortetracycline, Mr. Granger was able to increase his fluid intake moderately. He really enjoyed being able to have half a can of cola in the afternoon.

KEY POINTS AND CONCEPTS

- ADH secretion is very sensitive to changes in osmolality of as little as 1% to 2%.
- ADH secretion also is sensitive to changes in volume status of 10% to 15%.
- Trauma to or irritation of the neurohypophyseal unit may result in transient excess of ADH and in transient or permanent deficiency of ADH.
- States of excess ADH may be caused by CNS irritation, by tumor production of ADH, by stimulation of volume-sensing stretch receptors in the lung, by pneumonia or other lung conditions, or by potentiation of ADH effect by some medications.
- Treatment of ADH excess usually involves water deprivation and may include medications that antagonize the effects of ADH.
- ADH deficiency is the result of central hypothalamic or posterior pituitary damage.
- ADH insensitivity (nephrogenic diabetes insipidus) may be inherited or may be acquired, usually as a result of a condition or medication that impairs renal function.
- ADH deficiency may be treated with a long-lasting analogue, DDAVP.

SUGGESTED READING

Kovacs L, Robertson GL. Disorders of water balance—hyponatremia and hypernatremia. Clin Endocrinol Metab 6:107–127, 1992.

Robertson GL Differential diagnosis of polyuria. Annu Rev Med 39:425–442, 1988.

Seckl JR, Dunger DB. Diabetes insipidus: current treatment recommendations. Drugs 44:216–224, 1992.

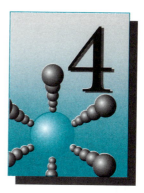

The Thyroid

Most metabolic functions are regulated by thyroid hormone. In addition to normal growth and development, a number of other basic functions also require the presence of normal levels of thyroid hormone. Although strides have been made in understanding the effects of thyroid hormone at physiologic levels, it is clinical observations of the effects of the extremes—high and low—of thyroid hormone concentration that have shaped our understanding of the vital role that the thyroid and its hormones play in the normal function of the human organism.

ANATOMY

The thyroid gland is the largest endocrine gland (Fig. 4-1). It is a bilobed structure derived from pharyngeal endoderm. During embryologic development, it descends from the pharynx through the thyroglossal duct to a position low in the anterior neck. The isthmus, a bridge of tissue connecting the right and left lobes of the thyroid gland, overlies the trachea at the level of the cricoid cartilage. In the adult, the entire thyroid gland weighs approximately 15 to 20 g, and the lobes measure approximately 4 cm in length, 2 to 2.5 cm in width, and 1 to 1.5 cm in thickness. Bilateral inferior, middle, and superior thyroid arteries, branches of the external carotid and subclavian arteries, provide a rich blood supply for the thyroid. Venous drainage is into the internal jugular and subclavian veins. The thyroid lies beneath the infrahyoid strap muscles of the anterior neck and medial to the sternocleidomastoid muscles and carotid sheaths. The parathyroid glands, usually four in number, are located directly behind the thyroid and derive their blood supply from the posterior capsule of the thyroid. The recurrent laryngeal nerves, branches of the vagus nerve, usually are found in the groove between the lobes of the thyroid and the trachea but can run through the substance of the thyroid. These nerves provide postganglionic motor innervation to the muscles of the vocal cords.

The follicle is the functional unit of the thyroid (Fig. 4-2). It consists of a spherical array of cells surrounding a noncellular center of proteinaceous material

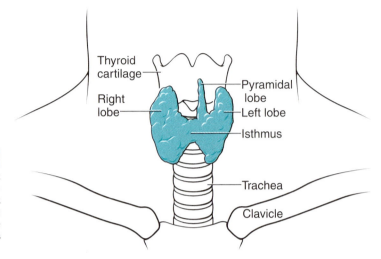

Figure 4-1. The normal thyroid gland. The thyroid gland is located low in the anterior neck. The right and left lobes are connected by the isthmus. A pyramidal lobe, a remnant of the embryologic descent of the thyroid from the base of the tongue to the anterior neck, sometimes is present.

that is referred to as colloid. The shape of the cells lining the follicle can vary, from cuboidal in conditions of little stimulation to columnar at times of more intense function. Fibrous tissue provides an endoskeleton upon which thousands of follicles are arranged and defines the shape and structure of the thyroid. Interspersed among the follicles are parafollicular cells, or C cells. These cells are the source of calcitonin (see Chapter 6) and appear to play no role in thyroid hormone physiology.

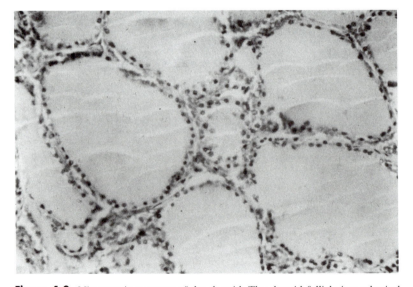

Figure 4-2. Microscopic anatomy of the thyroid. The thyroid follicle is a spherical array of cells surrounding a central mass of proteinaceous material, referred to as colloid. Parafollicular or C cells also are present in the thyroid.

CHEMISTRY

The thyroid follicular cell is shown in Figure 4-3. At the basal surface, the thyroid follicular cell actively pumps iodide molecules from the extracellular space into the cytoplasm (see Fig. 4-3). Although some molecules of iodide may passively diffuse back into the extracellular fluid, many are trapped in the follicular unit by the oxidation of iodide by thyroperoxidase, a process that occurs at the apex of the follicular cell. The oxidized iodine is covalently bound to a tyrosine molecule. The iodinated tyrosine residue is part of a large protein, thyroglobulin, that has multiple tyrosine residues available for iodination. Thyroglobulin is synthesized by the follicular cell and stored as a component of the colloid that fills the follicular lumen. Both oxidation and organification of iodine occur at the junction of the apex of the follicular cell and the colloid-containing lumen of the follicle. Each tyrosine molecule has two sites that can be iodinated.

The next step in the synthesis of thyroid hormone is the coupling of iodinated tyrosine residues within the thyroglobulin molecule. Coupling of two di-

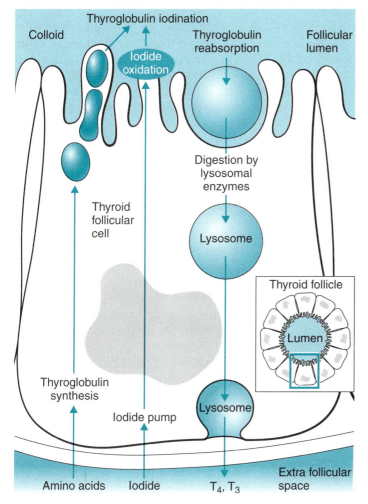

Figure 4-3. Thyroid hormone synthesis and release. Follicular cells trap and oxidize iodine. At the colloidal interface, thyroglobulin is iodinated, and eventually thyroid hormones are formed. Thyroglobulin is reabsorbed into the follicular cell and released after digestion by lysosomal enzymes.

iodinated tyrosine (DIT) residues results in the formation of thyroxine (T_4); similarly, the coupling of a mono-iodinated residue (MIT) with a di-iodinated residue results in the formation of triiodothyronine, or T_3.

Thyroid hormones (T_4 and T_3) are stored as part of the thyroglobulin molecule in the colloid portion of the follicle. Thyroid hormone is released into the extracellular space at the basal surface of the follicular cell after being brought back into the follicular cell from the colloid portion of the follicle by endocytosis. In preparation for release, endocytotic vesicles fuse with lysosomes, and thyroglobulin is degraded into T_4, T_3, MIT, DIT, and free amino acids. T_4 and T_3 are released at the basal surface of the cell into the extracellular space and, eventually, into the circulation.

Once secreted, thyroid hormone is bound extensively to circulating plasma proteins and has a half-life of approximately 7 days. Thyroid-binding globulin (TBG) binds about 75% of circulating hormone; transthyretin or thyroid-binding pre-albumin (TBPA) binds about 15%; and albumin binds about 10%. Circulating thyroxine is approximately 99.96% protein bound. Bound hormone is not available directly for metabolic activity but is in equilibrium with the 0.04% that is unbound. It is this free portion that is available for activation and eventual metabolic effect.

A large amount of T_4 is stored in the colloid of the many follicles of the thyroid. Although thyroxine is the principal product of the thyroid, it is not the active form of the hormone. The high nuclear receptor affinity for T_3 compared with T_4 makes T_3 a much more potent thyroid hormone. Under normal states of nutrition and thyroid function, approximately 15% of the circulating T_3 is derived from the thyroid gland. Most of the circulating T_3 is derived from the peripheral deiodination of T_4. Enzyme systems in the liver, kidney, and other tissues control the production of active T_3 or, depending on the presence of certain conditions or medications, may result in the production of an inactive form, reverse T_3 (rT_3). The structure of T_4 and the active (T_3) and inactive (rT_3) forms of T_3 are shown in Figure 4-4. Once released from the thyroid or produced by the peripheral monodeiodination of T_4, T_3 also is highly protein bound—99.3% by TBG and albumin. It has a half-life of 24 hours.

Unbound T_3 is actively transported across the cell membrane into the cytoplasm. At the nucleus, thyroid hormone binds to specific receptors—receptors in the same family of nuclear receptors that are involved in the action of steroid hormones and vitamin D. Binding on these receptors results in increased RNA transcriptional activity and the resultant production of various proteins. It also appears that there are posttranscriptional effects of thyroid hormone.

The metabolic functions of thyroid hormone are clear clinically when extreme excess or deficiency states are present. The intracellular basis for the metabolic effects of thyroid is less clear, but it includes increased Na^+-K^+ ATPase activity. The increased activity of this enzyme requires high levels of ATP and generates heat. The increased ATP requirement is supplied by oxidative phosphorylation in mitochondria. In states of excess thyroid hormone, there is increased oxygen demand, increased heat production, and increased metabolic fuel use that usually results in weight loss. When thyroid hormone deficiency is present, heat generation and oxygen demand decrease and metabolic fuels are burned less rapidly, resulting in weight gain. In addition, the activity of enzymes involved in the intermediary metabolism of carbohydrates, proteins, and fats is clearly affected by the level of thyroid hormone.

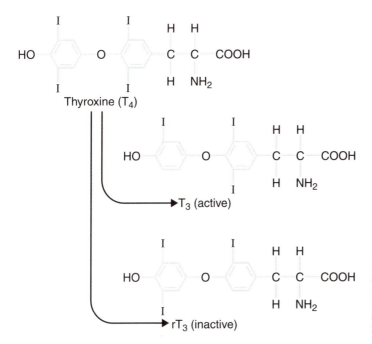

Figure 4-4. Metabolism of T_4. Monodeiodination of the outer ring of the thyroxine molecule results in activation of the hormone. Inner ring deiodination results in the production of an inactive form, rT_3.

REGULATION OF THYROID FUNCTION

The secretion of thyroid hormone from the thyroid gland is controlled by the anterior pituitary hormone, thyroid-stimulating hormone (TSH, thyrotropin) (Fig. 4-5). TSH is secreted by the thyrotroph cells of the anterior pituitary and stimulates both the synthesis and release of thyroid hormone. In addition, TSH stimulates the growth of the thyroid and increases vascularity. The secretion of TSH is controlled by the circulating level of thyroid hormone. TSH is a glycoprotein hormone with an alpha and a beta subunit. As is characteristic of protein hormones, it has a relatively short half-life of about 50 minutes. TSH shares the same alpha subunit with other glycoprotein hormones (i.e., LH, FSH, and hCG). Secretion of TSH by the anterior pituitary is facilitated by thyrotropin-releasing hormone (TRH), the hypothalamic-releasing hormone, distributed to the anterior pituitary from the hypothalamus by the portal system. The major factor controlling TSH synthesis and secretion is the T_3 concentration within the thyrotroph cell itself. T_3, whether derived from the circulation directly or from the intracellular deiodination of T_4 within the thyrotroph cell, inhibits gene transcription of both the alpha and beta subunits of TSH. High levels of T_3 shut off the production of TSH, and low levels enhance the production of TSH. This inhibition of TSH secretion and the resulting lack of thyroid stimulation complete the negative feedback loop. The end product of the system, T_3, controls its own production.

DISORDERS OF THE THYROID GLAND

Clinical disorders of the thyroid gland and of thyroid-related metabolic abnormalities fit into one of three categories: overactivity, underactivity, and abnormal anatomy. Anatomic abnormalities can at times be associated with overactivity

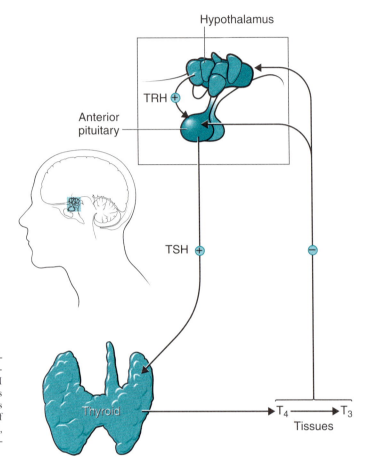

Figure 4-5. The hypothalamic–pituitary–thyroid axis. The active form of thyroid hormone, T_3, controls both TRH and TSH secretion. Although some T_3 is produced by the thyroid gland, most is derived from the monodeiodination of T_4, a process that occurs in many tissues, including the hypothalamus and the anterior pituitary.

or underactivity, but most are associated with normal function of the thyroid. Many aspects of thyroid disease are related to autoimmune phenomena and often are associated with other autoimmune processes involving the endocrine or other systems. Thyroid disorders occur more commonly in females and tend to cluster in families.

Although hypofunction of the thyroid can be the result of hypothalamic or pituitary disease, it is most commonly caused by failure of the thyroid gland itself. Autoimmune thyroiditis, often referred to as Hashimoto's thyroiditis, is the most common cause of thyroid gland failure, but viral infections, radiation-induced damage, and surgical removal are other mechanisms of thyroid gland failure. Because the thyroid has a very large functional reserve, destruction of the thyroid must be extensive before clinical hypothyroidism develops.

Hyperfunction of the thyroid is often the result of an autoimmune process. In Graves' disease, hyperfunction is mediated by an antibody that activates the TSH receptor and drives the thyroid in an unregulated, usually excessive, fashion. Autonomous function of a nodule or nodules of the thyroid is another cause of hyperfunction. The release of preformed, stored thyroid hormone caused by an inflammatory process is yet another mechanism by which thyroid hormone levels can be elevated. Only very rarely is thyroid hyperfunction due to pituitary disease or inappropriate TSH production.

Although most anatomic abnormalities of the thyroid are the result of benign conditions or processes, thyroid cancer does occur. For many patients, thyroid cancer is a rather unaggressive malignancy, but in a few it can be life-threatening, and all cases require careful evaluation and management.

CLINICALLY USEFUL TESTS OF THYROID FUNCTION AND ANATOMY

Serum Hormone Levels

Thyroxine (T_4) and Triiodothyronine (T_3). Clinical laboratories can, by various assay methods, accurately determine the total—including both bound and free hormone—concentrations of T_4 and T_3. The range of normal values for both T_4 and T_3 is quite wide: for T_4 it ranges from 5 to 12 μg/dL; for T_3 it ranges from 80 to 200 ng/dL. In addition, there can be significant variations in the measured concentrations of these hormones that are dependent on the concentration of binding proteins rather than on any abnormality of thyroid function. Alterations in binding protein concentration can make the interpretation of total T_4 or total T_3 concentrations difficult. Measurements of free T_4 and free T_3 do solve some of the problems and these tests are becoming more readily available.

T_3 Resin Uptake Test, Free Thyroxine Index, and Thyroid Hormone–Binding Ratio. The T_3 resin uptake test (T_3RU), the free thyroxine index (FTI), and the thyroid hormone–binding ratio (THBR) are designed to deal with variations in protein binding that may affect the interpretation of serum total T_4 and total T_3 levels. In these tests, the functional amount of binding protein present in the serum sample is measured using a competitive binding system. A radioactive tracer is attached to reagent T_3 molecules, which then are added to a mixture of patient serum and a resin that has affinity for T_3. After appropriate mixing and equilibration, the resin is separated from the serum, and the percent of isotope found on the resin is calculated. If binding sites on the patient's serum are filled, the resin uptake is higher than normal. A high resin uptake could, therefore, be seen either if the amount of binding protein were low or if the sites on normal levels of binding protein were already filled with large amounts of thyroid hormone. If the binding sites on the patient's serum were plentiful, however, a low resin uptake would be seen because the serum sites would take up significant amounts of the labeled T_3. Low resin uptake would be seen, therefore, in states of binding protein excess or in situations of thyroid hormone deficiency, with many open binding sites on normal levels of binding protein.

Multiplying the total T_4 concentration by the T_3RU yields the free thyroxine index. Elevations of T_4 that are not caused by binding protein increases are associated with a significantly elevated FTI (Table 4-1). When the T_4 elevation is the result of an increase in binding protein, the resultant decrease in the T_3RU results in a normal or near-normal FTI. Similarly, low levels of T_4 that are not the result of binding protein deficiency or abnormality are associated with very low FTI levels. The elevated T_3RU that results when binding proteins are decreased leads to an FTI in the normal range. The thyroid hormone–binding ratio, a variation of the T_3RU, is a mathematical rearrangement of this same information using 1 as the normal amount of thyroid hormone binding.

TABLE 4-1. *FREE THYROXINE INDEX*

CONDITION	T_4	T_3RU	FTI ($T_4 \times T_3RU$)
Hyperthyroxinemia	High	High	Very high
Elevated TBG	High	Low	Normal
Normal	Normal	Normal	Normal
Decreased TBG	Low	High	Normal
Hypothyroxinemia	Low	Low	Very low

TBG, thyroid-binding globulin.

Serum TSH. If pituitary function is normal and not affected by illness or medications, the serum TSH is an excellent test of thyroid function. A suppressed, below-normal value indicates excess levels of thyroid hormone. An elevated value indicates a deficiency of thyroid hormone. TSH levels have an inverse, log-linear relationship with thyroid hormone levels (Fig. 4-6). Small changes in thyroid hormone level, therefore, result in marked changes in serum TSH levels. Mild degrees of thyroid hormone excess, of either endogenous or exogenous origin, result in very low TSH concentrations. Similarly, small decreases in thyroid hormone level can result in large increases of TSH production and high levels of serum TSH. Long-term elevation of thyroid hormone levels can result in atrophy of TSH secreting ability that can last for several weeks or more. In addition, because several medications and illnesses can affect TSH secretion, the results of TSH testing must be interpreted carefully.

Serum Thyroglobulin Levels. Small amounts of thyroglobulin, the template upon which thyroid hormone synthesis occurs, are released into the circu-

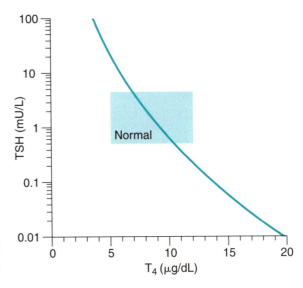

Figure 4-6. Serum TSH versus serum T_4. The scale of TSH is logarithmic, whereas the scale for T_4 is arithmetic. Small changes in T_4 can result in large changes in TSH.

lation with the secretion of thyroid hormone. Levels above normal can be seen in diseases in which the structural integrity of the thyroid follicle is altered (e.g., thyroiditis). Low levels are seen in situations of thyroid hormone excess that is of exogenous and not of thyroidal origin (e.g., surreptitious hormone use).

Radioactive Iodine Uptake. The uptake of a small tracer dose of radioactive iodine at 24 hours can be a very useful test of thyroid function. Twenty-four hours after the oral administration of ^{123}I, the uptake of the isotope by the thyroid is measured. The percentage of uptake is a function of the rate of iodine trapping by the thyroid and also of the size of the patient's iodine pool. The normal range is, therefore, highly dependent on the iodine content of the local diet and environment.

Table 4-2 illustrates how a patient's iodine status can affect the measurement of radioactive iodine uptake in different states of specific thyroid activity. When hyperthyroxinemia is associated with a high radioactive iodine uptake, the diagnosis and therapeutic options usually are quite clear. Hyperthyroxinemia with a low uptake is a more difficult diagnostic problem. Possibilities include iodine excess, thyroiditis, exogenous thyroid hormone use, or ectopic thyroid hormone production.

Radionuclide Scan. A functional picture of the thyroid can be made at the time of a radioactive iodine (^{123}I) uptake test or with technetium pertechnetate administered intravenousiy. A normal thyroid scan is shown in Figure 4-7. When the isotope is iodine, areas of the thyroid that are taking up and organifying the isotope are seen on the scan. Nonfunctional areas are not seen and are said to be "cold." With technetium scanning, the isotope is attached to a pertechnetate molecule that has the size and ionic charge of iodide. Because the pertechnetate is not organified, the image depends on the function of the iodine pump alone. Usually, areas of the thyroid that are "hot" to iodine are also "hot" when imaged with technetium. Similarly, areas that are "cold" usually do not take up either tracer.

Ultrasound Imaging of the Thyroid. Ultrasound imaging of the thyroid can be helpful in accurately measuring the size of the gland and nodules within

TABLE 4-2.	*RADIOACTIVE IODINE UPTAKE*		
RADIOACTIVE IODINE UPTAKE	**SPECIFIC THYROID ACTIVITY**		
	Elevated	**Normal**	**Decreased**
High	**Hyperfunction** (e.g., Graves' disease)	Iodine deficiency	Severe iodine deficiency
Normal	Iodine excess	**Normal**	Iodine deficiency
Low	Severe iodine excess	Iodine excess	**Hypofunction** (e.g., autoimmune or viral thyroiditis)

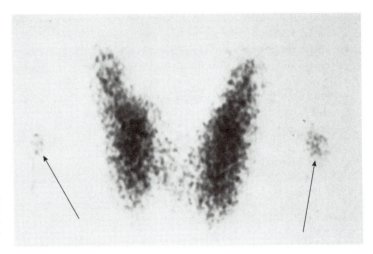

Figure 4-7. Normal thyroid scan. The small markers (*arrows*) on either side usually are 8 cm apart on the patient's neck and can be used to assess the size of the thyroid and of any abnormal areas seen in the thyroid.

it. An ultrasound image also can be useful in identifying fluid-filled or cystic nodules and to follow the size of thyroid nodules over time.

Needle Biopsy of the Thyroid. Although it often provides less than definitive diagnostic information, a simple aspiration biopsy of a thyroid mass can be very useful in the management of nodular thyroid disease. Usually, several (four to eight) passes are made with a fine-gauge (22-gauge) needle attached to a 10-mL syringe. Careful examination of the aspirated material by an experienced cytologist can detect clues to the underlying pathology. Finding evidence of a papillary or, more rarely, an anaplastic malignancy can lead to prompt, appropriate surgical therapy. Benign cytology results can allow careful follow-up rather than surgery as the next step in management. Normal-appearing follicles and follicular cells can be seen in follicular carcinoma of the thyroid. The criteria for a follicular malignancy—vascular or capsular invasion, or both—usually cannot be seen on aspirated material, and surgery usually is required for definitive diagnosis and management when a follicular lesion is found.

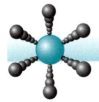

CASE PRESENTATION: CASE 1

Hyperthyroxinemia in a woman with a diffusely enlarged thyroid

Fatigue, a 15-pound weight loss, heat intolerance, palpitations, irritability, and 6 months of amenorrhea led Jane Jones to seek medical attention. She is 27 and works as a beautician. She and her husband, a computer repair technician, have two healthy children aged 2 and 4 years.

Although she was pleased by her weight loss, she was also surprised. At 5′4″, she felt that, at 135 pounds, she was too heavy. Mrs. Jones had not been very successful at dieting since the birth of her last child, but over the last 3 months, in spite of eating normally, her weight has dropped to 120 pounds. Fatigue is a major problem. Simple chores require major effort. In addition, she has become very irritable—upsetting her spouse, her children, and some of her customers. Her hands are very shaky, and she is no longer able to do some procedures at the beauty salon. She feels warm all the time and turns down the thermostat whenever possible.

Further questioning reveals frequent defecation with passage of small amounts of normal stool. Her menstrual periods resumed a few months after the birth of her last child but stopped suddenly about 4 months ago. Two home pregnancy tests have been negative.

Past Medical History

Illnesses:	No diabetes, tuberculosis, hepatitis, or hypertension
Operations:	Appendectomy at age 17
	Tonsillectomy at age 4
Medications:	Occasional aspirin
Allergies:	Penicillin–rash
Habits:	Coffee—4 cups per day
	Alcohol—2 drinks per week
	Tobacco—stopped 5 years ago—½ pack a day for 4 years prior

Family History

Father:	54, overweight, high blood pressure
Mother:	52, healthy, premature menopause at age 38
Siblings:	Sister, 29, healthy
	Brother, 23, healthy
Maternal aunt:	Thyroid condition, treated with surgery; has prominent eyes

Physical Examination

A thin, wide-eyed woman who is unable to sit still in the waiting room or office

Vital signs:	Blood pressure 140/60; pulse 110
Skin:	Warm, dry
HEENT:	Prominent eyes with lid lag and stare, sclerae injected, puffy lids. Media and fundi normal
Neck:	Easily visible and palpable thyroid approximately 2 to 3 times normal size. On auscultation there was a bruit over each lobe of the thyroid
Chest:	Clear
Heart:	Rapid rate, active precordium, easily palpable PMI, normal heart sounds
Abdomen:	Normal
Pelvic:	Normal
Rectal:	Normal
Extremities:	Normal
Neuro:	Normal except for irritability, very brisk deep tendon reflexes, and a fine tremor of her outstretched hands

Laboratory Studies

Test	Jane Jones	Normal
WBC	3100/mm^3	4300–10,800/mm^3
HCT	41%	37%–48% (female)
BUN	10 mg/dL	8–22 mg/dL
Creatinine	1.0 mg/dL	0.3–1.5 mg/dL
Alkaline phosphatase	150 U/L	30–120 U/L
Calcium	10.2 mg/dL	8.5–10.5 mg/dL
T$_4$	18.0 μg/dL	5–12 μg/dL
T$_3$RU	37%	25%–35%
TSH	<0.05 mU/L	0.3–5.0 mU/L
Radioactive iodine uptake	88% at 24 hrs	10%–25% at 24 hrs
hCG, beta subunit	Negative	Negative, not pregnant
Positive, pregnant

Thyroid scan: See Figure 4-8

While awaiting the results of the tests Mrs. Jones is started on propranolol, a beta-adrenergic blocking agent.

Weight loss in the face of adequate caloric intake and without evidence of malabsorption could be explained by an increased metabolic rate. Thyroid hormone is an important controller of metabolic rate and, when present in excess, may lead to a hypermetabolic state with increased nutrient use, increased oxygen requirements, and heat production. Palpitations and an el-

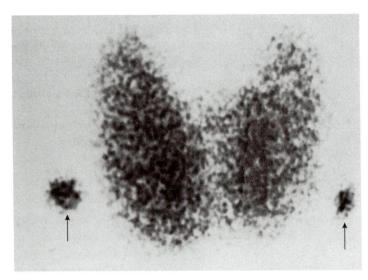

Figure 4-8. Thyroid scan: Jane Jones. The gland is significantly enlarged with isotope uptake distributed evenly. The markers (*arrows*) are 8 cm apart.

evated resting heart rate are among the most common symptoms of hyper-thyroxinemia. The increased oxygen demands of the hypermetabolic state require an increase in cardiac output that leads to an increased heart rate. The heart rate also is elevated by increased sensitivity of the heart to the effects of catecholamines when thyroid hormone levels are elevated. The wide pulse pressure—an elevated systolic pressure with a normal or low di-astolic pressure—is another cardiovascular manifestation of hyperthyroidism. Irritability, tremor, and hyperkinetic behavior are seen commonly in states of thyroid hormone excess. Gastrointestinal manifestations include hyper-defecation, with the frequent passage of small amounts of normal stool.

The amenorrhea of hyperthyroxinemia is related to a combination of factors, including weight loss and increased metabolic destruction of estro-gen, leading to inadequate endometrial stimulation for normal menstruation to occur.

The family history—an aunt with thyroid disease and a mother with premature menopause—points to a possible familial, autoimmune endocrine condition.

Mrs. Jones' physical examination is remarkable for tremor, tachycardia with a dynamic precordium, and wide pulse pressure. The obvious goiter (enlarged thyroid) gives a clue as to the source of the excess thyroid hor-mone. The bruit indicates increased blood flow in the neck, probably the result of a combination of increased carotid artery flow and increased thyroid perfusion.

Eye findings associated with thyroid disease include those seen with elevated hormone levels of any cause and those that are related to the spe-cific pathology of Graves' disease. Spasm of the levator palpebra muscles, which results in lid lag and stare, is seen in thyrotoxicosis of any source, whereas the proptosis (exophthalmos) seen in Graves' disease is caused by retro-orbital deposition of mucopolysaccharides.

In Mrs. Jones' case, the laboratory data confirm high levels of thyroid hormone. The high T_3RU, in the face of elevated T_4 and T_3 levels, indicates that the elevation in these total hormone levels is not caused simply by ele-vations in binding proteins. The diffusely enlarged thyroid with evidence of increased blood flow and markedly elevated radioactive iodine uptake sug-gest that Mrs. Jones' thyroid is being driven by a stimulating hormone. The TSH level is low, however—so low that it cannot be measured in the labo-ratory, even by a very sensitive assay. Either the thyroid is functioning auton-omously or something else that acts like TSH is driving the thyroid.

Mrs. Jones has Graves' disease. Described in 1835 by Robert James Graves, the condition can be seen sporadically but often is familial. Women are affected more commonly than men, by a ratio of about 4:1. The path-ophysiology is based on the abnormal production of an antibody (thyroid-stimulating immunoglobulin [TSI]) that activates the thyroid TSH receptor and results in enlargement of the gland along with overproduction and ex-cessive release of thyroid hormone. Although TSI levels can be measured, they usually are not needed in the diagnostic evaluation of a patient with thyrotoxicosis.

One week later, Mrs. Jones returned to discuss the test results. Her palpitations had lessened, and she felt calmer since starting on propranolol.

After reviewing the data, Mrs. Jones asked why she had this and what could be done about it. The pathophysiology of Graves' disease was reviewed, and therapy with the antithyroid drug propylthiouracil (PTU) was initiated.

Ideally, therapy for Mrs. Jones and other patients with Graves' disease would be directed at the abnormal immunoglobulin that is stimulating thyroid function. Because it is not possible to stop or attenuate the production of the abnormal thyroid-stimulating factor (TSI), therapy is directed at inhibition of thyroid hormone synthesis, release, or peripheral activation. Several possible points of intervention are shown in Figure 4-9. Beta-adrenergic blockade with propranolol or a similar agent can provide some immediate, symptomatic relief by decreasing heart rate and palpitations and by providing some reduction in anxiety and hyperkinetic symptoms. In addition to blocking adrenergic receptors, propranolol and similar beta-blocking agents also may help by decreasing the peripheral conversion of T_4 to T_3. A large amount of the circulating T_3 in active Graves' disease is, however, derived from direct secretion by the thyroid gland and not from the peripheral conversion of T_4 to T_3.

Antithyroid therapy with either propylthiouracil or methimazole inhibits the production of thyroid hormone by blocking the peroxidase reaction. The resultant decrease in the iodination of tyrosine residues results in decreased thyroid hormone production. Because the thyroid, especially the overstimulated thyroid of Graves' disease, has the ability to store large amounts of hormone, and because PTU and methimazole work very early in the biosynthetic pathway of thyroid hormone production, it may take a few weeks for these agents to have a significant effect on hormone levels and symptoms.

Both drugs, PTU and methimazole, have relatively short half-lives and have no apparent lasting effect on thyroid function. The side-effect profiles are very similar and include a metallic taste, rash, joint pains, and, most importantly, significant effects on granulocytes. A dose-dependent decrease in granulocyte count often is seen. The most worrisome side effect is an idiosyncratic agranulocytosis that occurs in about 1 per 1000 patients.

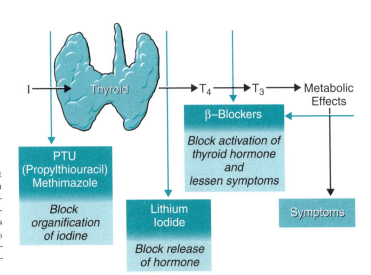

Figure 4-9. Nondestructive treatment of hyperthyroidism. Hyperthyroidism can be treated by drugs that block the organification of iodine or the release of thyroid hormone. Beta-adrenergic blockers block the conversion of T_4 to active T_3 and also decrease the symptoms associated with increased sensitivity to catecholamines.

A small percentage of patients with Graves' disease experience a remission without destructive therapy. Those with small glands and milder degrees of overactivity are more likely to have remissions. Because of this possibility of spontaneous remission—usually in the first year or two of the disease—antithyroid therapy with PTU or methimazole often is tried for 1 or 2 years. If the need for PTU or methimazole continues, or if there is difficulty controlling the thyrotoxicosis, destructive forms of therapy (e.g., radioactive iodine or surgery) are then tried.

More than 50 years of experience have showen that radioactive (^{131}I) iodine (RAI) is a safe and effective form of therapy for Graves' disease. Surgical removal of the thyroid may be preferred by some patients, especially very young patients with Graves' disease or those who plan a pregnancy in the very near future.

The likely and desired result of RAI or surgery in a patient with Graves' disease is hypothyroidism. Both modalities of destructive therapy usually result in permanent, lifelong hypothyroidism. If hypothyroidism occurs soon after therapy, replacement therapy can be started promptly, and clinical hypothyroidism can be avoided. Delayed hypothyroidism and recurrent hyperthyroidism are the possible disadvantages of less extensive destruction of the thyroid by either RAI or surgery. If a significant amount of thyroid tissue remains after surgery or RAI, TSI stimulation can result in growth of thyroid tissue and the return of thyrotoxicosis. On the other hand, atrophy of thyroid tissue over time can result in the gradual, unappreciated development of hypothyroidism.

Four weeks after starting PTU, Mrs. Jones returns for a follow-up visit. She is feeling quite a bit better. She has gained 3 pounds, and her pulse is down to 70 to 80 beats per minute. Arguments about the thermostat setting have stopped, and she is again able to groom eyebrows with a steady hand. She has not yet had a menstrual period. A metallic taste is the only side effect she has noted from the PTU.

Physical examination reveals a pulse of 74 and a blood pressure of 120/70. Her stare is less dramatic, and her thyroid is slightly smaller.

Laboratory Studies

Test	Jane Jones	Normal
WBC	3200/mm^3	4300–10,800/mm^3
Differential	Normal	Normal
T$_4$	13.2 μg/dL	5–12 μg/dL
T$_3$RU	34%	25%–35%
TSH	<0.5 mU/L	0.3–5.0 mU/L

Her medications are continued and she plans to return in 4 weeks for laboratory tests and a follow-up visit.

Mrs. Jones has responded well to antithyroid therapy. Soon it will be necessary to decrease the dose of PTU to avoid hypothyroidism from over-treatment.

Four weeks later, Mrs. Jones feels even better, with the exception of some morning nausea and breast tenderness. She has not had a menstrual period since starting the PTU.

Laboratory Studies

Test	Jane Jones	Normal
WBC	3800/mm^3	4300–10,800/mm^3
T$_4$	13.0 μg/dL	5–12 μg/dL
T$_3$RU	25%	25%–35%
TSH	<0.5 mU/L	0.3–5.0 mU/L
hCG, beta subunit	Positive	Negative, not pregnant Positive, pregnant

Mrs. Jones is surprised she is pregnant. She remembered the advice to use a barrier form of contraception until the Graves' disease was controlled and future pregnancies discussed. Because she wasn't having menstrual periods, however, she thought that she was unable to get pregnant.

Although the T$_4$ value is essentially unchanged, the decreasing T$_3$RU suggests an increased binding protein level, a situation seen in states of increased estrogen such as pregnancy. The free thyronine index is closer to normal than at the previous visit. Mrs. Jones' thyrotoxicosis is under control, but the unplanned pregnancy is a new, major problem. Pregnancy can exacerbate Graves' disease, and although only small amounts of thyroid hormone cross the placenta in either direction, maternal thyrotoxicosis and its treatment can have marked effects on the developing fetus. Maternal metabolic fuel requirements are increased during a normal, uncomplicated pregnancy. If the metabolic requirements are further increased by poorly controlled hyperthyroidism, nutritional deficiencies can occur in both the fetus and the mother. The antithyroid drugs PTU and methimazole cross the placenta and can affect neonatal thyroid function. High doses can result in neonatal hypothyroidism, cretinism, and goiter formation that can make vaginal delivery very difficult. TSI does cross the placenta, and, if present in high levels, can cause neonatal thyrotoxicosis.

Mrs. Jones does not want to consider terminating the pregnancy. She understands there are some risks, but she is willing to take them. After discussing the situation with her obstetrician, the plan is to follow her very carefully, using the lowest dose of PTU that will allow appropriate maternal weight gain and fetal development. A visit with a nutritionist is planned to be sure that Mrs. Jones fully understands her dietary needs with the combined requirements of pregnancy and hyperthyroidism. She and her obstetrician understand that her thyroid test results may not be "normal" because of the binding protein changes that occur as a result of the elevated estrogen levels of pregnancy.

At 38 weeks of gestation and after a 23-pound weight gain during the pregnancy, Mrs. Jones delivers a healthy 6-lb. 3-oz. boy. Postpartum, Mrs. Jones continues on PTU with good control of her thyroid function tests.

One year later, still requiring PTU, Mrs. Jones decides to have radioactive iodine therapy. A "window" or brief hiatus was placed in her PTU treatment to allow the radioactive iodine to be taken up and organified by the thyroid. A few days after the dose of radioactive iodine was administered, the PTU was restarted to allow control of her thyroid function while the effects of the radioactive iodine therapy take place. During the next 3 months, Mrs. Jones' PTU dose was tapered to 0. Two months later, thyroid function tests showed a TSH of 16.6 mU/L (normal 0.3 to 5.0 mU/L). Mrs. Jones felt well and was happy to be off medication completely but agreed to start T_4 therapy to prevent symptomatic hypothyroidism.

Luckily, Mrs. Jones' pregnancy was not complicated and the outcome was successful. Small amounts of PTU will appear in breast milk, which should be considered when breast-feeding is discussed.

Although for most patients it is a frightening concept, the use of radioactive iodine is an easy, effective way of managing Graves' disease.

CASE PRESENTATION: CASE 2

Hyperthyroxinemia and a "hot" nodule in a 52-year-old man with coronary artery disease

James Richardson is a 52-year-old man with known coronary artery disease who presents with increasing angina and a nodule in his left neck. He has no previous personal or family history of thyroid disease. His weight has been stable, and he denies heat intolerance or palpitations. Two years ago he underwent angioplasty of two coronary arteries, with marked improvement in his exercise tolerance. Recently, however, exercise-induced chest pain has returned, even more severely and with less exertion than before. His medications include a beta-blocker and a calcium channel blocker.

Physical Examination
Blood pressure 140/90, pulse 80
No lid lag or stare
Easily visible and palpable left-sided thyroid nodule

Laboratory Studies

Test	James Richardson	Normal
T_4	13.2 µg/dL	5–12 µg/dL
T_3RU	38%	25%–35%
TSH	<0.05 mU/L	0.3–5.0 mU/L
Radioactive iodine uptake	61% at 24 hrs	10%–25%

Thyroid scan: See Figure 4-10

Many of the symptoms of hyperthyroxinemia may be blocked by the beta-blocker therapy that Mr. Richardson uses for control of his heart disease. His increasing angina illustrates one effect thyrotoxicosis may have in a patient with coronary artery disease. Coronary artery disease limits the ability to increase myocardial oxygen delivery to meet the increased metabolic needs of the thyrotoxic state.

The functional anatomy of Mr. Richardson's thyroid, as depicted in his scan, reveals a pathophysiologic process very different from that seen in Graves' disease. Although the radioiodine uptake is increased, all the activity is concentrated in the palpable nodule. An autonomously functioning nodule rather than a TSH-like stimulating factor is the cause of Mr. Richardson's thyrotoxicosis.

Even though the pathophysiology and clinical situation are very different, the treatment options for Mr. Richardson are the same. Surgery to remove the toxic nodule would not be appropriate in this case because of the cardiovascular risks of a major surgical procedure. Radioactive iodine therapy would destroy the nodule, and because the remainder of the thyroid is functionally suppressed due to the lack of TSH, it is protected from the effects of radioactive iodine. This makes posttreatment hypothyroidism unlikely. The destruction of the hot nodule might, however, result in the inappropriate release of preformed thyroid hormone with worsening of the hypermetabolic state and anginal symptoms. Another treatment option would be to use PTU or methimazole to control the hyperthyroxinemia. After controlling the level of thyroid hormone and decreasing myocardial oxygen demands, treatment with radioactive iodine could be more safely undertaken.

Autonomous nodules appear to develop because of an inherent defect

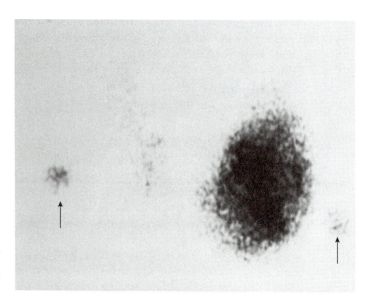

Figure 4-10. Thyroid scan: James Richardson. Virtually all of the isotope is concentrated in the globular structure of the patient's left side. The markers (*arrows*) are 8 cm apart.

that results in loss of normal physiologic control. In at least some cases a mutation of the TSH receptor gene results in continuous activation of the receptor in one group of cells.

CASE PRESENTATION: CASE 3

Hyperthyroxinemia in an elderly woman with a multinodular goiter

Mrs. Stark is an 82-year-old woman with failure to thrive who is brought in by her daughter. Although she has had a goiter for most of her adult life, thyroid tests as recently as 1 year ago were normal. Over the last 6 months, this previously active, talkative woman has become lethargic and withdrawn. Her weight has been essentially stable. A review of symptoms is unremarkable.

Physical Examination
  A lethargic, elderly woman who is detached, but cooperative
  Blood pressure 120–140/80–90; pulse 110, irregularly irregular
  Moderate temporalis muscle wasting
  No lid lag or stare
  Easily visible and palpable multinodular goiter

Laboratory Studies

Test	Joan Stark	Normal
T₄	14.8 μg/dL	5–12 μg/dL
T₃RU	38%	25%–35%
TSH	<0.05 mU/L	0.3–5.0 mU/L
Radioactive iodine uptake	48% at 24 hrs	10%–25%

EKG: Atrial fibrillation, ventricular response rate 102
Thyroid scan: See Figure 4-11

In elderly patients the usual symptoms of thyrotoxicosis may not be present. Apathy and cardiovascular effects may be the only manifestations. The new onset of atrial fibrillation should raise the question of hyperthyroidism because this is a common cardiovascular manifestation of thyrotoxicosis. In an elderly patient the ventricular response rate in atrial fibrillation may be slower than expected because of age-related changes in the conducting system of the heart. Autonomous function of multiple nodules explains the laboratory findings in this patient. The TSH is appropriately suppressed by the high levels of thyroxine and T₃. Antithyroid drug therapy and eventual radioactive iodine therapy would be appropriate for her. It is usually difficult to correct the atrial fibrillation until the thyrotoxicosis is controlled.

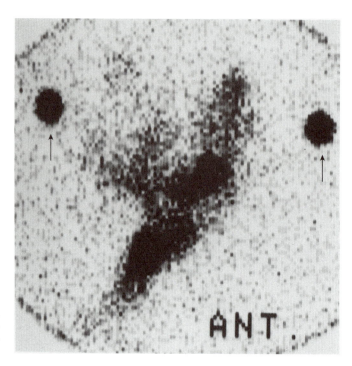

Figure 4-11. Thyroid scan: Joan Stark. The gland is enlarged, with a very patchy distribution of the isotope. The markers (*arrows*) are 8 cm apart.

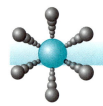

CASE PRESENTATION: CASE 4

Hyperthyroxinemia in a 25-year-old woman on oral contraceptives

Alice Avery is a 25-year-old woman on oral contraceptives who was found to have an elevated T_4 on routine screening tests done when she started a new job. She feels well and has no personal or family history of thyroid disease.

Physical Examination
Blood pressure 110/70; pulse 64
Thyroid is normal to inspection and palpation

Laboratory Studies

Test	Alice Avery	Normal
T_4	13.2 μg/dL	5–12 μg/dL
T_3RU	22%	25%–35%
TSH	2.0 mU/L	0.3–5.0 mU/L
Radioactive iodine uptake	16% at 24 hrs	10%–25%

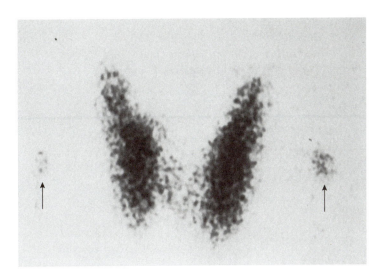

Figure 4-12. Thyroid scan: Alice Avery. The scan shows a thyroid of normal size with normally distributed uptake. The markers (*arrows*) are 8 cm apart.

Thyroid scan: **See Figure 4-12**

Although the total T_4 is elevated, Alice Avery's thyroid function is entirely normal. The estrogen component of the oral contraceptives she is taking has increased hepatic production of thyroid-binding globulin. The increased concentration of thyroid-binding globulin results in increased binding of T_4 in the serum, which leads to a transient fall in T_4 levels. The lowering of T_4 levels transiently stimulates TSH secretion by the pituitary and increases thyroid hormone synthesis and release by the thyroid. After this short-lived adjustment to the change in the level of binding protein, a new equilibrium is reached. The normalcy of Ms. Avery's thyroid status also is demonstrated by a normal free thyroxine index, the normal TSH, and the normal radioactive iodine uptake and scan. A normal TSH alone would have confirmed her normalcy; the scan and uptake were clearly unnecessary. No treatment is indicated.

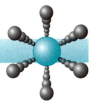

CASE PRESENTATION: CASE 5

Hyperthyroxinemia in a 30-year-old woman with a sore neck

Marian Masters is a 30-year-old third grade teacher who presents with weight loss, palpitations, and a very sore anterior neck. The pain radiates into her ears. The symptoms developed after a severe head cold and during a time when her classroom contained 24 sniffling, sneezing, coughing youngsters.

Physical Examination
Vital signs: Blood pressure 130/60; pulse 110
HEENT: No lid lag or stare; ears normal
Neck: Very tender, slightly enlarged thyroid

Laboratory Studies

Test	Marian Masters	Normal
Erythrocyte sedimentation rate	112 mm/hr	0–20 mm/hr
T_4	16.4 μg/dL	5–12 μg/dL
T_3RU	38%	25%–35%
TSH	<0.05 mU/L	0.3–5.0 mU/L
Radioactive iodine uptake	0% at 24 hrs	10%–25%

Thyroid scan: See Figure 4-13

Although the classic findings of thyrotoxicosis—weight loss, palpitations, T_4 elevation, and TSH suppression—are present in this patient, the mechanism of the excess thyroid hormone is not immediately clear. The radioactive iodine uptake is 0, suggesting that, if she is not iodine overloaded, her gland is not at all active. Although an exogenous source of T_4 cannot be completely excluded, the elevated sedimentation rate and the tender gland most likely are the result of viral infection of the thyroid, a condition referred to as *subacute thyroiditis*. The specific virus causing this inflammation of the thyroid usually is unclear, but the large pool of potential viral candidates in the classroom makes a virus the likely source.

Viral infection and destruction of follicular cells result in the inappropriate release of preformed hormone and development of the symptoms of thyrotoxicosis. Recovery after 6 to 8 weeks is the usual outcome. After the inappropriately released hormone has cleared, transient, mild hypothyroidism occurs. Suppressed TSH levels become elevated in response to low levels of thyroid hormone. Follicular cells by then have recovered and respond to the increasing TSH levels with thyroid hormone synthesis and release. Long-term thyroid problems usually are not seen.

Figure 4-13. Thyroid scan: Marian Masters. Between the markers, which are 8 cm apart, there is no evidence of any uptake of isotope.

CASE PRESENTATION: CASE 6

Toxic effects of exogenous thyroid hormone in a 38-year-old man

Walter "Tiny" Griswald is a 38-year-old retired professional basketball player who has been offered the opportunity to return to the court by the management of a new expansion team. The $1 million contract will allow him to settle his debts with the Internal Revenue Service and pay off his mortgage. Since his retirement 2 years ago, Mr. Griswald has gained 60 pounds. In an effort to get his weight down and improve his performance, he has consulted a "sports medicine" expert who took care of several athletes at the recent Olympics. He was given a prescription for Cytomel (triiodothyronine [T_3]), 50 μg three times a day. After 3 weeks on this medication, he has lost 20 pounds, but he has become irritable and shaky and has marked dyspnea with exertion. He had to be taken out of his first scrimmage after only 4 minutes because of extreme dyspnea. He now presents for evaluation.

His past medical history is unremarkable.

Physical Examination
A large, moderately overweight man
Blood pressure 160/80, pulse 110
No lid lag or stare, no palpable thyroid
Fine tremor of outstretched hands

Laboratory Studies

Test	Walter Griswald	Normal
T_4	0.8 μg/dL	5–12 μg/dL
T_3RU	25%	25%–35%
TSH	<0.05 mU/L	0.3–5.0 mU/L
T_3 (total)	356 ng/dL	80–200 ng/dL
Radioactive iodine uptake	0% at 24 hrs	10%–25%

Scan: **no image possible**

Exogenous thyroid hormone in excess can have significant metabolic effects. The exogenous T_3 taken by this basketball player is an especially potent form of thyroid hormone. It is directly active and does not require deiodination to become effective. Although excess exogenous T_4 may have significant metabolic effects, the magnitude of its effect is diminished by the fact that T_4 is a prohormone that requires a specific form of deiodination for it to be effective.

Tiny's elevated T_3 levels have shut off endogenous T_4 production. Thyroid function and a normal metabolic state will return several weeks after discontinuation of Cytomel.

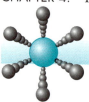

CASE PRESENTATION: CASE 7

Hypothyroxinemia in a 32-year-old woman with menorrhagia and an enlarged thyroid gland

Six months of irregular, heavy menstrual bleeding led Susan Gilman to see her gynecologist. Her periods had always been regular, except when she was pregnant. She is 32 years old and has two healthy children, aged 4 and 7 years old. In the past year she has been more tired and has gained about 14 pounds. Constipation also has become a major problem.

Physical Examination
A moderately overweight woman
Blood pressure 150/90, pulse 58
Full neck with an enlarged (1.5 to 2 times normal) thyroid
Deep tendon reflexes are "hung up"

Laboratory Studies

Test	Susan Gilman	Normal
T_4	2.8 μg/dL	5–12 μg/dL
T_3RU	20%	25%–35%
TSH	94.3 mU/L	0.3–5.0 mU/L

Weight gain, constipation, and menorrhagia can all be symptoms of hypothyroidism. Mild hypertension, goiter, and delayed relaxation of deep tendon reflexes are some of the common physical findings in hypothyroidism. Decreased metabolic rate results in less caloric combustion and slower gastrointestinal peristalsis. Menorrhagia is caused by a decrease in the metabolism of estrogen, resulting in estrogen levels that are inappropriately high and leading to excessive stimulation of the endometrium, with the possible development of endometrial hyperplasia and "breakthrough" bleeding.

The mechanism of Mrs. Gilman's hypothyroidism is end-organ or thyroid gland failure. The elevated TSH indicates an appropriate pituitary and hypothalamic response to the low levels of thyroid hormone. Her thyroid is not responding to TSH with the expected rise in thyroid hormone production. Autoimmune thyroiditis, often referred to as Hashimoto's thyroiditis, is the most common cause of this condition. Like most other thyroid problems, it is more common in women and tends to cluster in families.

Treatment involves replacement of thyroid hormone. Luckily, thyroid hormone is fairly well absorbed from the gastrointestinal tract. Although animal thyroid gland has been used for more than 100 years, most patients currently are treated with synthetically produced T_4. After absorption from the gastrointestinal tract, thyroxine is converted to active hormone, T_3, or to an inactive form, rT_3. The goal of therapy, in addition to relieving symptoms, is to normalize the TSH level. The lowest dose of thyroid hormone needed to normalize TSH is the correct dose.

The clinical effectiveness of thyroid hormone replacement is seen over weeks and months. Most, if not all, the symptoms should improve.

CASE PRESENTATION: CASE 8

Thyroid nodule found during a routine physical examination in a 32-year-old man

During a routine physical examination, a 1.5-cm nodule was found on the right side of Mark Cohen's neck. The nodule moved well with swallowing and seemed to be at the lower pole of the right hemithyroid. Mr. Cohen is 32 years old, and his past medical history is unremarkable. He works as a manager in a large automobile dealership. He has no previous personal or family history of thyroid disease. He is not aware of any significant radiation exposure.

Physical examination reveals a 1.5-cm nodule in the right lobe of the thyroid. The nodule is smooth, firm, and moves well with swallowing. There is no palpable lymphadenopathy. The remainder of his physical examination is normal.

Laboratory Studies

Test	Mark Cohen	Normal
T_4	8.0 μg/dL	5–12 μg/dL
T_3RU	28%	25%–35%
TSH	1.1 mU/L	0.3–5.0 mU/L
Radioactive iodine uptake	20%	10%–25% at 24 hrs

Thyroid scan: **See Figure 4-14**

Mr. Cohen presents with an asymptomatic thyroid nodule and normal thyroid function tests. The scan shows that the area that corresponds to the palpable nodule does not concentrate the radioactive iodine. If the nodule did take up iodine, the chance of malignancy would be very, very low, and, unless there were evidence of hyperfunction, nothing more, other than careful follow-up examinations, would be necessary.

The fact that the nodule is ''cold''—i.e., does not take up and concentrate iodine—is associated with a chance of malignancy of between 5% and 10%. There are four types of thyroid cancer (Table 4-3).

An ultrasound study of the neck could be performed to determine whether the palpable nodule is solid or cystic and whether other nonpalpable nodules are present. A cystic lesion is less likely to be malignant but still requires further evaluation.

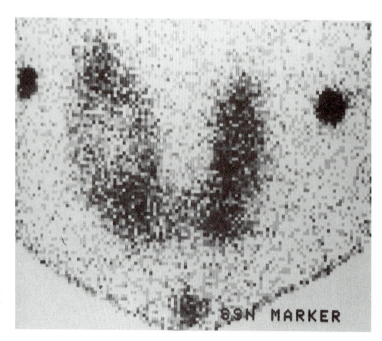

Figure 4-14. Thyroid scan: Mark Cohen. A cold area is present in the patient's right thyroid lobe. This area of decreased isotope uptake corresponds with the palpable nodule. The markers are 8 cm apart.

After discussing the test results and the possible next steps, Mr. Cohen agrees that a fine-needle biopsy of the nodule should be done.

After alcohol preparation of the neck, six passes were made with a 22-gauge, 1.5-inch needle attached to a 12-mL syringe. Each of the aspirations produced a small amount of bloody material that was spread on a slide and immediately fixed. The syringe was rinsed in cytology preparation fluid and sent for analysis.

Even without any anesthesia, Mr. Cohen tolerated the procedure well and returned to work with only a Band-Aid to cover the biopsy site.

TABLE 4-3. *THYROID CANCER*	
TYPE OF THYROID CANCER	**CHARACTERISTICS**
Anaplastic	Rapidly growing, locally invasive, poor prognosis.
Medullary	A differentiated tumor of the parafollicular or C cells of the thyroid that produce calcitonin; may occur sporadically or may be part of a familial syndrome (see Chapter 11); can be associated with pheochromocytoma and hyperparathyroidism.
Follicular	Normal-appearing thyroid follicular cells that can spread hematogenously to lung and bone; prognosis is fairly good.
Papillary	An indolent malignancy with a characteristic cellular pattern that tends to spread locally; prognosis usually is very good.

Because only small amounts of tissue are obtained through fine-needle aspiration, the cytology must be reviewed and interpreted very carefully. Anaplastic lesions and medullary carcinoma have a characteristic pattern, as does papillary carcinoma of the thyroid. Follicular lesions—nodules that have the usual architecture of normal thyroid tissue—may be very hard to evaluate by fine-needle techniques. The criteria for detecting malignancy in follicular lesions are based on evidence of vascular or capsular invasion, information that usually is not available from fine-needle aspiration techniques. Surgical removal and careful examination of multiple cut sections of a follicular nodule usually are necessary to make a diagnosis of follicular thyroid carcinoma.

The biopsy specimen showed psammoma bodies and fronds of papillary tissue. These findings indicate that the nodule is very likely to be a papillary carcinoma.

Three weeks later Mr. Cohen had surgery to remove the right lobe of his thyroid and the adjacent isthmus. The left lobe appeared normal, and there was no lymphadenopathy noted at the time of surgery. The pathological examination of the material removed confirmed the diagnosis of papillary carcinoma. It was, however, well encapsulated.

Postoperatively, Mr. Cohen recovered well. He was started on thyroxine (T$_4$) to suppress his TSH level. One week postoperatively Mr. Cohen was back to work, relieved that he would not need any more tests or procedures for a while. He will have an ultrasound study in 6 months to look for any nodules that may be developing on the left side and to look for lymphadenopathy. He understands that he may need radioactive iodine therapy or more surgery if there is evidence of recurrence.

Mr. Cohen's prognosis is quite good. Animal models of thyroid cancer indicate improved outcomes if TSH is suppressed by the administration of exogenous thyroid hormone. It has become common practice to suppress TSH to nonmeasurable levels in patients with a history of thyroid cancer. Radioactive iodine also can be used to treat thyroid cancer, even if, as in Mr. Cohen's case, the initial lesion did not concentrate iodine. For radioactive iodine to be useful in such cases, any remaining normal thyroid tissue must be removed surgically or destroyed by radioactive iodine. After this has been completed, and if the TSH is allowed to rise for a brief period of time, some iodine uptake can sometimes be seen. This identifies the presence and location of residual or recurrent tissue and allows radioactive iodine to be a possible therapeutic tool.

KEY POINTS AND CONCEPTS

- Thyroid hormone has multiple metabolic effects.
- The thyroid contains large amounts of preformed hormone.
- Hyperthyroxinemia may occur with:
  - Overstimulation, as in Graves' disease.
  - Autonomous function, as in toxic adenoma and toxic multinodular goiter.
  - Inappropriate release of preformed hormone.
  - Excess exogenous hormone intake.

- Overproduction of TSH by the pituitary is a very rare cause of thyrotoxicosis.
- Treatment of hyperthyroxinemia depends on the cause but can include antithyroid drugs (e.g., PTU, methimazole), beta-blockers, radioactive iodine, and surgery.
- Hypothyroidism may occur with:
  - End-organ or thyroid gland failure (primary hypothyroidism), as in Hashimoto's thyroiditis.
  - Pituitary (secondary hypothyroidism) or hypothalamic (tertiary hypothyroidism) failure.
  - Less common causes, including iodine deficiency and drug-induced gland failure.
- Treatment of hypothyroidism involves oral replacement with thyroid hormone, monitoring clinical response, and, in primary hypothyroidism (the most common cases), normalizing TSH.
- Goiter and thyroid nodules:
  - An enlarged gland may function normally, or it may be hyper- or hypofunctional.
  - Malignancy is rare in a nodule that concentrates iodine.
  - Cold nodules, nodules that do not concentrate iodine, have a 5% to 10% chance of malignancy. Fine-needle aspiration or surgery may be needed to evaluate a cold nodule.

SUGGESTED READING

Brent GA. The molecular basis of thyroid hormone action. N Engl J Med 331:847–853, 1994.

Burrow GN, Fisher DA, Larsen PR. Maternal and fetal thyroid function. N Engl J Med 331:1072–1078, 1994.

Surks MI, Sievert R. Drugs and thyroid function. N Engl J Med 333:1688–1694, 1995.

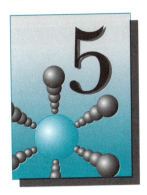

CHAPTER 5

The Adrenal Cortex

The adrenal cortex is the source of three distinct types of steroid hormones: glucocorticoids, mineralocorticoids, and androgens (Table 5-1). Glucocorticoids, in addition to having many other effects, play a vital role in the body's ability to tolerate intermittent food intake. Mineralocorticoids control renal potassium excretion and help maintain normal blood volume and blood pressure. Androgens are male sex steroid hormones and are produced by the gonad as well. The adrenal medulla, a source of catecholamine hormones, is located in the inner part of each adrenal gland (see Chapter 10).

ANATOMY

The adrenal cortex is derived from mesodermal tissue. Neural crest tissue supplies the adrenal medulla, which joins the developing cortex early in the embryologic process. In the fetus, the adrenal cortex is clearly developed by 2 months. It becomes relatively large—about the size of the fetal kidney—during midgestation. Most of the enlargement during fetal development occurs in what is called the fetal zone. The enzymes of steroid biosynthesis present in the fetal adrenal produce significant amounts of dehydroepiandrosterone (DHEA) and

TABLE 5-1.	*STEROID HORMONES*
TYPE	**HORMONES**
Glucocorticoid	Cortisol (hydrocortisone)
Mineralocorticoid	Aldosterone
Androgen	Dihydroepiandrosterone (DHEA), DHEA-sulfate, androstenedione

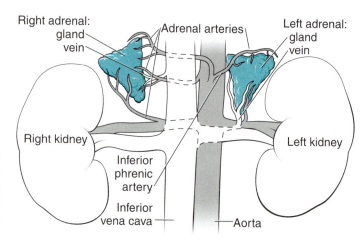

Figure 5-1. Gross anatomy of the adrenal glands. The adrenal glands are located above and medial to the kidneys. Each gland is well supplied with arterial blood. Venous drainage is into the vena cava on the right and into the renal vein on the left.

DHEA-sulfate, which serve as precursors for placental estrogen production. After birth the fetal zone regresses, and during the first 3 years after birth, the three zones of the adult adrenal cortex—the glomerulosa, fasciculata, and reticularis—develop. The outer glomerulosa zone lacks the 17-hydroxylase enzyme needed to make cortisol and androgens and is the principal site of aldosterone production. The fasciculata and reticularis do not have the 18-hydroxylase enzyme required for the production of aldosterone, but they do have the enzyme systems needed to produce cortisol and androgens.

In the adult, the total weight of both adrenal glands is about 8 to 10 g. The adrenal medulla accounts for about 10% of the weight of each adrenal. The adrenals are located in the retroperitoneal space above and slightly medial to the kidneys (Fig. 5-1). Each adrenal has three separate arterial blood supplies and one vein. The right adrenal vein empties directly into the vena cava, whereas the left adrenal vein drains into the left renal vein.

CHEMISTRY

Steroid hormones are modified cholesterol molecules (Fig. 5-2). Synthesis of these hormones starts with cholesterol, which is derived largely from the circulation but also can be made from acetate in the adrenal cortex. The cascade of steroid hormone biosynthesis is shown in Figure 5-3. The rate-limiting step in adrenal steroidogenesis is the conversion of cholesterol to pregnenolone. The transformation of cholesterol to pregnenolone occurs at the mitochondria and involves a side chain cleavage and two hydroxylations. Molecular oxygen and a pair of electrons are required. Pregnenolone, once produced, leaves the mitochondria, and 17-hydroxylation occurs on the endoplasmic reticulum. 3β-hydroxysteroid dehydrogenase isomerase, also working at the endoplasmic reticulum, results in further changes, yielding 17-hydroxyprogesterone. The process continues at the mitochondria, with 21- and 11-hydroxylation resulting in the final production of cortisol. Cortisol also is called hydrocortisone. The suffix *-one* of corti*sone* refers to the ket*one* group at the 11 position. When an OH group is present at the 11 position, the molecule is called hydrocortisone or cortisol.

Aldosterone and adrenal androgens are produced by a similar cascading sequence of enzymatically controlled reactions that share many of the same com-

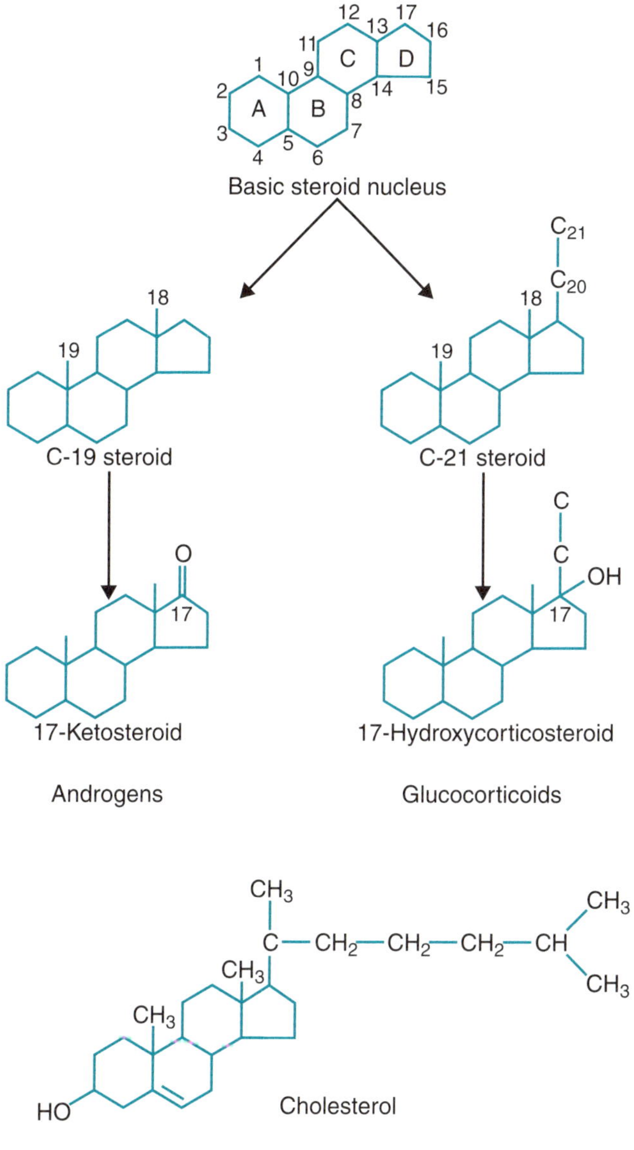

12 13 17 16
11 C D
1 10 9 14 15
2 A B 8
3 5 6 7
4

Basic steroid nucleus

18
19

C-19 steroid

18 C21 C20
19

C-21 steroid

O
17

17-Ketosteroid

Androgens

C
C
OH
17

17-Hydroxycorticosteroid

Glucocorticoids

CH3
C — CH2 — CH2 — CH2 — CH
CH3 CH3
CH3
HO Cholesterol

Figure 5-2. Cholesterol and basic steroid molecules. Steroid hormones are modified cholesterol molecules. A ketone at the 17 position is associated with androgen effects. Glucocorticoids have an alcohol group and side chain at the 17 position.

ponents as the cortisol synthesis pathway. The interdependence of steroid hormone biosynthesis is seen most clearly when enzyme deficiencies in this cascade result in overproduction of precursor molecules, some of which may have biologic effects or provide increased substrate for conversion to other active hormones.

Once secreted, cortisol is transported by plasma proteins—cortisol-binding globulin (CBG) and albumin. Approximately 10% of the circulating cortisol is free, 75% is bound to CBG, and 15% is bound to albumin. The plasma half-life of cortisol is 70 to 90 minutes, but the duration of biologic effects often is very much longer. Other steroid hormones are variably bound to plasma proteins. In general, steroid hormones are metabolized by the liver. The metabolites and small amounts of the hormones themselves are excreted by the kidney.

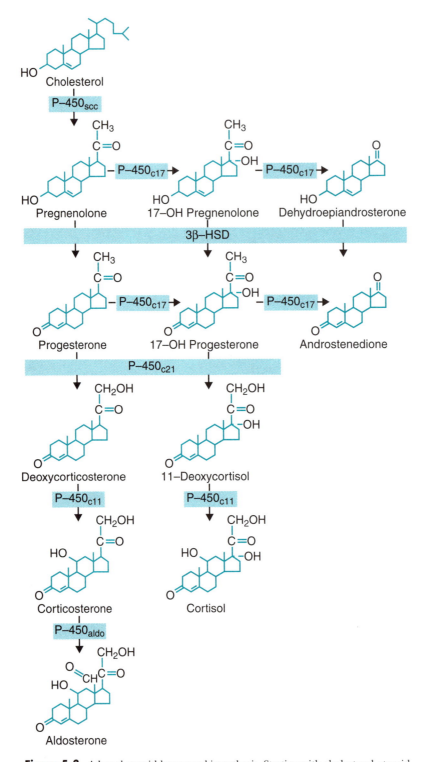

Figure 5-3. Adrenal steroid hormone biosynthesis. Starting with cholesterol, steroid hormones are synthesized by a series of enzymatically controlled reactions. P-450$_{scc}$ cleaves the side chain from the 20 position of the cholesterol molecule. P-450$_{c17}$ catalyzes first hydroxylation and then side chain removal and ketone formation at the 17 position. 3-hydroxysteroid dehydrogenase (3-HSD) converts the 5,6 double bond to a 4,5 double bond with formation of a ketone group at the 3 position. P-450$_{c21}$ and P-450$_{c11}$ allow hydroxylation at the 21 and 11 positions, respectively. In the zona glomerulosa of the adrenal cortex P-450$_{aldo}$, an enzyme very similar to P-450$_{c11}$, converts corticosterone to aldosterone.

CORTISOL

Cortisol is the principal glucocorticoid hormone. Glucocorticoid receptors are found in virtually all tissues. In most tissues—the liver is an important exception—glucocorticoids inhibit the synthesis of DNA, RNA, and many proteins and increase protein catabolism. Glucocorticoids, like other steroid hormones, exert their effects by binding to nuclear chromatin, which results in altered protein synthesis (Table 5-2).

Cortisol has multiple effects on intermediary metabolism; all of them tend

TABLE 5-2.	*EFFECTS OF GLUCOCORTICOIDS*
TISSUE/FUNCTION	**GLUCOCORTICOID EFFECT**
Liver/hepatic glucose production	Increases gluconeogenesis, directly and by increasing effects of other gluconeogenic hormones. Increases availability of gluconeogenic substrates.
Peripheral glucose metabolism	Decreases glucose uptake in muscle and adipose tissue.
Adipose tissue	Increases lipolysis and release of glycerol and free fatty acids.
Connective tissue	Excess causes inhibition of fibroblast activity.
Bone	Excess causes inhibition of bone formation with decreased synthesis of collagen, protein, and hyaluronidate.
Calcium metabolism	Excess decreases calcium absorption by GI tract (anti–vitamin D effect) with secondary hyperparathyroidism, increases urinary calcium excretion.
Growth	Necessary for normal growth. Excess inhibits growth in children (decreases GH, decreases somatomedin).
Blood cells	Excess increases circulating granulocytes—increases release from bone marrow, increases $t_{1/2}$ of granulocytes, decreases release from vascular compartment and migration of inflammatory cells. Excess decreases lymphocytes, eosinophils, monocytes in peripheral circulation.
Immunologic effects	Excess decreases antigen processing, decreases antibody production and impairs release of effector substances.
Cardiovascular function	Maintains cardiac output and vascular tone, augments the effects of vasoconstrictors.
Renal function	Maintains GFR. Excess causes hypokalemia.
Central nervous system	Glucocorticoids freely enter the brain. Excess causes euphoria, irritability, depression, emotional lability. Deficiency causes apathy, depression, irritability.
Gonadal	Excess inhibits gonadal function by inhibiting gonadotropin secretion.

GFR, glomerular filtration rate; GH, growth hormone.

to result in an increase in glucose availability. Cortisol decreases glucose uptake by adipose and other tissues and increases glucose synthesis by the liver. The increased production of glucose by the liver is the result, in part, of glucocorticoid-induced breakdown of muscle protein, which results in an increased supply of amino acids. In adipose tissue, cortisol decreases lipogenesis and increases lipolysis, which provides additional gluconeogenic substrates for the liver.

In addition to multiple metabolic effects, cortisol and related molecules have potent antiinflammatory effects. Antiinflammatory effectiveness parallels glucocorticoid effectiveness. Cortisol and its synthetic analogues often are used in clinical medicine for their antiinflammatory effects. Glucocorticoids decrease the delivery of inflammatory cells to injured areas and inhibit the release of inflammatory cytokines. Unfortunately, significant side effects often result from the inseparable metabolic and anatomic effects of glucocorticoids. The constellation of effects induced by excess glucocorticoids is called Cushing's syndrome (discussed later in this chapter).

REGULATION OF CORTISOL SECRETION

Some of the factors that control cortisol secretion are shown in Figure 5-4. In response to several types of input, the hypothalamus secretes corticotrophin-releasing hormone (CRH). CRH is delivered via the hypothalamic–pituitary portal system to the anterior pituitary, where it stimulates production and secretion of ACTH by the corticotroph cells of the anterior pituitary. Vasopressin (ADH), when secreted in large amounts, also can stimulate the secretion of ACTH.

In addition to stimulating the adrenal cortex to produce and release steroid hormones, ACTH stimulates DNA, RNA, and protein synthesis in the adrenal cortex. When present in excess, ACTH causes hypertrophy of the adrenal cortex. Atrophy occurs when ACTH is deficient.

ACTH binds to cell surface receptors in the adrenal cortex and activates adenylate cyclase. The resultant increase in cyclic adenosine monophosphate (cAMP) activates phosphoprotein kinases, stimulating the conversion of cholesterol to pregnenolone and beginning the cascade of steroid hormone production. The phosphoprotein kinases also activate cholesterol ester hydrolase, resulting in increased availability of free cholesterol for steroid synthesis.

At least four mechanisms of control of the hypothalamic–pituitary–adrenocortical axis have been described:

Circadian rhythm
Stress
Feedback inhibition by cortisol
Stimulation by inflammatory cytokines

Under ordinary, nonstressed conditions, the hypothalamic–pituitary–adrenal axis operates in a diurnal fashion. An increased frequency of pulses of ACTH secretion is seen during the hours from 4 a.m. to 8 a.m. The resulting rise in cortisol production and secretion results in a rise in plasma cortisol levels that peaks toward the end of this period (Fig. 5-5). The lowest values of ACTH and cortisol are seen between midnight and 4 a.m. The rhythm of cortisol secretion is influenced by a number of factors, including sleep cycles, activity schedule, and light exposure. Some aspects of jet lag probably are caused by the time it takes to reset this and other rhythms to a new time zone.

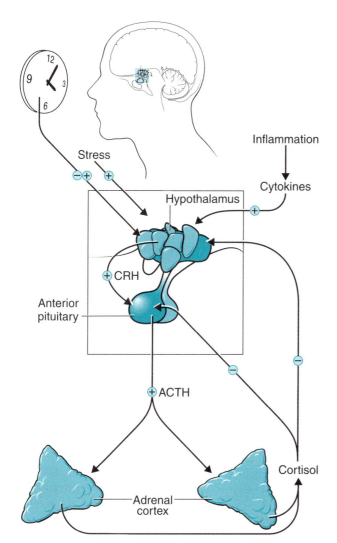

Figure 5-4. The hypothalamic–pituitary–adrenal axis. In addition to negative feedback by the end product of the axis, a number of other factors influence the regulation of cortisol production. Time of day, level of stress, and the presence of inflammatory cytokines all have important effects on the control of cortisol secretion.

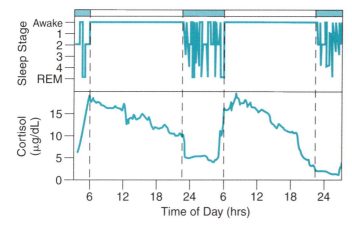

Figure 5-5. Diurnal variation in cortisol levels. Cortisol levels are highest between 5 and 7 a.m. Stress—emotional or physical—can override this diurnal variation.

The diurnal rhythm of ACTH and cortisol secretion can, at any time, be overridden by stress. The stress that stimulates the axis may be physical—e.g., hypoglycemia, fever, or hypotension—or psychological. Input from higher centers and from the sympathetic nervous system result in increased secretion of CRH and ADH. Although both CRH and ADH can stimulate ACTH secretion, the effect when both are present is not merely additive; rather, the release of ACTH and the subsequent release of cortisol are magnified.

As with most physiologic feedback loops, the end product of the system, in this case cortisol, is a potent inhibitor of the system. Cortisol, if present in adequate amounts, dampens or obliterates both diurnal and stress-induced stimulation of ACTH. When exogenous glucocorticoids (e.g., cortisol or one of its synthetic analogues) are administered, there is a prompt decrease in CRH and ACTH production and release. Long-term administration of exogenous glucocorticoids or autonomous, unregulated, endogenous overproduction of cortisol can result in functional and anatomic atrophy of the axis. Disuse atrophy, induced by exogenous steroids, is a function of both dosage and time. No clear threshold for suppression of the axis has been defined, but high doses for a relatively short period of time (days to weeks) and lower, near-physiologic doses for longer periods (months to years) have been shown to result in functional atrophy of the axis.

Inflammatory cytokines, tissue necrosis factor (TNF), and interleukins increase CRH and AVP secretion, resulting in increased ACTH secretion and, thereby, increased cortisol levels. Cortisol suppresses the inflammatory response and the release of inflammatory cytokines. These recently developed findings suggest an additional feedback loop that participates in the control of cortisol secretion.

ALDOSTERONE

Aldosterone circulates in an unbound state and is degraded by the liver. In the distal nephron, the distal tubule and the cortical collecting ducts, aldosterone stimulates the reabsorption of Na^+ and the excretion of K^+ and H^+ into the tubular fluid. Aldosterone increases the number of channels that allow sodium ions to be reabsorbed from the tubular fluid. Apical epithelial cell potassium conductivity increases, as does synthesis of an Na^+-K^+ ATPase, which results in an electrochemical gradient that drives the ionic exchange stimulated by aldosterone. The net result of the effect of aldosterone is the exchange of Na^+ ions for K^+ and H^+ ions at a ratio of 3 Na^+ ions for 2 K^+ ions and one H^+ ion.

The cellular mechanism of aldosterone effect, as with other steroid hormones, occurs at the level of the nucleus. Curiously, the nuclear receptor for mineralocorticoid effect is equally responsive to both aldosterone and cortisol. Although cortisol usually is present in much higher concentrations, it usually does not activate the mineralocorticoid receptor. In mineralocorticoid-sensitive cells, cortisol is converted to cortisone by 11β-hydroxysteroid dehydrogenase (Fig. 5-6). The presence of a ketone group at the 11 position of the molecule results in inactivation of the cortisol molecule. This intracellular inactivation of cortisol in mineralocorticoid-sensitive cells allows aldosterone, even though present in low concentration, to control sodium reabsorption and potassium excretion. Elevated levels of cortisol may override this degradative enzyme system and result in a cortisol-induced mineralocorticoid effect.

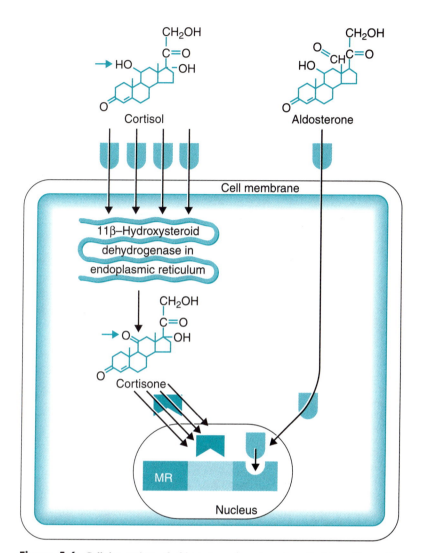

Figure 5-6. Cellular action of aldosterone. In mineralocorticoid-sensitive cells, both cortisol and aldosterone can activate the mineralocorticoid receptor. A specificity-conferring enzyme system, 11-hydroxysteroid dehydrogenase, present in the endoplasmic reticulum, inactivates cortisol. Inactivation occurs when the OH group at the 11 position of cortisol is converted to a ketone group (*arrows*), forming cortisone, a molecule that cannot activate the mineralocorticoid receptor. This allows aldosterone, which is present in a much lower concentration, to regulate sodium resorption and potassium and hydrogen ion secretion. (Modified from White PC. Disorders of aldosterone biosynthesis and action. N Engl J Med 331:250–258, 1994.)

Three mechanisms control aldosterone secretion (Fig. 5-7). The serum potassium level and the activity of the renin-angiotensin system are the principal regulators of aldosterone secretion. The mechanism by which potassium stimulates aldosterone secretion is unclear, but a rising potassium level is a potent stimulus to aldosterone secretion. Low levels of potassium, however, do not appear to inhibit aldosterone secretion stimulated by the renin-angiotensin system or ACTH. Although the synthesis and secretion of aldosterone can be stimulated by ACTH, ACTH plays a relatively small role in controlling aldosterone secretion.

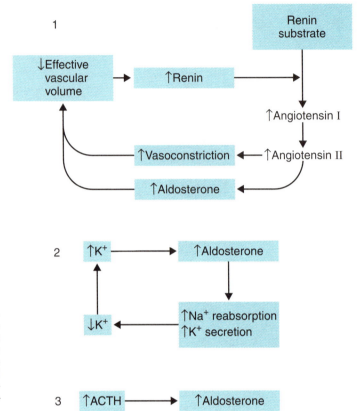

Figure 5-7. Control of aldosterone secretion. The activity of the renin-angiotensin system and the level of potassium in the extracellular fluid space are the principal controllers of aldosterone secretion. ACTH stimulation of the adrenal cortex does lead to aldosterone secretion, but this is a minor aspect of aldosterone regulation.

Renin is a proteolytic enzyme released by the granular cells of the juxtaglomerular apparatus of the kidney. Release occurs in response to volume depletion, hypotension, and beta$_1$-adrenergic stimulation. The decreased distal nephron sodium delivery that occurs with volume contraction results in increased renin release. Renin catalyzes the splitting of hepatically produced angiotensinogen or renin substrate into a 10-amino-acid polypeptide, angiotensin I. This prohormone is cleaved by angiotensin-converting enzyme (ACE) to the potent vasoconstrictor, as its name implies, angiotensin II. In addition to provoking vasoconstriction and a number of other effects, angiotensin II is a potent secretogogue for aldosterone.

Excessive, uncontrolled production of aldosterone results in hypertension and in hypokalemia. Edema can be seen initially in states of uncontrolled aldosterone excess, but subsides (the escape phenomenon) as other mechanisms for sodium excretion come into play. Aldosterone deficiency usually is seen with deficiency of cortisol. Hypotension, hyponatremia, and hyperkalemia are the usual findings.

ADRENAL ANDROGENS

Dehydroepiandrosterone, its sulfate, and androstenedione are androgenic steroids produced by the adrenal cortex. All are weak androgens, but they can be converted in the periphery to testosterone, which is a powerful androgen. In addition, adrenal androgens can be converted in the liver and in adipose tissue to estrone, an estrogenic compound.

TABLE 5-3. *MECHANISMS OF CORTISOL EXCESS*	
NON–ACTH-DEPENDENT	**ACTH-DEPENDENT**
Iatrogenic—exogenous steroids	Ectopic ACTH production
Adrenal adenoma	Cushing's disease—pituitary-based Cushing's syndrome
Adrenal cortical carcinoma	Ectopic CRH production

ACTH, adrenocorticotrophic hormone; CRH, corticotropin-releasing hormone.

Although ACTH stimulates the production of adrenal androgens, there must be other important factors. In young children, levels of adrenal androgens are low, but early in puberty—at andrarche—the levels increase. During late adulthood, levels of adrenal androgens fall without any clear change in ACTH dynamics. The contribution of adrenal androgens to the adult male androgen pool is small in comparison with the androgen effect of testosterone produced by the testis, but in the adult female the adrenal cortex is a major source of androgens.

Excessive adrenal androgen production in the female results in hirsutism and, when overproduction is extreme, in virilization. In the adult male, adrenal androgen overproduction usually is not associated with any clinical findings because of the major androgen effect of testosterone produced by the testicle. Adrenal androgen deficiency is not clinically apparent in men with normal testicular function. In women, adrenal androgens play a role in the maintenance of normal axillary and pubic hair and possibly in libido.

OVERVIEW OF ADRENOCORTICAL PATHOLOGY

Cushing's syndrome is the clinical manifestation of excess glucocorticoid effect. The mechanisms of cortisol excess can be divided into ACTH-dependent and non–ACTH-dependent (Table 5-3).

Overproduction of other adrenocortical hormones, aldosterone and adrenal androgens, also can occur and also may be classified as ACTH-dependent or ACTH-independent.

Syndromes of adrenocortical insufficiency also can be assessed in regard to ACTH levels (Table 5-4). Primary end-organ adrenal insufficiency is associated with

TABLE 5-4. *MECHANISMS OF CORTISOL DEFICIENCY*		
	ACTH ABSENT	**ACTH PRESENT**
Diagnosis	Secondary adrenal insufficiency	Primary adrenal insufficiency
Causes	Exogenous steroids, hypothalamic disease, pituitary disease	End organ—adrenocortical—failure; autoimmune, hemorrhagic
Features	Normokalemia/normal aldosterone function	Hyperkalemia/aldosterone deficiency, hyperpigmentation

elevated ACTH levels, whereas ACTH deficiency caused by hypothalamic–pituitary disease or suppression by previously elevated glucocorticoid levels results in secondary adrenal insufficiency. In addition, a helpful clinical finding is the preservation of normal aldosterone function in states of secondary adrenal insufficiency.

Combinations of adrenal steroid hormone deficiency and hormone overproduction can be seen in syndromes of congenital adrenal hyperplasia (CAH). Deficiencies in any of the several enzymes involved in steroid biosynthesis may result in anatomic hyperplasia of the adrenal cortex and in overproduction of the precursor molecules upstream from the enzyme block.

CLINICALLY USEFUL TESTS OF ADRENOCORTICAL FUNCTION AND ANATOMY

Ordering and interpreting tests of adrenocortical function requires a clear understanding of the dynamic function of the hypothalamic–pituitary–adrenocortical axis. Because the overlap of levels seen in pathologic states and among healthy people is large, random serum or plasma hormone levels rarely are definitively diagnostic. A definitive diagnosis almost always requires a dynamic test, either a stimulation test for suspected states of insufficiency or a suppression test for suspected cases of hyperfunction.

Plasma Levels

Cortisol. Plasma levels of cortisol vary in a diurnal fashion during the day (see Fig. 5-5). Interpretation of cortisol levels requires careful attention to the clinical setting, e.g., time of day and level of stress. A low cortisol value in the face of severe stress—e.g., fever, pneumonia, hypotension, hypoxia—indicates hypofunction of the axis, while an elevated value in the same situation would be reassuring that the axis is functioning properly. Intermediate values are much more difficult to interpret.

ACTH. Because of its shorter half-life, levels of ACTH vary even more widely than do cortisol levels. The ACTH assay is more expensive and less readily available than are assays of cortisol. Elevated values of ACTH in the face of low cortisol levels point to end-organ adrenocortical failure. High levels in the face of elevated cortisol levels and clinical evidence of hypercortisolism point to Cushing's disease or ectopic ACTH production by a tumor.

Aldosterone. Aldosterone levels vary widely, depending on salt intake, position, and a number of other factors. Low levels of aldosterone in the face of hypotension, volume contraction, or hyperkalemia suggest adrenal insufficiency.

Potassium. In the setting of normal renal and gastrointestinal function and normal potassium intake, the serum potassium concentration often can be used as a rough gauge of aldosterone activity. Hypokalemia is seen in states of aldosterone excess and hyperkalemia in states of aldosterone deficiency.

Renin Activity. Measurement of plasma renin activity (PRA) can be helpful in assessing abnormal aldosterone levels. In the absence of hyperkalemia, a low PRA paired with an elevated aldosterone level suggests that the aldosterone elevation is the result of autonomous overproduction. Elevated levels of PRA are seen in renovascular and malignant hypertension.

24-Hour Urine Testing.
Measurement of the excretion of cortisol, other steroid hormones, and their metabolites in timed—usually 24-hour—collections of urine can be extremely helpful in assessing adrenocortical function. The urine collection process essentially integrates the area under the curve of plasma levels

during the time of collection. Because there is a great overlap between excretion levels in people with deficiency syndromes and in healthy people, 24-hour urine testing is not useful in the diagnosis of adrenal axis insufficiency. Urine collections can be very useful, however, in identifying and defining syndromes of steroid hormone excess.

24-Hour Urinary Cortisol Excretion (Urinary Free Cortisol). Small amounts of cortisol are filtered through the glomerulus and are excreted in the urine. Values in excess of 100 μg per 24 hours are seen in Cushing's syndrome. This test provides one of the best screening tests for the presence of Cushing's syndrome because it is not affected by changes in cortisol-binding protein and is not distorted by obesity and abnormalities in hepatic function.

24-Hour 17-Hydroxycorticosteroid Excretion. 17-hydroxycorticosteroids are metabolites of steroid molecules that are hydroxylated at the 17 position. Cortisol is the principal contributor to the excretion of 17-hydroxycorticosteroids. The test is similar to urinary free cortisol testing. Many standard tests of adrenocortical axis function have been based on dynamic changes in 17-hydroxycorticosteroid excretion.

24-Hour 17-Ketosteroid Excretion. Metabolites of adrenal androgens retain a ketone group at position 17, which allows differentiation of androgen metabolites from the metabolites of cortisol and aldosterone. Mild elevations in 17-ketosteroid excretion can be seen in adrenal hyperfunction of any cause, but high values suggest the possible presence of an adrenocortical carcinoma. Relative enzyme deficiencies in such tumors may lead to a preponderance of precursor molecules and their by-products, often adrenal androgens.

DYNAMIC TESTING FOR SYNDROMES OF POSSIBLE CORTISOL EXCESS

Screening Tests

When clinical findings of cortisol excess or Cushing's syndrome are present (e.g., hypertension, hypokalemia, glucose intolerance, centripetal weight distribution, and striae), a screening test should be done. A normal *24-hour urinary free cortisol* excretion effectively rules out Cushing's syndrome. An elevated or equivocal value could be repeated or could lead to more definitive testing.

An *overnight dexamethasone suppression test (ONDST)* is another screening procedure that is less specific but is more easily conducted than the 24-hour urine collection for free cortisol. The patient takes 1 mg of dexamethasone between 11 p.m. and midnight. The plasma cortisol concentration at 8 a.m. should be less than 5 μg/dL. Dexamethasone is a potent analogue of cortisol and should provide sufficient glucocorticoid effect to suppress the expected morning rise of both CRH and ACTH, which should result in suppression of the serum cortisol at 8 a.m. A false lack of suppression is seen in some obese patients, in depressed patients, in patients on estrogen or anticonvulsants, and in some who may have been significantly stressed during the period just before phlebotomy.

Definitive Diagnostic Testing

When screening tests point to excess cortisol production, definitive diagnostic testing is indicated. These tests are designed to confirm the presence of excess cortisol production and to determine the source and likely pathologic mechanism.

Cushing's syndrome can occur from glucocorticoid excess of either exoge-

TABLE 5-5. EVALUATION OF CUSHING'S SYNDROME WITH SIMULTANEOUS CORTISOL AND ACTH LEVELS		
8 a.m. CORTISOL	**8 a.m. ACTH**	**POSSIBLE DIAGNOSIS**
High	Low	Non–ACTH-dependent cortisol production—adrenal adenoma, or exogenous steroid ingestion
Normal or high	"Normal" or slightly increased	Cushing's disease
High	High	Ectopic ACTH or CRH

ACTH, adrenocorticotrophic hormone; CRH, corticotropin-releasing hormone.

nous or endogenous origin. ACTH levels in patients with Cushing's syndrome often give an indication of the pathophysiologic mechanism involved. Cortisol excess in the face of low ACTH levels is seen when the source is either exogenous or an autonomously functioning adrenal adenoma or, rarely, an adrenocortical carcinoma. ACTH-stimulated (or -dependent) cortisol excess is seen in pituitary-based Cushing's syndrome, referred to as Cushing's disease, or in syndromes of ectopic ACTH or CRH production. Evaluation of mild cases of Cushing's syndrome caused by Cushing's disease can reveal only slight elevations of cortisol and ACTH and usually require additional dynamic studies for complete evaluation (Table 5-5).

Very low levels of ACTH (<25 pg/mL) in the face of cortisol excess point to an adrenal tumor or exogenous steroids as the culprit. In syndromes of ectopic production of ACTH by tumors, ACTH values tend to be significantly elevated, usually greater than 100 pg/mL, but the overlap in ACTH levels seen in patients with pituitary-based Cushing's syndrome is great. In patients with pituitary-based cortisol excess (e.g., those with Cushing's disease), ACTH values may be deceptively normal (i.e., measurable), although they should be low in the face of cortisol excess.

High-Dose Versus Low-Dose Dexamethasone Suppression Testing

When screening tests suggest cortisol excess, low-dose dexamethasone suppression testing is used to provide definitive evidence of endogenous cortisol overproduction (Table 5-6). This test is a more rigorous version of the ONDST.

Although ACTH levels may provide a diagnostic clue, some patients can benefit from high-dose dexamethasone testing. After establishing the presence of abnormal cortisol production, high-dose dexamethasone suppression testing can evaluate the possible presence of Cushing's disease. Table 5-6 presents the expected outcomes of low- and high-dose dexamethasone suppression testing. ACTH and cortisol secretion in pituitary-based Cushing's syndrome (i.e., Cushing's disease) often can be suppressed, at least partially, by significantly supraphysiologic doses of dexamethasone. A dexamethasone dose of 8 mg per 24 hours (about 10 times the physiologic dose) suppresses almost all patients with pituitary-based Cushing's syndrome. This finding suggests that the major problem in this form of Cushing's syndrome is an abnormal set-point for cortisol feedback. Like a ther-

| | TABLE 5-6. | *DEXAMETHASONE SUPPRESSION TESTING* |

TEST FORMAT	SERUM CORTISOL	URINARY 17-OH STEROID EXCRETION
Low-dose dexamethasone (2 mg/24 hr)	Cortisol <5 μg/dL at 8 a.m. after 2 days of dexamethasone	17-OH steroids <4 mg/24 hr
High-dose dexamethasone (8 mg/24 hr)	Reduction of 8 a.m. cortisol to less than 50% of baseline	50% or more reduction in 24-hr 17-OH steroid excretion

mostat set for a higher temperature, the cortisol feedback mechanism in these patients requires a higher dose of glucocorticoid effect to inhibit ACTH production. The higher level of cortisol required results in the metabolic and anatomic changes of Cushing's syndrome.

TESTING FOR SYNDROMES OF POSSIBLE CORTISOL DEFICIENCY

As opposed to the evaluation of adrenocortical excess, syndromes of possible deficiency demand immediate and definitive testing. There should be no screening process. When suspected, this potentially life-threatening condition should be formally evaluated and treated while awaiting the results of testing. Adrenal insufficiency should be suspected when hypotension, hyponatremia, hyperkalemia, and poor response to stress are present. Especially in the presence of metastatic disease, autoimmune disease, and systemic infection, adrenal insufficiency should always be considered as a possible factor. Pituitary disease and previous exposure to glucocorticoid therapy should raise the possibility of secondary adrenal insufficiency. The possibility of inadequate function of the hypothalamic–pituitary–adrenal axis can be approached in several different ways. Tests available for assessing adrenal responsiveness are listed in Table 5-7.

| | TABLE 5-7. | *TESTS FOR ADRENAL INSUFFICIENCY* |

TEST	PHYSIOLOGIC BASIS/COMMENTS
ACTH stimulation test (cosyntropin test)	Evaluates ability of the end organ (the adrenal cortex) to respond.
Metyrapone	By blocking the 11-hydroxylation of 11-deoxycortisol, the feedback loop is not satisfied and the entire axis is stimulated.
Insulin-induced hypoglycemia	Tests the entire axis in the stress-response mode.

ACTH, adrenocorticotropic hormone.

ACTH Stimulation Test. Adrenocortical function can be tested by administration of exogenous ACTH and assessment of the response of the adrenal cortex. The short version, or cosyntropin test, involves the use of a fully active, synthetic form of ACTH that includes the first 24 of the 39 amino acids of the native ACTH molecule. The cortisol level is measured before administration of ACTH and at 30 and 60 minutes after administration. A rise of at least 10 μg/dL or a value of 18 μg/dL or higher at any point indicates adequate end-organ function. Lack of response is seen in primary adrenal failure or Addison's disease but also can be seen in most forms of secondary adrenal insufficiency. Table 5-8 outlines the possible responses to the cosyntropin test.

As shown in Table 5-8, there is an aldosterone response in cases of secondary adrenal insufficiency, but not in primary end-organ failure, because aldosterone secretion is not solely dependent on ACTH and aldosterone secretory ability does not atrophy when ACTH is absent. Another testing strategy is to use repeated infusions of ACTH over a period of several days in an effort to reverse the functional and anatomic atrophy that develops in secondary adrenal insufficiency.

Metyrapone Testing. The cortisol feedback component of the control of the hypothalamic–pituitary–adrenal axis is the basis for metyrapone testing, an integrated test of axis function. Metyrapone blocks the final step of cortisol biosynthesis, 11-hydroxylation (see Fig. 5-3), and thereby lowers cortisol levels significantly. The low cortisol level results in increased CRH and ACTH secretion and stimulation of the entire axis up to the point of the metyrapone-induced enzyme blockade. Measurement of cortisol (to ensure adequate production blockade), its precursor, 11-deoxycortisol, and ACTH allows an assessment of hypothalamic–pituitary–adrenocortical axis function. If the expected rise in ACTH and 11-deoxycortisol is not seen in the face of adequate cortisol deficiency, axis dysfunction is present and the level of malfunction can be identified. An ACTH response without an increase in 11-deoxycortisol indicates end-organ failure, whereas a deficient ACTH and 11-deoxycortisol response indicates hypothalamic–pituitary failure.

Insulin Tolerance Testing. Perhaps the best test of the hypothalamic–pituitary–adrenal axis is responsiveness to stress. With insulin-induced hypoglyce-

TABLE 5-8. *RESPONSE TO COSYNTROPIN TEST OR "RAPID" ACTH STIMULATION TEST*			
CORTISOL	**ALDOSTERONE**	**DIAGNOSIS**	**COMMENTS**
Increased	Increased	Normal	
Decreased	Decreased	Primary adrenal insufficiency	End-organ failure (Addison's disease)
Decreased	Increased	Secondary adrenal insufficiency	Exogenous steroids, pituitary disease, hypothalamic disease
Increased	Decreased	Isolated aldosterone deficiency	Very rare

ACTH, adrenocorticotropic hormone.

mia as the stress, cortisol and ACTH levels can be followed to assess responsiveness and isolate the basis of an inadequate response. The test, however, has significant risks. The hypoglycemia and the catecholamine discharge it stimulates can pose a serious threat to patients with coronary artery or cerebrovascular disease. Careful monitoring and good intravenous access for rescue with intravenous glucose must be available.

ANATOMIC TESTING

Both MRI and CT scanning can be used to assess adrenal and pituitary anatomy. Hormonally inactive, unimportant, benign adenomas or "incidentalomas" of both the adrenal and pituitary often are present, which can make interpretation of anatomic test results very difficult. Anatomic testing, therefore, should be only done after dynamic chemical testing points to the need for an anatomic collaboration of the biochemical results.

INVASIVE TESTING

Simultaneous catheterization of the right and left adrenal veins with hormonal sampling of the venous effluent is accomplished relatively easily and may provide very valuable data. When an adrenal adenoma is suspected as the source of adrenal steroid excess, venous sampling can provide important anatomic and functional confirmation.

Bilateral petrosal sinus catheterization with measurement of ACTH levels in the venous effluent draining the pituitary is much more difficult and less readily available. This test can be done with or without the administration of CRH to magnify the levels of ACTH. In the setting of suspected pituitary-based Cushing's syndrome (Cushing's disease), this procedure can be used to verify that the pituitary is the source of the abnormally elevated ACTH and, in addition, may provide some data with regard to the localization of the adenoma within the pituitary.

CASE PRESENTATION: CASE 1

Truncal obesity, striae, hypertension, and glucose intolerance in a 39-year-old man

Charles Denney's visit to the local emergency room was prompted by a nasty coffee burn. He was driving his delivery van through a complicated intersection, shifting gears and balancing a cup of very hot coffee, when the spill occurred. The burn extended over his anterior thighs and upper abdomen and quickly blistered.

The physician in the emergency room was more impressed by Mr. Denney's appearance than by the burns. At age 39, Mr. Denney's past medical history was largely unremarkable, but he had noticed some changes over the past couple of years. His weight had gone up about 30 pounds, most of it distributed in his trunk and face. He also had noted some purple stretch marks on his abdomen, mild but continuing facial acne, and a slightly scaly patchy discoloration of his chest and back. He always looked red-faced, as if he had been out in the sun or wind. His muscle strength had decreased. Loading and unloading his van was more difficult, and he even had difficulty getting out of his easy chair, needing to use his hands to push himself up.

On physical examination he was found to be a plethoric, red-faced male with a protuberant abdomen, and relatively thin extremities.

Vital signs:	Blood pressure 160/100; pulse 98
Skin:	Tinea versicolor of the upper chest and back
	Second-degree burns of the upper abdomen and mid-thighs bilaterally
	Violaceous pigmented striae of the abdomen
	Mild facial acne
HEENT:	Normal
Chest:	Normal
Heart:	Normal
Abdomen:	Protuberant without palpable organomegaly
Genitals:	Normal penis and testes
Extremities:	Thin compared to body size, no edema

Laboratory Studies

Test	Charles Denney	Normal
CBC	Normal	Normal
Serum sodium	140 mEq/L	135–145 mEq/L
Serum potassium	3.1 mEq/L	3.5–5.0 mEq/L
Glucose (random)	162 mg/dL	70–110 mg/dL, fasting
Creatinine	0.9 mg/dL	0.3–1.5 mg/dL
BUN	10 mg/dL	8–22 mg/dL

Excess levels of glucocorticoids, of either exogenous or endogenous origin, result in a clinical constellation of findings referred to as Cushing's syndrome. In addition to the common clinical problems of hypertension, obesity, and glucose intolerance, Cushing's syndrome can include a large number of other clinical findings.

Clinical Features of Cushing's Syndrome

Centripetal obesity	Striae
Hypertension	Acne
Facial fullness	Emotional lability
Hirsutism	Bruising
Menstrual disorders	Edema
Hypertension	Diabetes mellitus
Muscular weakness	Hypercalciuria
Back pain	Hypokalemia

Mr. Denney has a number of findings consistent with Cushing's syndrome, and further evaluation clearly is necessary.

The burn was evaluated and dressed with an antibiotic ointment, and Mr. Denney was given a tetanus shot. The emergency room physician added a cortisol level to the lab work already done and referred Mr. Denney to a primary care physician for further evaluation. The referral form outlined the clinical suspicion and called attention to the pending laboratory result.

Mr. Denney returned fasting the next morning for a check of the burn and a dressing change. On examination, his blood pressure was 158/92. The burn was not any worse. A new dressing was applied, and instructions for home care were given.

Laboratory Studies

Test	Charles Denney	Normal
Glucose, fasting	143 mg/dL	70–110 mg/dL, fasting
Cortisol (10 a.m.)	29 µg/dL	8 a.m.: 5–25 µg/dL
		4 p.m.: 3–12 µg/dL

Mr. Denney's history, his physical examination, the elevated fasting blood glucose, the persistent hypertension, the hypokalemia, and the relatively high cortisol level all suggest Cushing's syndrome, but the data at this point are not definitive and do not offer a pathophysiologic mechanism.

One week later Mr. Denney was seen by his new primary care physician, who reviewed the data, confirmed the physical findings, and agreed that Cushing's syndrome is an important possibility. Some additional studies were ordered.

Test	Charles Denney	Normal
Cortisol (8 a.m.)	39 µg/dL	8 a.m.: 5–25 µg/dL
		4 p.m.: 3–12 µg/dL
ACTH (8 a.m.)	62 pg/mL	8 a.m.: <80 pg/mL
24-hr urinary free cortisol	425 µg/d	20–70 µg/d

The significant elevation of urinary cortisol excretion provides strong evidence of Cushing's syndrome. The 8 a.m. plasma cortisol clearly is elevated, but the ACTH level is within the normal range. These values do not provide definitive information but do suggest that the ACTH level is inappropriately elevated or, alternatively, not appropriately suppressed.

As an outpatient, Mr. Denney began a series of 24-hour urine collections and 8 a.m. blood tests to measure responsiveness of his hypothalamic–pituitary–adrenal axis to varying doses of dexamethasone:

Day	Condition	8 a.m. Cortisol	Urinary Free Cortisol/24 hrs	17OH-Steroids mg/24 hrs
	Normal	5–25 µg/dL	20–70 µg/d	3–10 mg/d
1	Baseline	39	425	22.8
2	Baseline	42	389	18.9
3	Low-dose dex (2 mg/24 hrs)	38	392	19.6
4	Low-dose dex	39	402	20.1
5	High-dose dex (8 mg/24 hrs)	19	227	16.4
6	High-dose dex	9	147	15.9

dex, dexamethasone.

On the basis of these results, cortisol excess clearly is documented, and some function of the cortisol feedback mechanism is demonstrated by the response to high-dose dexamethasone. These data are consistent with pituitary-based Cushing's syndrome, or Cushing's disease.

After reviewing the dexamethasone suppression data with Mr. Denney, an MRI of the pituitary was ordered. It showed a 1.8-cm pituitary adenoma.

Mr. Denney's laboratory studies and the imaging study all point to a pituitary origin for the Cushing's syndrome. There is a remote possibility that the pituitary lesion could be an incidental finding, a nonfunctional adenoma that is unrelated to his clinical syndrome. Some clinicians might suggest that a petrosal sinus catheterization study be performed to be absolutely sure that the excess ACTH is indeed coming from the pituitary fossa.

The therapeutic options for the treatment of pituitary-based Cushing's syndrome include surgery with removal of the pituitary adenoma, hopefully sparing the nonadenomatous portion of the pituitary. This usually provides very effective control of the hypercortisolism. The return to normal hypothalamic–pituitary–adrenocortical axis function, however, may take several months because of suppression of the remaining normal, ACTH-secreting, corticotroph cells of the anterior pituitary. Radiation therapy also can be used, but it may take several months or more for the effect to be significant. In some patients, bilateral adrenalectomy is required to control cortisol production. Unilateral or subtotal adrenalectomy might provide a temporary decrease in cortisol production, but the continued stimulation by ACTH usually results in functional hypertrophy of the remaining tissue that makes a less than total adrenalectomy a short-lived solution to the problem.

When bilateral adrenalectomy is used in the treatment of Cushing's disease, one problem—Cushing's disease—is exchanged for another—Addison's disease, or adrenal end-organ insufficiency. For some patients, this is a reasonable exchange. Adrenal insufficiency can be managed with fewer long-term complications than are associated with continued Cushing's syndrome. A small proportion of patients who undergo adrenalectomy as therapy for Cushing's disease develop a significant, ACTH-secreting pituitary tumor. This condition, referred to as Nelson's syndrome, provides support for the set-point abnormality concept of Cushing's disease. Physiologic replacement doses of cortisol are not high enough to suppress ACTH secretion and inhibit the continued growth of corticotrophs.

After completing the tests, Mr. Denney underwent successful transsphenoidal hypophysectomy with removal of the adenoma seen on MRI. Pathology studies revealed a benign tumor with histologic and staining characteristics consistent with an ACTH-secreting adenoma.

Perioperatively Mr. Denney was "covered" with "stress steroids," and postoperatively his steroid dose was tapered down to a physiologic dose. After a few weeks of physiologic replacement, he was tapered gradually to no exogenous cortisol. Over the next several months his body weight decreased by about 20 pounds, his facial redness decreased, his blood pressure improved, and glucose intolerance was no longer present. The stretch marks are still there, but they are less colorful and in general Mr. Denney feels quite a bit better. His muscle strength has improved significantly. By 6 months postoperatively his morning cortisol level was normal, at 23 µg/dL.

At some point it would be useful to test Mr. Denney's hypothalamic–pituitary–adrenal axis for stress responsiveness, to be sure that full, stress-responsive function of the system has returned.

CASE PRESENTATION: CASE 2

Fatigue, hypokalemia, and a lung mass in a 65-year-old man

William Atkinson had smoked cigarettes for most of his adult life, at least two packs a day. He retired about 5 years ago, at age 65, from his work as a pipe fitter and now enjoyed working in his garden and spending time with his grandchildren. His past medical history was largely unremarkable. He is on no medications.

Over the last several weeks he has become increasingly fatigued and has noted significant polyuria and polydipsia. Although he was not due to see his physician for another 6 months, he decided to make a visit sooner.

Physical examination revealed a barrel-chested man with a blood pressure of 160/100.

Skin:	**Normal, no striae**
HEENT:	**Normal**
Chest:	**Increased AP diameter and prolonged expiration phase with fair air movement and no evidence of consolidation**
Heart:	**Distant heart sounds**
Abdomen:	**Unremarkable**
Extremities:	**Moderate atrophy of quadriceps muscles, bilaterally**

Laboratory Studies

Test	William Atkinson	Normal
Serum sodium	145 mEq/L	135–145 mEq/L
Serum potassium	2.9 mEq/L	3.5–5.0 mEq/L
Glucose (random)	287 mg/dL	70–110 mg/dL, fasting

Chest X-ray:	**Right upper lobe lung nodule, measuring approximately 3 cm in diameter with mediastinal adenopathy**

The new onset of diabetes, the hypokalemia, and the chest mass all require further evaluation. Hypokalemia in a normally nourished person who is not on any medications and who is not having diarrhea or vomiting suggests mineralocorticoid excess. Although cortisol at physiologic levels does not have a significant mineralocorticoid effect, it does have an aldosterone-like effect when present in larger amounts. Glucose intolerance is not an unusual clinical finding, but in this case it could be related to hypokalemia in at least two ways. Hypokalemia decreases the secretion of insulin, with resultant effects on glucose metabolism. In addition, if the hypokalemia is the result of adrenocortical hyperfunction, the contra-insulin and gluconeogenic effects of excess cortisol also could be a significant factor in the development of glucose intolerance. The lung lesion is a possible source of ACTH that stimulates excess cortisol excretion.

Mr. Atkinson returned to discuss the chest X-ray, the laboratory studies, and the new onset of diabetes with his doctor. Additional studies were ordered that included the following:

Test	William Atkinson	Normal
Cortisol (4 p.m.)	52 μg/dL	8 a.m.: 5–25 μg/dL 4 p.m.: 3–12 μg/dL
ACTH (4 p.m.)	357 pg/mL	8 a.m.: <80 pg/mL

The extremely high cortisol and ACTH levels in this patient with a lung lesion are essentially diagnostic of an ACTH-producing lung cancer. Although Mr. Atkinson does not have the classic physical findings of Cushing's syndrome, he clearly has significant cortisol excess. It may take many months for the physical findings of Cushing's syndrome to develop, but the metabolic effects—hypokalemia, glucose intolerance, and hypertension—occur much more quickly. Although dexamethasone suppression testing could be done, it is not indicated in this clinical setting. A tissue diagnosis of the lung lesion should be made and appropriate treatment started.

Biopsy of the lung lesion revealed oat cell carcinoma of the lung, and Mr. Atkinson was started on appropriate chemotherapy, with significant improvement in his diabetes and hypokalemia. His muscle strength also improved.

Six months later, however, hypokalemia, hyperglycemia, and proximal myopathy returned. Further chemotherapy was not successful, and Mr. Atkinson died after developing an aggressive pneumonia.

Management of cortisol overproduction in this clinical situation can be done in several ways. Bilateral adrenalectomy, followed by physiologic cortisol and aldosterone replacement, is possible, but the operative procedure is major and might not be well tolerated. Metyrapone, the drug that blocks 11-hydroxylation of cortisol, can be used to decrease cortisol production with benefit in some patients. Aminoglutethimide and ketoconazole also offer inhibition of steroid hormone production and can be useful in some clinical situations. Successful treatment of the ACTH-producing tumor can decrease steroid production, and, in the rare cases when the lung tumor can be cured, the Cushing's syndrome also is corrected.

CASE PRESENTATION: CASE 3

Fatigue, hyperpigmentation, and hyperkalemia in a 38-year-old woman

Anne Darlington is a 38-year-old woman who complains of malaise and fatigue. Her past medical history has been largely unremarkable, but recently she noted a 10-pound, unintentional weight loss. In addition, she feels very dizzy when she stands up. She has not had a menstrual period in about 4 months and does not think she could be pregnant. Her skin color has changed. She is now deeply tanned, in spite of the fact that it is midwinter and she has not been in the sun in several months. She has also noted a curious craving for potato chips and pickles. She is on no medications.

Physical examination reveals a thin, tanned woman with a supine blood pressure of 90/50 that falls to 80/30 on standing. Her pulse goes from 90 to 120.

Skin:	Diffuse hyperpigmentation, very darkly pigmented nipples and palmar creases of both hands, small patches of decreased pigmentation of left thigh and right mid-back	
HEENT:	Normal	
Neck:	Normal, no thyroid enlargement	
Chest:	Clear	
Heart:	Normal	
Abdomen:	Normal	
Extremities:	Thin, no edema	
Neuro:	Normal	

Laboratory Studies

Test	Anne Darlington	Normal
Serum sodium	124 mEq/L	135–145 mEq/L
Serum potassium	5.8 mEq/L	3.5–5.0 mEq/L
Glucose, random	55 mg/dL	70–110 mg/dL, fasting
Creatinine	1.2 mg/dL	0.3–1.5 mg/dL
BUN	32 mg/dL	8–22 mg/dL

Inability to maintain a normal blood pressure with change in posture suggests significant volume depletion. In the absence of medications, diarrhea, vomiting, or increased sweating, postural hypotension indicates a malfunction of either volume maintenance or cardiovascular reflexes. The rise in Ms. Darlington's pulse rate is a normal cardiovascular response to the hypotension. Hypotension and hyperkalemia are potentially life-threatening, and the combination points to possible failure of mineralocorticoid function. The mild elevation of BUN in the face of a normal creatinine also is consistent with a prerenal or volume-depleted state. The hyperkalemia suggests a decreased ability to excrete potassium. The low serum sodium indicates an inability to excrete free water. The low glucose concentration raises the possibility that Ms. Darlington may have a problem maintaining her glucose level.

Clinical Features of Addison's Disease: End-Organ Adrenal Insufficiency
 Weakness, fatigue
 Anorexia
 Weight loss
 Nausea, loose stools
 Hypoglycemia
 Hypotension
 Hyponatremia
 Salt craving
 Hyperkalemia
 Hyperpigmentation

Based on these initial findings, adrenal insufficiency was suspected, and a cosyntropin stimulation test was done. The results are tabulated below.

Shortly after the testing was completed, Ms. Darlington was started on hydrocortisone and intravenous saline. Six hours later she felt quite a bit better. Her blood pressure was 110/70 and fell to only 100/60 when she stood up. Her pulse was down to 74 and rose to 82 when she went from lying to standing.

Cosyntropin Stimulation Test

Time	Cortisol (µg/dL)	Aldosterone (ng/dL)
0 min	4	3
30 min	3	4
60 min	4	5

The following additional morning laboratory values were obtained:

Test	Anne Darlington	Normal
Serum sodium	131 mEq/L	135–145 mEq/L
Serum potassium	4.9 mEq/L	3.5–5.0 mEq/L
Glucose, fasting	82 mg/dL	70–110 mg/dL, fasting
Creatinine	1.0 mg/dL	0.3–1.5 mg/dL
BUN	18 mg/dL	8–22 mg/dL

Ms. Darlington was begun on hydrocortisone replacement and instructed to take 20 mg in the morning and 10 mg in the early afternoon. In addition, fludrocortisone, an orally administered analogue of aldosterone, was added to the regimen to replace mineralocorticoid function.

On a follow-up visit 10 days later, the initial ACTH level was available: ACTH at 5 p.m.: 555 pg/mL (normal range, 0 to 80 pg/mL at 8 a.m.).

Ms. Darlington is feeling very much better. She has gained 7 pounds and no longer is dizzy when she gets up. She was instructed to wear an identifying bracelet and to take additional doses at times of illness or significant stress to meet increased needs for glucocorticoid.

Although definitive diagnostic information is provided by the results of the ACTH stimulation test, evidence of ACTH insensitivity and end-organ adrenocortical failure clearly were present in Ms. Darlington's history and on her physical examination. The high ACTH level indicates that Ms. Darlington had, in effect, already done her own ACTH stimulation test. There was inadequate response of the adrenal cortex to either endogenous or ex-

TABLE 5-9.	*MECHANISMS OF ADRENAL INSUFFICIENCY*
PRIMARY	**SECONDARY**
Autoimmune	Exogenous steroids
Infection	Hypothalamic or pituitary disease
Hemorrhage	Tumor—primary or metastatic
Infarction	Infiltrative disease
Infiltrative disease	Trauma
Metastatic disease	Infarction
Congenital enzyme deficiencies	
Drugs that inhibit steroid production	

ogenous ACTH. The hyperpigmentation is due to the presence of excess MSH, a by-product of excessive ACTH production, and serves as an endogenous bioassay of ACTH secretion. Appropriate treatment with exogenous cortisol should not only make Ms. Darlington feel better, but it also should decrease ACTH production and thereby decrease her hyperpigmentation.

Hyperkalemia is a potent stimulus of aldosterone secretion. The release of aldosterone in response to hyperkalemia does not require the presence of ACTH. In the face of normal renal function, the aldosterone secreted should work to correct the elevated potassium level. The presence of hyperkalemia, therefore, strongly supports the possibility that end-organ adrenal failure is the basis of Ms. Darlington's clinical findings.

The cause of the adrenal insufficiency in this case is most likely autoimmune adrenal destruction. Some of the possible mechanisms of adrenal insufficiency are listed in Table 5-9.

Hormonal replacement for Addison's disease is done in a fashion that roughly mimics the normal diurnal variation of cortisol secretion, with additional doses at times of increased need such as illness and other stresses. The normal, non-stressed secretion of hydrocortisone over a 24-hour period is between 20 mg and 30 mg. Wearing an identification bracelet or a similar form of identification can lead to the administration of life-saving stress doses of glucocorticoids and volume replacement at times of injury or illness.

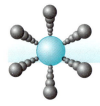

CASE PRESENTATION: CASE 4

The problems of exogenous steroid in a 48-year-old woman

Marjorie Young is 48 years old and has had ulcerative colitis for the past 7 years. Crampy abdominal discomfort and explosive diarrhea led to the diagnosis, which was confirmed by an endoscopic study with biopsies. The disease was only partially controlled on azulfidine or its analogues, and

eventually treatment with glucocorticoids was started. The relief that came with prednisone was significant, but it required at least 20 mg per day to control her symptoms, a dose that is roughly 4 times physiologic.

After several months of daily prednisone therapy at 20 mg/day, Mrs. Young developed mild hypertension—150/90. Her face became round and full, and she began to have mild facial acne, a problem she had not had in many years. Her abdomen became more protuberant, and she lost about 1″ in height. In addition, she has had several episodes of significant thoracic back pain.

Physical examination reveals a kyphotic, cushingoid-appearing woman with a round red face, mild facial acne, very thin extremities, and a protuberant abdomen. Her blood pressure is 150/100.

Mrs. Young has Cushing's syndrome caused by exogenous steroids. The antiinflammatory effects of glucocorticoids can be very helpful for the management of a number of conditions, but, unfortunately, the catabolic side effects are inseparable from the antiinflammatory effects. The loss of height and the back pain are caused by significant osteoporosis with multiple compression fractures of the thoracic spine. Glucocorticoids in pharmacologic doses accelerate bone loss and can cause osteoporosis. The mild hypertension and proximal myopathy also are the result of steroid excess.

Each of the previous three or four attempts to lower the prednisone dose has resulted in a significant flair of the ulcerative colitis. However, the back pain, the loss of height, and now the hypertension really worry Mrs. Young. "The treatment is worse than the disease!"

Mrs. Young has always dreaded the thought of a colectomy and the "ostomy" that would result, but now she finds herself wondering if the steroids she has to take may be even more of a problem. After a full discussion, Mrs. Young and her physician decide on one more try to taper her prednisone dose. If the disease flares, she is resigned to having a colectomy but hopes that it can be done in conjunction with one of the new procedures that might allow her to avoid an ileostomy.

In spite of tapering the prednisone slowly, by the time she got to a dose of 15 mg/day (about 2 to 3 times physiologic), frequent, bloody, mucoid stools and crampy abdominal pain returned. The prednisone dose was increased to 40 mg each day, with marked improvement, over the next 10 days. As a result of this failure to taper off steroids, Mrs. Young consulted the surgeon she had tried to avoid for the past 7 years.

In preparation for surgery Mrs. Young was started on clear liquids and a bowel-cleansing antibiotic regimen. Additional preoperative orders included methylprednisolone hemisuccinate, 20 mg IV every 12 hours, to start 12 hours before surgery.

The procedure went well, and by 2 days postoperatively her steroid dose was decreased to 16 mg of the steroid every 12 hours.

The flare of an underlying inflammatory disease during a steroid taper, even a slow taper, often is seen and usually leads to the resumption of steroid therapy at levels that are as high as or higher than those at the start of the taper. An additional problem for Mrs. Young and other patients treated with supraphysiologic steroid doses is the suppression of the hypothalamic–pituitary–adrenocortical axis (HPA) that occurs with significant steroid therapy. Alternate-day steroid therapy occasionally can control some inflammatory conditions with less suppressing impact on the HPA axis, but most significant inflammatory processes require daily steroid therapy to achieve reasonable control.

Because no parenteral form of prednisone is available, Mrs. Young's glucocorticoid therapy was switched to an equivalent dose of a water-soluble analogue of prednisone and cortisol—methylprednisolone hemisuccinate—that is available for intravenous administration. Neither prednisone nor methylprednisolone has significant mineralocorticoid effect. Mrs. Young's ability to secrete aldosterone in response to hyperkalemia and volume depletion should be intact because her adrenal insufficiency is secondary, not primary.

Postoperatively her steroid dose can be tapered but will need to be tapered slowly. Rapid taper of glucocorticoids, even to levels that are considered supraphysiologic, can result in a withdrawal syndrome characterized by fever, joint pain, malaise, and mucous membrane desquamation. A slow, gentle taper prevents this problem.

In addition, Mrs. Young needs adequate glucocorticoid levels to deal with the stress of her recent surgery and recovery. Maximal cortisol output, as might be seen during and immediately following a major operation, is about 10 mg/hour. Physiologic stress dose coverage schedules usually call for 300 mg of hydrocortisone or its equivalent per 24 hours (10 mg/hr × 24 hr + approximately 25% for safety margin). Table 5-10 lists the equivalent doses of various glucocorticoids preparations.

Mrs. Young's recovery was uncomplicated, and she left the hospital on the 8th postoperative day on prednisone, 10 mg twice a day. She was disappointed that she is still on prednisone, but understands that it will take several months for her adrenal cortex and pituitary to recover function fully.

After 3 weeks she has tapered down to 8 mg of prednisone per day. Her blood pressure is down to 130/80, and her face is less round. The next step is to taper off prednisone completely. Mrs. Young begins a schedule

TABLE 5-10. *GLUCOCORTICOID DOSE EQUIVALENTS*[a]		
GLUCOCORTICOID	**EQUIVALENT DOSE**	**GLUCOCORTICOID EFFECT AS % OF HYDROCORTISONE**
Hydrocortisone (cortisol)	20 mg	100%
Cortisone	25 mg	80%
Prednisone	5 mg	400%
Methylprednisolone	4 mg	500%
Dexamethasone	0.75 mg	2500%

[a] Compared to hydrocortisone.

that reduces her daily prednisone dose by 1 mg each week over the next 8 weeks. She is instructed to call if she gets ill or feels significant stress.

After 4 weeks of this tapering process, at a dose of 4 mg/day of prednisone, Mrs. Young developed the same symptoms her 4-year-old grandson had recently—nausea, vomiting, and diarrhea. On the way to the bathroom for the fourth time in the past 2 hours, Mrs. Young lost consciousness but quickly regained it, finding herself on the cold, hard bathroom floor. Her family called an ambulance and she was brought to the local emergency room.

On examination in the emergency room, her blood pressure was 90/60 supine, 60/40 sitting; and her pulse was 110 supine and 134 sitting.

Laboratory Studies

Test	Marjorie Young	Normal
Serum sodium	130 mEq/L	135–145 mEq/L
Serum potassium	3.4 mEq/L	3.5–5.0 mEq/L
Glucose	52 mg/dL	70–110 mg/dL, fasting
Creatinine	1.0 mg/dL	0.3–1.5 mg/dL
BUN	26 mg/dL	8–22 mg/dL

Postural hypotension and reflex tachycardia suggest volume depletion or inadequate cardiovascular response or both. In Mrs. Young, both are present. The gastroenteritis has resulted in some volume depletion. In addition, her inability to absorb the extra doses of prednisone may have resulted in significant glucocorticoid deficiency with loss of vascular smooth muscle reactivity.

Intravenous fluid and 20 mg of methylprednisolone intravenously lead, in about 2 hours, to marked improvement in blood pressure and in Mrs. Young's overall condition. After 8 hours in the emergency room, Mrs. Young was well enough to go home, feeling a lot better, but disappointed that getting off prednisone is such a difficult project.

After the episode of gastroenteritis, Mrs. Young resumed her taper and in 6 weeks was off prednisone completely. Six months later the following test results were obtained:

8 a.m. cortisol: 17 μg/dL (normal range is 5 to 25 μg/dL)

ACTH Stimulation Test

Time	Cortisol
0 min	12 μg/dL
30 min	24 μg/dL
60 min	26 μg/dL

Mrs. Young feels well. Her blood pressure is normal, and her face is almost back to its pre-prednisone shape. She remains kyphotic and shorter by 2 inches than she was before the prednisone, but is happy to be free of prednisone and its side effects.

She is taking supplemental calcium and vitamin D in an effort to minimize further bone loss. Although she is very leery about taking any more medications, she is considering postmenopausal estrogen replacement and a bisphosphonate (see Chapter 6) to minimize further bone loss.

Recovery of the suppressed HPA axis extends over 6 to 12 months (Fig. 5-8). Hypothalamic recovery followed by pituitary recovery leads eventually to adrenocortical recovery and the resumption of normal function. Mild adrenal insufficiency or cortisol deficiency during the process cannot be avoided because it is the stimulus for recovery.

Accurately assessing recovery of the axis is difficult. Although a low 8 a.m. cortisol indicates that recovery has not yet occurred, a normal value does not provide any data about the stress responsiveness of the axis. A good response to ACTH, as in Mrs. Young's case, although not specifically testing the function of her hypothalamic–pituitary unit, does provide reassuring information when the response is normal. A brisk response to exogenous ACTH suggests that the adrenal cortex has recovered from suppression, an event that would have occurred only via recovery of hypothalamic and pituitary function. Insulin-induced hypoglycemia and metyrapone testing are other, more cumbersome, and potentially more dangerous ways of assessing the functional reserve of the axis.

Patients who have taken potentially suppressing doses of exogenous steroids within the previous year are at some risk of adrenal insufficiency in stressful situations. Unless testing that documents recovery of function is available, such patients should be ''covered'' with stress doses of glucocorticoids for surgery and major injuries and illnesses.

Figure 5-8. Recovery of the hypothalamic–pituitary–adrenal axis from suppression. Several months are required for normal secretion of cortisol to return after suppression by excess levels of exogenous or endogenous steroids. Recovery of hypothalamic and pituitary function is followed by reversal of adrenocortical atrophy.

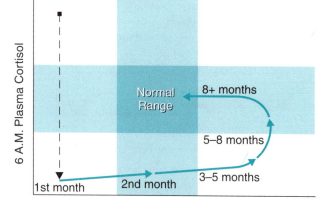

6 A.M. Plasma Cortisol

Normal Range

8+ months

5–8 months

3–5 months

1st month 2nd month

6 A.M. Plasma ACTH

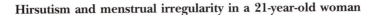

CASE PRESENTATION: CASE 5

Hirsutism and menstrual irregularity in a 21-year-old woman

Ever since age 13, when she started to have menstrual periods, Alison Rossiter has been plagued by increasing facial and body hair. She has used waxes, depilatory creams, and bleach, and has even had electrolysis, but she finds that she is facing a constant battle and spends a number of hours each week dealing with the problem.

Her childhood development was normal, and her general health has been excellent. Although Alison was the tallest girl in her class in the second grade when she was 7, she was now, at age 21, one of the shortest students in her class in college. Her menstrual periods have never been regular. She has experienced short episodes of mild bleeding on an unpredictable basis every few months. Alison has not been sexually active but worries about her sexuality—both about her attractiveness and about her ability to have children in the future.

Alison is on no medications, and other than some caffeine in coffee and in soda, she does not use any drugs or medications. Her parents are healthy, and neither her mother nor her older sister has had problems with hirsutism.

Physical examination reveals a healthy-appearing young woman.

Vital signs:	Blood pressure 130/74; pulse 78
Height:	5'1"
Weight:	104 lbs
Skin:	Increased pigmented coarse facial, forearm, presternal, and periareolar hair. Pubic hair extends in the midline up to the umbilicus. Legs and thighs show evidence of recent shaving
HEENT:	Normal
Chest:	Clear
Heart:	Normal
Abdomen:	Normal
Genital/pelvic:	Mild clitoromegaly, normal vagina, healthy-appearing cervix. Bimanual examination is unremarkable

Laboratory Studies

Test	Alison Rossiter	Normal Values
CBC	Normal	Normal
Serum sodium	140 mEq/L	135–145 mEq/L
Serum potassium	3.6 mEq/L	3.5–5.0 mEq/L
LH	5 mU/mL	*Female:* Prepubertal: <5 mU/mL Pre- or postovulatory: 5–25 mU/mL Ovulatory surge: 12–30 mU/mL Postmenopausal: >30 mU/mL

FSH	5	Female: Prepubertal: <5 mU/mL Pre- or postovulatory: 5–20 mU/mL Ovulatory surge: 12–30 mU/mL Postmenopausal: >30 mU/mL
Testosterone (total)	154	Adult Female: 20–90 ng/dL
DHEA-sulfate	842	Adult Female: 80–443 μg/dL
Prolactin	12	5–25 ng/mL

Hirsutism can be a devastating problem for many women. Medications (e.g., phenytoin, minoxidil, phenothiazines) can cause increased hair growth. Ethnic and genetic factors also may result in more facial and body hair than is desired. In some cases the cause of hirsutism is undiscovered and occurs in the face of normal hormonal function (idiopathic), possibly as a result of increased hair follicle sensitivity to normal androgen levels. When hirsutism is associated with abnormal menstrual function or with evidence of masculinization, increased androgen levels may be present, and further evaluation is indicated.

Alison's family history and her medical history offer no explanation for the hirsutism. The male pattern of Alison's hair growth and the slight enlargement of the clitoris suggest significant androgen excess. Her testosterone level is slightly high, as is the level of DHEA-sulfate, an adrenal androgen. Steroid hormones can be synthesized in only two tissues—the adrenal cortex and the gonad. These two glands must, therefore, be considered when clinical and laboratory findings suggest steroid hormone overproduction. Normal gonadotropin levels together with a normal pelvic exam make polycystic ovary syndrome (PCO) unlikely (see Chapter 9). Because DHEA and its sulfate are principally of adrenal origin, further evaluation of Alison's problem should focus on her adrenal function.

After reviewing the initial laboratory studies and discussing the results with Alison, further studies were ordered:

Test	Alison Rossiter	Normal
17-hydroxyprogesterone	6.7 μg/L	Female: Follicular: 0.1–1.0 μg/L Luteal: 0.5–3.5 μg/L
17-ketosteroid excretion (24-hr urine)	18 mg/24 hrs	Female: 3–15 mg/24 hrs
Cortisol (8 a.m.)	16 μg/dL	8 a.m.: 5–25 μg/dL

Although the urinary excretion of 17-ketosteroids is elevated, it is not in the markedly elevated range seen in adrenocortical carcinoma. The elevation does, however, suggest that there is overproduction of steroid hormones, with a ketone group at the 17 position. These compounds usually are androgenic steroids of varying strength. The elevated 17-hydroxyprogesterone, an intermediary compound in the biosynthetic cascade of adrenal steroid production (see Fig. 5-3), provides a clue to the cause of Alison's problem. An enzyme deficiency in the sequence of adrenal steroid production can result in the buildup of precursors such as 17-hydroxyprogesterone. Because the levels of the end product of the cascade, cortisol and aldosterone, are controlled by active feedback mechanisms, the production of these hormones is maintained. A complete or near-complete enzyme deficiency would result in severe deficiency of end product, but milder deficiencies could be compensated by adrenal hyperplasia stimulated by ACTH and the renin-angiotensin system. The resulting increase in volume of the adrenal cortex results in normal or near-normal end product production, but there is an overproduction of precursors above the level of the enzyme block. This increase in substrate availability may lead to increased production of other steroid hormones.

In Alison's case, a partial deficiency of 21-hydroxylase could explain her clinical presentation and laboratory findings (Fig. 5-9). Although her cortisol level was normal when measured, it is normal by virtue of adrenocortical hyperplasia and a significant buildup in steroid molecules above the enzyme deficiency, including 17-hydroxyprogesterone (see Fig. 5-9). These abundant precursors spill over into the androgen portion of the cascade and result in overproduction of adrenal androgens. These androgens result in increased hair growth, interference with menstrual function, and mild masculinization with clitoromegaly. Increased production of androgen during her childhood may explain Alison's increased height at age 7 because androgens stimulate bone growth. At the same time, the effect of the androgens over time is to close epiphysial growth plates, which, in Alison's case, may have limited her growth potential and accounts for her current relatively short stature.

At least five syndromes of deficiencies of steroid hormone synthesis enzymes have been described. They are categorized as syndromes of congenital adrenal hyperplasia and can present, as shown in Table 5-11, with a wide variety of clinical findings depending on which enzyme is deficient and the degree of deficiency. Deficiencies of enzymes along the cascade of steroid biosynthesis can result in relative decrease in cortisol or aldosterone. The resulting deficiency of the end product of hormone biosynthesis triggers the feedback loop, which results in stimulation of the adrenal cortex, both anatomically and functionally. There is both hyperplasia of the glands and overproduction of steroid molecules above the enzyme deficiency. Gonadal tissue, the other site of steroid hormone biosynthesis, also may be affected in some of the syndromes. Forms of CAH that result in severe mineralocorticoid deficiency may result in neonatal death, an outcome that can be avoided with early detection of volume depletion and careful perinatal care for babies at risk for these conditions.

Evaluation of patients with possible CAH may include ACTH stimula-

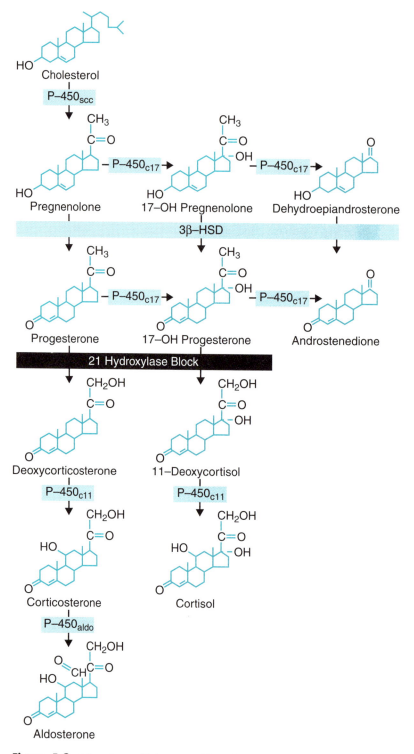

Figure 5-9. Adrenal steroid hormone biosynthesis—21-hydroxylase deficiency. A complete absence of 21-hydroxylase activity would result in failure of both glucocorticoid and mineralocorticoid production and is fatal unless detected and treated shortly after birth. Less severe forms of 21-hydroxylase deficiency may not present until later in childhood or in early adulthood and are associated with androgen excess. In an effort to produce normal amounts of cortisol and aldosterone, precursors above the enzyme block are synthesized in amounts much higher than normal.

TABLE 5-11. *SYNDROMES OF CONGENITAL ADRENAL HYPERPLASIA*	
DEFICIENT ENZYME	**CLINICAL FINDINGS**
Side chain cleavage (SCC)	Salt wasting, cortisol deficiency, sex steroid deficiency.
17-hydroxylase	Hypertension caused by increased mineralocorticoid production, decreased androgen production.
3-beta-ol-dehydrogenase	Increased androgen production, variable deficiency of aldosterone production.
21-hydroxylase	Most common. Androgen excess in the female results in hirsutism, amenorrhea, masculinization. Three different forms are described. Degree of salt wasting and age of onset vary.
11-hydroxylase	Hypertension and increased androgen production.

Shading indicates deficiency in both adrenal and gonadal tissue.

tion testing. ACTH administration magnifies the effects of the enzyme block and can, with measurement of the appropriate precursor molecules, pinpoint the deficiency.

Treatment usually consists of cortisol and, if necessary, mineralocorticoid replacement. Treatment must be tailored to the specific deficiency and the age and sex of the individual. Gonadal steroid production also may be involved. An exogenous glucocorticoid supply satisfies physiologic needs for cortisol and decreases ACTH secretion. The lowering of ACTH results in a decrease in the production of the steroid precursor molecules and thereby ameliorates the syndrome developed by the overproduction of the intermediary steroid compounds. When enzyme deficiencies block the production of aldosterone, mineralocorticoid replacement also is necessary.

Although she was not sure she understood the problem, Alison was relieved to hear that there might be something that will help her. She began dexamethasone, 0.5 mg each day. After about 2 months she noted a significant decrease in her hair growth, and she had two menstrual periods. The second menstrual period was very different from any she had had before. It was preceded by breast tenderness and was associated with heavier flow and cramps. She was not happy about the cramps, but it was reassuring for her to have a more normal menstrual cycle.

Alison still needs to use depilatories and has an occasional electrolysis treatment, but she is spending less time with better results then ever before. She wears an ID bracelet that lists her diagnosis and her medication. In addition, there is a toll-free number to call for more information about Alison and her treatment.

Alison has had the expected response to the glucocorticoid therapy. The development of an ovulatory menstrual cycle, as suggested by the breast tenderness and the cramps, and the improvement in her hirsutism indicate that her androgen production has decreased significantly. Unfortunately, once a hair follicle is established, it may continue to be active even if the hormonal stimulus to its initial development is removed. The rate of hair growth may decrease, however, and electrolysis can be used to destroy the follicle.

Treatment with glucocorticoids suppresses ACTH production. This is the goal of therapy in this case and in other cases of congenital adrenal hyperplasia. The condition itself and treatment with exogenous steroids are associated with decreased stress-responsive production of adrenocortical steroids. Alison will, at times of significant physical and, perhaps, emotional stress, need to increase her steroid dose; hence the need for a medical ID bracelet. In many ways the management is similar to the management of a patient with Addison's disease.

KEY POINTS AND CONCEPTS

- Three classes of steroid hormones are produced by the adrenal cortex:
  - Glucocorticoids (e.g., cortisol)
    - Function: helps maintain glucose levels during fasting and stress; required for normal vascular responsiveness; anti-inflammatory effects
    - Control: synthesis and secretion are stimulated by ACTH and regulated by the following factors:
      - Circadian rhythm
      - Stress
      - Feedback inhibition by cortisol
      - Stimulation by inflammatory cytokines
  - Mineralocorticoids (e.g., aldosterone)
    - Function: maintains blood volume by promoting sodium retention; promotes potassium excretion
    - Control:
      - Potassium (K^+) stimulates secretion
      - Renin-angiotensin system stimulates secretion; angiotensin II is a potent stimulator of aldosterone secretion
      - ACTH is a less important stimulator of aldosterone secretion
  - Androgens (e.g., DHEA, DHEA-sulfate, androstenedione)
    - Function: in females, provides a significant portion of total androgen; in males, the contribution to the androgen economy is very small
    - Control: poorly understood; stimulated by ACTH and possibly by other factors
- Elevated steroid hormone levels:
  - Cushing's syndrome (cortisol)
  - Hypertension, hypokalemia (aldosterone)
  - Hirsutism and masculinization (androgens)
  - Causes:
    - Exogenous steroids
    - Ectopic ACTH or CRH production

- Abnormal set-point of feedback control (Cushing's disease)
- Autonomous adrenal function (adenoma or, rarely, carcinoma)
- Congenital adrenal hyperplasia
- Treatment: focused on mechanism; may include surgery, radiation, and medication to block or replace steroid production
- Deficient steroid production:
  - Causes:
    - Adrenocortical failure—Addison's disease, usually autoimmune, but may be caused by other destructive processes
    - Secondary failure caused by lack of ACTH
      - Pituitary or hypothalamic failure
      - Suppression of the axis with exogenous steroids
  - Treatment:
    - Replacement steroids
      - Cortisol for both primary and secondary adrenal insufficiency
      - Aldosterone, usually required in addition for primary adrenal insufficiency

SUGGESTED READING

Chrousos GP. The hypothalamic-pituitary-adrenal axis and immune-mediated inflammation. N Engl J Med 332:1351–1362, 1995.

Orth DN. Cushing's syndrome. N Engl J Med 332:791–803, 1995.

White PC. Disorders of aldosterone biosynthesis and action. N Engl J Med 331:250–258, 1994.

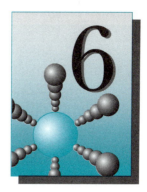

CHAPTER

6

Calcium Metabolism

The concentration of calcium in extracellular fluid is closely controlled within very narrow limits. Calcium is found principally in the extracellular space. The intracellular concentration of calcium is about 1/10,000 of the extracellular concentration. The proper concentration of calcium, both inside the cell and out, is vital for the normal function of a number of physiologic systems. Nerve conduction, muscle contraction, and blood clotting are critically dependent on normal levels of calcium. Calcium serves as a cofactor in many enzymatic reactions and as the coupling agent between muscle excitation and contraction. In addition, the strength and structure of the skeletal system depend on the presence of calcium salts deposited on the protein matrix of bone.

In the circulation, calcium is present in an ionized state (Ca^{2+}) and also is bound to proteins and chelated by various negatively charged compounds. About 50% of the total calcium concentration measured is made up of the free or ionized form. It is this ionized form that is the biologically active moiety, the form that plays a key role in normal neuromuscular and clotting function. The extracellular ionized calcium also is in equilibrium with the storage form of calcium—the bone. In the human adult, more than 1000 g of calcium are stored in bone, which serves both a structural and a storage function.

Normal bone is constantly undergoing remodeling with breakdown and rebuilding. The resulting demineralization and remineralization process places the calcium salts of bone in a dynamic equilibrium with calcium in the extracellular fluid space. Along with phosphate, the principal anion of the mineral portion of bone, calcium is constantly being liberated from and reprecipitated in bone. Although not a static, test-tube environment, there is an important relationship between the extracellular fluid concentrations of calcium and phosphate. The solubility product of these two ions is roughly maintained. As calcium rises, mineralization tends to increase, with a resultant decrease in phosphate concentration. When the extracellular fluid calcium falls, demineralization is favored and the phosphate rises.

The mechanisms involved in the maintenance of a normal extracellular ionized calcium concentration include control of gastrointestinal absorption, control

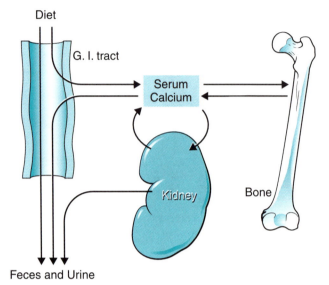

Diet

G. I. tract

Serum
Calcium

Kidney

Bone

Feces and Urine

Figure 6-1. Overview of calcium metabolism. In the presence of vitamin D, calcium is absorbed from the gastrointestinal tract. A significant amount of ingested calcium passes through unabsorbed, and a small amount is added to the GI tract in digestive fluids. Calcium in the extracellular fluid space is in equilibrium with calcium stored in bone. Some of the calcium filtered at the glomerulus is reabsorbed.

of renal excretion, and exchange with bone, the storage site for calcium (Fig. 6-1). The body defends itself against hypocalcemia by increased gastrointestinal absorption, decreased renal excretion, and increased bone breakdown with demineralization. High concentrations of calcium in the extracellular space result in decreased gastrointestinal abosrption, increased renal excretion, and increased bone mineralization.

PARATHYROID HORMONE

Parathyroid hormone (PTH) is a protein hormone secreted by the parathyroid glands in response to a low ionized calcium concentration in the extracellular fluid. When present in the circulation, PTH promotes entry of calcium into the extracellular fluid in three ways: increased gastrointestinal absorption, increased renal reabsorption, and increased bone resorption and demineralization.

Most humans have four separate parathyroid glands, each of which is less than 5 mm in diameter and weighs between 15 and 75 mg. The parathyroid glands are embryologically derived from the third and fourth branchial pouches and are made up of chief cells, the cells that produce parathyroid hormone, and oxyphil cells, the function of which is unknown. Located immediately behind the thyroid gland, the parathyroid glands derive their arterial supply from the posterior capsule of the thyroid. Venous drainage is into the cervical plexus of veins. There is significant functional reserve in the parathyroid system. Normal calcium balance can be maintained with only one-half of one of the four glands. Some decline in function appears to be a normal concomitant of aging but rarely becomes clinically important.

A calcium receptor on the surface of the parathyroid cell regulates the secretion of PTH. The receptor is a member of the G protein–coupled superfamily of receptors. The PTH molecule that is released in response to stimulation by low calcium levels is synthesized as part of a larger 115-amino-acid precursor molecule, pre-proparathyroid hormone. This precursor molecule is split into a smaller precursor molecule, proparathyroid hormone, containing 90 amino acids. Proparathyroid hormone is enzymatically cleaved yet again to yield the active, 84-amino-acid PTH molecule. Once in the circulation, PTH has a half-life of about 10 minutes and is cleaved in peripheral tissues into smaller forms. The only active forms are the intact PTH molecule and possibly some of the fragments with an amino terminal configuration.

PTH has multiple effects on calcium metabolism. In each case the effect of PTH is to increase the concentration of calcium in the extracellular fluid.

Effects of PTH
Renal tubular reabsorption of calcium is increased, lessening urinary excretion of calcium and increasing extracellular calcium.
Renal tubular reabsorption of phosphate is decreased, increasing urinary phosphate excretion and decreasing extracellular phosphate. This tends to increase extracellular calcium.
Vitamin D is activated by stimulation of the 1-hydroxylation of 25-hydroxyvitamin D (see Vitamin D, later in this chapter). Gastrointestinal calcium absorption is thereby increased.
Bone turnover is activated by stimulation of osteoblastic activity. The increase in osteoclastic activity that is paired with osteoblast function allows bone calcium to be available to the extracellular calcium pool.

PTH is quickly released by the parathyroid glands in response to a fall in extracellular calcium. Its effects on the renal handling of calcium and phosphate and on bone demineralization are almost immediate. The effects of PTH on vitamin D metabolism and the resultant vitamin D–mediated effects on calcium absorption occur over longer periods of time. The short half-life of PTH results in prompt reversal of the calcium-raising effects of the hormone when normocalcemia has been attained.

The mechanism of action of PTH is similar to that of many other peptide hormones. PTH action begins with binding to a membrane-bound adenylate cyclase system that results in the intracellular production of cyclic adenosine monophosphate (cAMP). This second messenger leads to the biologic effect at the cellular level in both the kidney and the bone.

VITAMIN D

Along with PTH, vitamin D is an important regulator of mineral metabolism. Vitamin D is a fat-soluble molecule similar to cholesterol (Fig. 6-2). It is available from dietary sources and also can be synthesized in the skin when it is exposed to ultraviolet radiation. Many foods, especially dairy products, are fortified with vitamin D. Intestinal absorption of vitamin D parallels fat absorption and is affected by the same factors that influence dietary fat absorption. The form of vitamin D (vitamin D_3, or cholecalciferol) that is available from most dietary sources and that is made by ultraviolet radiation of the skin is a relatively inactive precursor of the most active form of the vitamin (calcitriol—1,25-dihydroxyvitamin D_3). Activation of vitamin D occurs when the basic molecule (cholecalciferol, vitamin D_3) is hydroxylated at the 25 position by enzyme systems in the liver and also hydroxylated at the 1 position by enzyme systems in the kidney. The renal 1-hydroxylation of vitamin D is stimulated by the action of PTH and, in addition, is enhanced in the presence of hypophosphatemia.

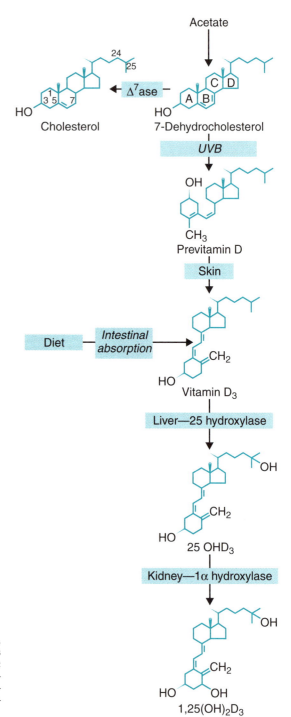

Figure 6-2. Synthesis of vitamin D. Starting with acetate, vitamin D can be synthesized through a synthetic process that requires ultraviolet radiation and several enzymatic steps that activate the molecule. Diet and supplements provide vitamin D_3, which, like endogenously produced vitamin D_3, requires 25-hydroxylation by the liver and 1-hydroxylation by the kidney to be fully active.

The mechanism of action of vitamin D at the cellular level is similar to the mechanism of action of thyroid hormone and steroid hormones. After traversing the cell membrane, vitamin D is bound to an intracellular receptor. The resulting complex binds to an intranuclear chromosomal site. Changes in protein production that lead to the biologic effects of vitamin D follow.

In the gastrointestinal tract, vitamin D stimulates the production of a calcium-binding molecule that mediates the absorption of calcium. Phosphate absorption also is enhanced in the presence of vitamin D. Bone resorption and the closely coupled formation of new bone also are stimulated by vitamin D. This increase in bone turnover provides increased opportunity for exchange of bone stores of calcium and phosphate with the extracellular pool of these ions. The fat solubility of vitamin D results in a storage system that means most individuals can tolerate wide variations in vitamin D intake and ultraviolet light exposure without developing vitamin D deficiency.

CALCITONIN

Calcitonin is a 32-amino-acid peptide secreted by the parafollicular or C-cells of the thyroid. Calcitonin is secreted in response to elevations in the ionized calcium concentration in the extracellular fluid. The principal effect of the hormone is to inhibit osteoclasts and thereby decrease osteoclastic bone resorption. This results in less demineralization and a decrease of calcium outflux from bone. As with other protein hormones, the half-life of calcitonin is short. The physiologic significance of calcitonin in calcium regulation is unclear because normal calcium balance is maintained in individuals who are unable to produce calcitonin. Similarly, high unregulated levels of calcitonin, such as are seen in medullary carcinoma of the thyroid, a C-cell tumor, usually do not result in significant changes in calcium metabolism.

Calcitonin used pharmacologically, however, does have important effects on calcium metabolism and bone turnover. In Paget's disease of bone, a condition in which there is a marked increase in osteoclastic activity, calcitonin can be used to decrease the rate of osteoclastic activity. Other uses include the treatment of hypercalcemia of malignancy and osteoporosis.

GASTROINTESTINAL CALCIUM ABSORPTION

A number of foods—dairy products, tofu, sardines, and dark green vegetables—contain significant amounts of calcium. The average dietary intake of calcium ranges from 0.6 to 1.5 g per day. Calcium absorption from the gastrointestinal (GI) tract occurs principally in the proximal small bowel, the jejunum, and is directly related to the activity of vitamin D. The absorption of calcium also is significantly influenced by the presence of dietary components that bind calcium and can thereby alter the availability of calcium for absorption. Only about 50% to 75% of ingested calcium is absorbed. Although some secretion of calcium into the GI tract in the form of hepatic and pancreatic secretions may occur, the GI tract is the site of calcium absorption, not an avenue for significant calcium excretion or reduction in total body calcium content.

RENAL EXCRETION OF CALCIUM

Renal excretion of calcium is controlled by changes in the amount of calcium that is reabsorbed from the glomerular filtrate. In the steady state, the amount of calcium excreted by the kidney—100 to 400 mg per day—is equal to the amount absorbed from the GI tract. The glomerular filtration of calcium is a function of the serum concentration of ionized calcium and the filtration rate. In the presence of PTH, tubular reabsorption of calcium is enhanced and less calcium is excreted in the final urine. At the same time, the action of PTH increases the renal excretion of phosphate, resulting in a decrease in the serum and extracellular phosphate levels. This tends to increase the serum calcium level (see the section on Phosphate Metabolism). Changes in the renal handling of calcium and phosphate can significantly affect the excretion of these minerals, but renal mechanisms cannot lead to any increase in the content of calcium or phosphate in the body.

BONE

Normal bone is constantly being remodeled. Specialized cells—osteoclasts and osteoblasts—that are present in bone mediate this remodeling process. Osteoclastic and osteoblastic activity are tightly coupled and extremely interdependent. When osteoclasts are active, bone is broken down. The resulting demineralization liberates calcium and phosphate into the extracellular fluid. Osteoblastic activity, on the other hand, results in formation of new bone. The mineralization that occurs with new bone formation leads to significant movement of calcium from the extracellular space into the newly formed bone. Osteoclasts do not have receptors for either PTH or vitamin D, but they do have receptors for calcitonin. Osteoblasts, however, have receptors for both PTH and vitamin D. The coupling of osteoclastic and osteoblastic activity is such that stimulation of osteoblastic activity by PTH results in increased osteoclastic activity. The mechanism of this coupling is unclear.

PHOSPHATE METABOLISM

The concentration of phosphate is less tightly controlled than that of calcium. About 600 g of phosphorus is present in the adult human, most of it in the form of inorganic phosphate and most of that in the skeleton. The intracellular concentration of phosphate is about half that found in the extracellular space. The transfer of phosphate across the cell membrane appears to be passive and to be largely determined by the flux of calcium. Phosphate molecules play a key role in energy transfer within the cell, serve as modifiers of enzymatic function, and are an important component of cell membranes.

In the serum, a small amount of phosphate is protein bound; the remainder is ultrafilterable and is either in an ionized form or complexed with calcium or another cation. At the normal pH of serum the majority of phosphate is present in the divalent form, HPO_4^{-2}.

The regulation of phosphate homeostasis is closely related to the factors that control calcium balance. Gastrointestinal absorption of phosphate is enhanced by vitamin D but is otherwise essentially unregulated. The average diet contains about 1500 mg of phosphorus, an element found in a wide variety of foods. Renal excretion of phosphate is the principal regulation point of phosphate metabolism. Low levels of phosphate result in enhanced bone demineralization, increased activation of vitamin D by the kidney, and increased tubular reabsorption of phosphate. These three processes result in an increase in the phosphate concentration. Hyperphosphatemia, on the other hand, leads to a decrease in calcium concentration. The resultant stimulation of PTH causes a decrease in the tubular reabsorption of phosphate and increased renal excretion of phosphate.

Disorders of phosphate metabolism usually are directly related to the renal handling of phosphate. Phosphate depletion can occur in states of extreme diuresis, as in the patient with diabetic ketoacidosis, and in various forms of malnutrition.

DISORDERS OF CALCIUM AND PHOSPHATE METABOLISM

Hypercalcemia is a life-threatening problem that requires prompt treatment and careful diagnostic study. Bone destruction resulting from metastatic disease, parathyroid gland overactivity, or the secretion of a PTH-like protein by a tumor accounts for many cases. The initial treatment of hypercalcemia—hydration and pharmacologic intervention to decrease bone demineralization—is the same for all causes of hypercalcemia. In most cases the clinical setting and the associated phosphate level give a clue to the cause of the hypercalcemia, but further studies usually are warranted and are helpful in clinical management.

Hypocalcemia also is an important clinical problem. It is seen in the face of renal failure, inadequate PTH secretion (hypoparathyroidism), insensitivity to PTH (pseudo-hypoparathyroidism), magnesium depletion, and vitamin D deficiency. Although calcium infusion may be needed acutely, definitive therapy for hypocalcemia is tailored to the specific cause.

Abnormalities of calcium concentration often can be initially assessed by considering the concomitant phosphate and alkaline phosphatase levels (Table 6-1). Additional studies to confirm the diagnosis and to direct further management usually are appropriate.

CLINICALLY USEFUL TESTS OF CALCIUM METABOLISM

Serum Calcium Concentration. Most serum calcium measurements determine the concentration of all forms of calcium in the serum. In usual circumstances, about half of the total calcium concentration is accounted for by the active moiety, ionized calcium. The rest of the calcium is either protein bound or chelated to various ligands. Alterations in the concentration of calcium, therefore, must be carefully

TABLE 6-1. *ABNORMAL CALCIUM CONCENTRATION: DIAGNOSTIC POSSIBILITIES*

SERUM CALCIUM	SERUM PHOSPHATE	SERUM ALKALINE PHOSPHATASE	DIAGNOSIS
Elevated	Elevated	Normal	Vitamin D intoxication
Elevated	Decreased	Normal or slightly elevated	Hyperparathyroidism
Elevated	Normal or elevated	Elevated	Metastatic bone disease
Decreased	Elevated	Normal or elevated	Renal failure (elevated BUN and creatinine)
Decreased	Elevated	Normal	Hypoparathyroidism
Decreased	Decreased	Elevated	Vitamin D deficiency

interpreted in light of the concentration of the principal protein binding calcium, albumin. Each gram of albumin binds about 88 mg of calcium. Other factors (e.g., pH) may change the binding affinity of protein for calcium and result in shifts in the concentration of the biologically active ionized form without any change in the measured total calcium concentration. In the setting of the alkalosis that might result from hyperventilation, for example, more calcium is protein bound and less is in the ionized form, but the total concentration of calcium is normal and unchanged. The lowered concentration of the ionized calcium results in the symptoms of tingling and muscular irritability that are seen in hyperventilation.

The range of normal in most laboratories is 8.5 to 10.5 mg/dL. Elevated values suggest excess PTH, excess vitamin D, or increased bone breakdown. Lower than normal levels are seen in PTH deficiency, renal failure, and vitamin D deficiency.

Ionized Calcium. Although it is a more expensive and less readily available test, the ionized calcium concentration can be useful in assessing some problems of calcium metabolism. Abnormalities of protein concentration and pH are factored out, and a direct measurement of the active moiety can, in certain situations, be helpful in assessing a clinical problem.

Phosphate Concentration. Serum phosphate levels are readily available and may be useful in assessing calcium metabolism. The normal range is 3 to 4.5 mg/dL. PTH, vitamin D, and the serum calcium level itself have important effects on the phosphate concentration. In addition to states of phosphate depletion, low levels of phosphate are usually seen when PTH levels are elevated. High phosphate levels and low calcium levels are present in renal failure and in hypoparathyroidism. Vitamin D deficiency results in low phosphate levels, whereas higher phosphate levels are seen in vitamin D intoxication.

Magnesium Concentration. Because deficiency of magnesium can result in significant parathyroid dysfunction and in decreased effectiveness of PTH, a serum magnesium level may be helpful in assessing a problem of calcium metabolism. Some clinical problems that appear to be caused by PTH deficiency are, in fact, primarily the result of magnesium deficiency.

Parathyroid Hormone Concentration. Radioimmunoassay techniques are available to measure the intact PTH molecule. Assays that detect various fragments of PTH with different metabolic effects and different half-lives are available and may be useful in unusual circumstances. The intact molecule, double-antibody, immunoradiometric assay is both specific and sensitive enough for clinical use. Interpretation of the results of PTH testing can be done only with accurate information about the concomitant serum calcium level. The results often are provided in a nomogram or chart, similar to the one presented in Figure 6-3, that correlates PTH levels with various calcium concentrations.

If the serum calcium is low, the PTH levels should be elevated. Conversely, if the serum calcium is elevated from a non–PTH-mediated condition, the PTH level should be very low. A "normal" PTH level may, in fact, be high or low, depending on the serum calcium level.

Vitamin D Concentration. Although expensive and slow to be reported, vitamin D levels can be measured. The level of calcitriol (1,25-dihydroxyvitamin D_3), the most active form of the hormone, fluctuates and may not give a good approximation of body stores of vitamin D. A more helpful measure of body stores can be made by determining the concentration of calcifediol (25-hydroxyvitamin

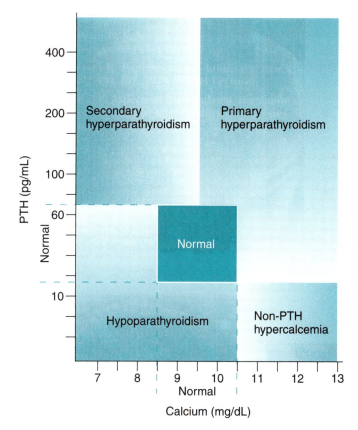

Figure 6-3. Nomogram for PTH versus calcium. Simultaneous measurement of the serum PTH and calcium levels can be a first step toward understanding the pathophysiology of calcium disorders. When both PTH and calcium are elevated or when both are low, a disorder of parathyroid function is present. When one is elevated and the other low, a non–PTH-mediated disorder is present. A high PTH in the presence of a low calcium level (secondary hyperparathyroidism) is the expected response of the parathyroid glands. A low PTH would be expected in the face of a non–PTH-mediated cause of hypercalcemia.

D₃). Low values are seen in dietary deficiency, malabsorption, and liver disease, whereas elevated values are seen in states of vitamin D intoxication.

Alkaline Phosphatase Concentration. Bone and liver are the primary sources of alkaline phosphatase in the serum. When liver function tests are normal, the source of an elevated serum level of this enzyme probably is the bone. Alkaline phosphatase is produced in bone by osteoblasts and is elevated during periods of increased osteoblastic activity—normal growing, a healing fracture, and other states of increased bone turnover. Because osteoclastic and osteoblastic activity are tightly coupled, any increase in bone turnover usually results in an increase in the level of alkaline phosphatase.

Bone Density Studies. Conventional X-rays of bones may show fractures or, occasionally, other abnormalities that are helpful in assessing calcium metabolism, but X-rays rarely are helpful in providing the definitive diagnosis of a metabolic bone problem. Bone density may be subjectively assessed on plain X-rays, but more information can be obtained by bone densitometry. Although various techniques are available (e.g., computed tomographic [CT] scan, single photon absorptiometry), dual X-ray absorptiometry (DXA) provides reproducible measurements of bone density with little radiation exposure and relatively low cost (shown later in Fig. 6-11). Bone density usually is measured in the lumbar spine or femur and can be followed over time to assess bone status. Lower values of bone density are associated clinically with a higher risk of fracture.

Bone Scan. A modified phosphate molecule, labeled with a gamma ray–emitting isotope, technetium 99m, can be used as a bone scanning agent. The radiolabeled molecule is deposited in bone in proportion to the rate of mineralization or new bone formation. Blood flow and mineral turnover are important determinants of isotope distribution. Focal increases in uptake are seen in areas of fracture and metastatic disease. A generalized increased uptake is seen in metabolic bone diseases such as hyperparathyroidism.

Parathyroid Imaging or Localizing Studies. When hyperparathyroidism is suspected, imaging studies may be used to locate the abnormal gland or glands. Various techniques are available, including magnetic resonance imaging (MRI), ultrasound, venous catheterization with PTH sampling, and several nuclear medicine procedures that can be helpful in visualizing or localizing PTH-secreting tissue.

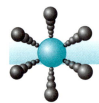

CASE PRESENTATION: CASE 1

Urolithiasis and hypercalcemia in a 54-year-old woman

Agnes Allen had never had pain this intense before. It started suddenly, just after playing three sets of tennis in the hot sun. The pain came in waves, and although she had trouble localizing it at first, it was clearly now in her right flank and radiating into her groin. Matters were made even worse when she passed very red urine. Now she was really worried.

Agnes Allen is 54 years old and has been in excellent health. She works as an administrative assistant for a startup biotech company and lives with her husband, who manages a local supermarket. Their two children are married and live nearby.

When her menstrual periods stopped about 4 years ago, she discussed menopausal hormonal replacement with her doctor and decided not to take estrogen. She would take some calcium supplementation and maintain her active life as a way to decrease her risk of osteoporosis. Other than an uncomplicated urinary tract infection several years ago, she has no history of kidney or bladder problems.

Past Medical History
Illnesses:	No diabetes, tuberculosis, hepatitis, or hypertension
Surgery:	Appendectomy at age 30
	Tonsillectomy and adenoidectomy at age 7
Allergies:	None known
Habits:	Nonsmoker
	Small amounts of alcohol
	Moderate amounts of coffee
	No recreational drugs
Medications:	None
Prescription:	OTC: Calcium supplement 600 mg with vitamin D, 100 units three times a day; TUMS and Maalox for occasional heartburn

Family history:	Father, 84, healthy
	Mother, 82, osteoporosis
	3 siblings, healthy
	2 children, healthy

Review of Systems

General:	Feels well
Skin:	Negative
HEENT:	Negative
CR:	Negative
Gastrointestinal:	Heartburn, occasional constipation, increasing recently
Genitourinary:	See HPI
Musculoskeletal:	Occasional knee pain and swelling
Neuro:	Negative
Psychiatric:	Stressed at work, slightly depressed

Physical Examination

Healthy-appearing woman

Vital signs:	Blood pressure 150/90; pulse 88
Skin:	Normal
HEENT:	Normal
Neck:	Normal
Chest:	Clear
Heart:	Normal
Abdomen:	Normal
GYN:	Normal
Extremities:	Normal
Neuro:	Normal

Laboratory Studies

Test	Agnes Allen	Normal
WBC	5600/mm^3	4300–10,800/mm^3
HCT	39%	37%–48% (female)
Calcium	11.3 mg/dL	8.5–10.5 mg/dL
Phosphate	1.8 mg/dL	3–4.5 mg/dL
Alkaline phosphatase	199 U/L	30–120 U/L
Albumin	4.1 g/dL	3.5–5.5 g/dL
Urinalysis:		
Color	Amber, cloudy	Yellow, clear
Specific gravity	1.012	1.001–1.020
Blood	+ 4	Negative
Glucose	Negative	Negative
Ketones	Negative	Negative
Nitrite	Negative	Negative
Microscopic	TNTC (too numerous to count) red cells	<4/high-power field

Colicky flank pain radiating into the groin strongly suggests a kidney stone. The hematuria further supports and really clinches the clinical diagnosis. An imaging study of the urinary tract—either an IVP, an ultrasound, or a CT scan—should be done, looking for evidence of ureteral obstruction.

The mild dehydration that developed while Mrs. Allen was playing tennis increased urinary solute concentration. The resultant rise in the ion solubility product in the urine allowed crystals to precipitate and a stone to form. The pain and hematuria result from stretching and damage to the collecting system.

Hypercalcemia also played a significant role in the formation of Mrs. Allen's stone. Her total serum calcium concentration is elevated, and, because her albumin is normal, her ionized calcium level is high. This results in an increased amount of calcium filtered at the glomerulus. The increased filtered load of calcium increases renal tubular fluid calcium content and concentration—a situation that favors the precipitation of calcium-containing stones.

Hypercalcemia is an important clinical problem that can, at high levels, be life-threatening. In Mrs. Allen's case, the elevated calcium is seen in the face of a low phosphate. This combination of findings strongly points to an unregulated excess of PTH as the mechanism of her hypercalcemia. Ordinarily, a high calcium level would result in suppression of PTH with a resultant decrease in calcium absorption from the GI tract, increased renal excretion of calcium, decreased renal excretion of phosphate, and increased bone mineralization. Autonomous overproduction of PTH (i.e., production that is not inhibited by high levels of calcium) results in elevation of serum calcium.

One of the renal effects of PTH is to decrease the tubular reabsorption of phosphate. The increase in urinary phosphate excretion that follows lowers the serum phosphate concentration. The elevated alkaline phosphatase level is also consistent with hyperparathyroidism. When an elevated alkaline phosphatase is of bony origin, it indicates increased osteoblastic activity, a phenomenon that is seen when bone turnover is stimulated by PTH or other factors. Normally, a high serum calcium concentration would result in suppression of PTH secretion, but in Mrs. Allen's case there is evidence of PTH activity (low phosphate, increased phosphatase) in spite of an elevated calcium concentration.

With narcotics, the pain came under control, and Mrs. Allen was able to increase her fluid intake. She also began to strain all her urine through a filter she got from the emergency room. An intravenous pyelogram (IVP) X-ray confirmed the presence of a kidney stone on the right. The calcified stone was 5 mm in diameter, "hung up" at the right ureterovesicular junction, and associated with a moderate degree of hydronephrosis on the right side. Other than a 3-mm calcified stone in the left renal pelvis, the IVP was normal.

Two hours after the IVP Mrs. Allen had another brief episode of more pain and more hematuria. On her next voiding she found 2 pieces of brown, irregular hard material that were each about 2 to 3 mm in size.

Stone analysis: Calcium oxalate = 100%

Laboratory Studies

Test	Agnes Allen	Normal
Calcium	11.0 mg/dL	8.5–10.5 mg/dL
PTH	110 pg/mL	10–65 pg/mL

Nomogram: See Figure 6-4

The IVP and stone analysis confirm the original clinical evaluation of Mrs. Allen's problem. The PTH level is elevated and clearly inappropriate for the serum calcium level. The excess PTH has resulted in increased vitamin D activation with increased intestinal absorption of calcium. In addition, the calcium and vitamin D supplementation, although intended to prevent osteoporosis, provided even more resources for increased GI calcium absorption. Increased bone turnover stimulated by PTH resulted in increased bone demineralization and increased flux of calcium into the extracellular space. The rise in ultrafiltrable calcium markedly increased the filtered load of calcium entering the proximal renal tubule. Even though the tubular reabsorption of calcium is elevated by PTH, the huge filtered load of calcium

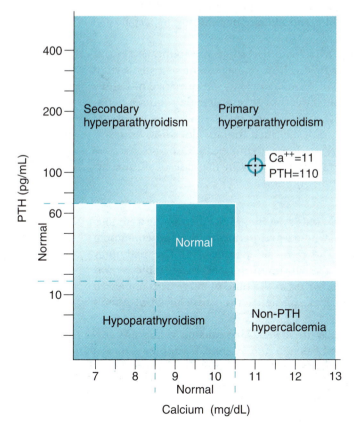

Figure 6-4. Nomogram of PTH versus calcium: Agnes Allen. The elevated serum calcium level has not suppressed the PTH level, a finding that points to primary hyperparathyroidism.

results in the excretion of large amounts of calcium in the final urine. This increase in renal calcium excretion magnifies the risk of stone formation.

It is likely that Mrs. Allen has had mild hyperparathyroidism for a few years. The calcium and vitamin D supplementation and the dehydration precipitated both a stone and an evaluation that led to the diagnosis. In addition to kidney stones, hyperparathyroidism can cause a number of other problems. Calcium stimulates gastric acid secretion, and elevated concentrations may result in acid-peptic symptoms. Some of Agnes Allen's heartburn may be caused by the hypercalcemia. Over time, the increased bone turnover can result in a significant decline in bone mass and an increased risk of fractures.

Mrs. Allen is now free of pain, and her urine is free of blood. She has stopped all calcium and vitamin supplementation. In addition, she has been drinking at least 2 or 3 quarts of fluid a day, more when she is active and in hot weather. She is, however, concerned about her bones, especially in view of her mother's osteoporosis. The possibility of another episode of renal colic—after all, there is a remaining stone on the left—also is very troubling.

Although she may have had mild, relatively asymptomatic hyperparathyroidism for a few years, Mrs. Allen clearly is no longer asymptomatic. Primary hyperparathyroidism almost always is a benign condition of parathyroid overactivity. An adenoma of a single gland accounts for about 90% of cases; diffuse hyperplasia and hyperfunction of all four glands account for the remainder of cases. Parathyroid gland malignancy causing hyperparathyroidism is very rare.

Many cases of asymptomatic hyperparathyroidism are found as a result of routine screening tests. Although the best management of truly asymptomatic patients with hyperparathyroidism is unclear, the presence of kidney stones, bone disease, or the systemic effects of hypercalcemia requires definitive therapy. Increased phosphate intake can, by affecting the solubility product, decrease the serum calcium level. Such therapy does not, however, decrease the risk of kidney stones or bone demineralization. Surgical removal of the adenoma or a ⅞ parathyroidectomy in the case of diffuse hyperplasia is required to manage the condition.

Four months after passing the kidney stone, Mrs. Allen underwent successful surgical neck exploration. An enlarged parathyroid gland containing an adenoma was removed from the right side, inferiorly. The pathology showed a chief cell adenoma with a small rim of normal tissue. A biopsy was performed on the right upper parathyroid at the time of surgery. It appeared normal, which ruled out diffuse hyperplasia as the cause of Mrs. Allen's hyperparathyroidism.

Postoperatively, Mrs. Allen has done well. Her calcium values are normal, and she has carefully restarted calcium and vitamin D supplementation in hopes of rebuilding the bone she probably lost during her hyperparathyroidism. Although one stone remains on the left side, she hopes she'll never experience that pain and worry again.

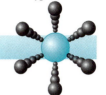

CASE PRESENTATION: CASE 2

Coma and hypercalcemia in an older man

Although he usually loved to walk on the beach in the sun, this summer Clarence Hamilton found himself with less and less energy. On a hot August afternoon he was found by his grandson in a comatose state in his urine-soaked bed.

In the emergency room, he was barely responsive and clearly volume depleted. Physical examination revealed a supine blood pressure of 110/70 that fell to 90/60 when he was propped up. His pulse went from 90 to 120 with that maneuver. His mucous membranes were dry. His general physical examination was otherwise unremarkable, except for the neurologic exam, which revealed an obtunded man who could barely respond to simple questions. He was able to move all extremities on command.

Laboratory Studies

Test	Clarence Hamilton	Normal
Glucose	88 mg/dL	70–110 mg/dL
Toxic screen	Negative	Negative
Calcium	13.6 mg/dL	8.5–10.5 mg/dL
Phosphate	5.9 mg/dL	3–4.5 mg/dL
Albumin	5.0 g/dL	3.5–5.5 g/dL
BUN	55 mg/dL	8–22 mg/dL
Creatinine	2.0 mg/dL	0.3–1.5 mg/dL
Alkaline phosphatase	65 U/L	30–120 U/L

Mr. Hamilton has life-threatening hypercalcemia. If measured, an ionized calcium would be significantly elevated. Even though the cause of the hypercalcemia is not clear, the magnitude is significant. The immediate treatment, no matter what the cause, is vigorous hydration. Hypercalcemia and dehydration often coexist. Because renal excretion of calcium is an important mechanism for lowering elevated calcium values, any decline in renal function, such as might be seen with volume depletion and the resultant decline in the glomerular filtration rate, tends to impede the excretion of calcium. In addition, hypercalcemia of any cause decreases the concentrating ability of the kidney, often making matters even worse. The nephrogenic diabetes insipidus induced by hypercalcemia results in further volume depletion and further decline in renal function and in the ability to excrete calcium.

Although a malignancy making a PTH-like substance (PTH-related protein [PTHrP]) or leading to the destruction of bone with the release of large amounts of calcium and phosphate into the circulation is a possible cause of Mr. Hamilton's hypercalcemia. Hypercalcemia usually is not the initial manifestation of those malignant processes.

After 6 hours and 3.5 liters of intravenous saline, Mr. Hamilton's blood pressure and his mental status dramatically improved. He was able to relate his past medical history, which was remarkable for significant osteoarthritis, principally involving his knees. Mr. Hamilton was somewhat vague about what medications, if any, he was taking.

Later in the day his grandson came to visit and brought with him a bag full of medications that he had found in his grandfather's bathroom. In addition to aspirin, acetaminophen, and ibuprofen, a number of vitamin supplements were found. When the contents of the bag were reviewed with Mr. Hamilton, he indicated, rather sheepishly, that he had, in fact, been taking a large number of the items in the bag. The salesman at the health food store had been quite convincing. "BONEALL" contained everything that would be needed for strengthening bones and might help with the osteoarthritis that had plagued him for years. Although the directions clearly stated that only one should be taken daily, Clarence Hamilton did as he often did with medications. He took them when and as often as he wanted to. He thought that the BONEALL was really helping and ended up taking 16 to 20 of the large tablets each day. Both BONEALL and several of the other vitamin preparations contained vitamin D.

Further laboratory values revealed the following:

Test	Clarence Hamilton	Normal
Calcium	11.6 mg/dL	8.5–10.5 mg/dL
Phosphate	5.2 mg/dL	3–4.5 mg/dL
BUN	21 mg/dL	8–22 mg/dL
Creatinine	1.7 mg/dL	0.3–1.5 mg/dL
PTH	< 10 pg/mL	10–65 pg/mL
25-OH-vitamin D_3	352 mg/mL	Summer: 15–80 ng/mL Winter: 14–42 ng/mL

Nomogram: See Figure 6-5

The low PTH in the face of an elevated calcium is a normal finding. PTH synthesis and secretion should be intensely inhibited by the elevated calcium level. The elevation of both the calcium and the phosphate levels also suggests a non-PTH mechanism for the hypercalcemia because elevated PTH levels decrease tubular reabsorption of phosphate, which usually results in a decrease in serum phosphate levels. The lack of bone pain and the normal alkaline phosphatase level make a malignant process very unlikely. The history of vitamin ingestion, with the possibility of some further vitamin

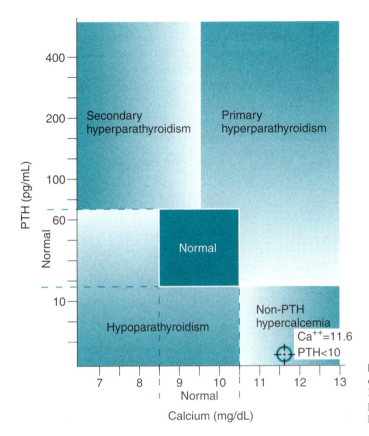

Figure 6-5. Nomogram of PTH versus calcium: Clarence Hamilton. Because Mr. Hamilton's PTH level is appropriately suppressed, a non-PTH mechanism for his hypercalcemia is present.

D production by beachside ultraviolet irradiation, all point to vitamin D intoxication. The diagnosis is confirmed by the elevated levels of the long–half-life form of vitamin D: 25-hydroxyvitamin D_3.

Vitamin D stimulates the gastrointestinal absorption of both calcium and phosphate. The resultant increase in calcium influx decreases PTH levels, which tends to further increase phosphate levels. Increased renal excretion of calcium occurs because of the reduced tubular reabsorption of calcium that is seen in the face of low PTH levels. Although increased renal excretion of calcium can compensate to a limited extent, when calcium influx significantly exceeds outflux, hypercalcemia results. If volume depletion develops, renal excretion of calcium—the only significant mechanism available to decrease total body calcium—declines and the level of calcium in the extracellular space rises, often to a critical level.

Although hydration should improve Mr. Hamilton's situation acutely, the potential for further problems with hypercalcemia may continue for months—even after stopping the vitamin D supplements. Vitamin D is fat soluble, and large amounts are stored in body fat. Glucocorticoids antagonize the effect of vitamin D and can be used in severe cases. Less severe cases can be managed by increased intake of fluids and sodium. Increased salt intake results in increased urinary sodium excretion and increased calcium excretion.

Clarence Hamilton is no longer taking any of the pills in the bag or anything from the health food store. His calcium level is slightly elevated, but controlled by the three or four quarts of fluid he drinks each day and the extra salt he adds to his food. After several months the vitamin D level is still elevated, but closer to normal, and his serum calcium usually is at the upper end of the normal range.

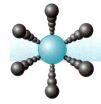

CASE PRESENTATION: CASE 3

Lethargy and hypercalcemia in a 68-year-old woman with metastatic breast cancer

Emma Watson has been dealing with breast cancer for the past 6 years. She has had surgery, radiation, and chemotherapy. Her most recent bone scan showed significant uptake in her spine, in her ribs, and in both femurs. She is in significant pain and just cannot get comfortable. In addition, she has developed polyuria and polydipsia and has difficulty keeping up with her thirst. Although her family knows that she hates to go to the hospital, she is now too lethargic to object and they bring her to the emergency room.

On physical examination she is cachectic and volume depleted. Her mouth is dry. Her blood pressure is 90/50, and her pulse is 120.

Laboratory Studies

Test	Emma Watson	Normal
Calcium	13.9 mg/dL	8.5–10.5 mg/dL
Phosphate	5.0 mg/dL	3–4.5 mg/dL
Albumin	4.2 g/dL	3.5–5.5 g/dL
BUN	28 mg/dL	8–22 mg/dL
Creatinine	1.3 mg/dL	0.3–1.5 mg/dL
Alkaline phosphatase	560 U/L	30–120 U/L
PTH	<10 pg/mL	10–65 pg/mL

Nomogram: See Figure 6-6

Hypercalcemia in the face of hyperphosphatemia points to a non–PTH-mediated abnormality in calcium metabolism. When renal function is normal, an elevated PTH level usually is associated with a lower than normal phosphate level. The elevated alkaline phosphatase indicates increased bone turnover. The history and laboratory findings are consistent with metastatic disease involving and breaking down bone. The ability of the kidney to excrete the increased load of calcium entering the extracellular space is rate limiting. The impairment of renal concentrating ability that occurs with hypercalcemia further decreases renal calcium excretion. A vicious cycle of hypercalcemia leading to further hypercalcemia develops.

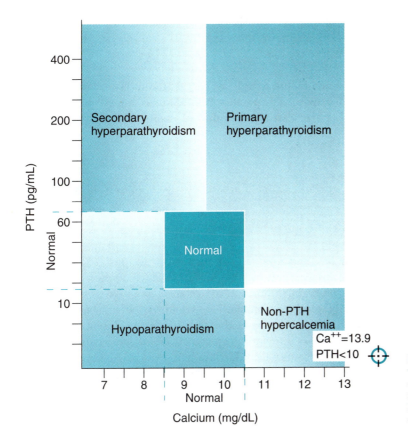

Figure 6-6. Nomogram for PTH versus calcium: Emma Watson. Because Ms. Watson's PTH level is appropriately suppressed, a non-PTH mechanism for her hypercalcemia is present.

The hypercalcemia of metastatic bone disease, like hypercalcemia of other causes, initially is treated with hydration. Improving renal calcium excretion with hydration often can result in marked improvement in the calcium level and decrease in calcium-related symptoms.

After 5 L of intravenous saline Ms. Watson is much improved. The thirst is finally under control, and she is much less lethargic. A new pain medication regimen is underway and she is much more comfortable.

Follow-up Laboratory Studies

Test	Emma Watson	Normal
Calcium	11.2 mg/dL	8.5–10.5 mg/dL
BUN	20 mg/dL	8–22 mg/dL
Creatinine	0.6 mg/dL	0.3–1.5 mg/dL

Calcitonin also can be used to decrease osteoclastic activity and to decrease calcium liberation from the bone. As an added benefit, calcitonin also can decrease bone pain. In addition, drugs from the bisphosphonate group (e.g., etidronate, alendronate, pamidronate) can be used to decrease the ability of osteoclasts to demineralize bone. The presence of these pyrophosphate-like molecules in the bone matrix inhibits osteoclastic function and decreases bone demineralization.

Increased fluid intake and two doses of calcitonin have made Ms. Watson much more comfortable. The pain is under control, her calcium is nearly normal, and she is hopeful that a new round of chemotherapy will stem the course of her breast cancer.

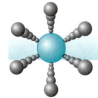

CASE PRESENTATION: CASE 4

Hypocalcemia and bone pain in a 50-year-old woman

Maria Renaldi has had nontropical sprue for the past 15 years. The diarrhea and weight loss caused by this condition started when she was 35 years old. Although she had a number of office visits and tests, it took several months before the diagnosis was made. The treatment wasn't easy: she had to avoid all wheat products. She was unable to tolerate any gluten, the protein of wheat. When she followed her diet rigorously, her diarrhea stopped, and she gained weight and felt quite well. Her Italian heritage, however, was part of the problem. Pasta and bread in any form were forbidden. Even some tomato sauces might have a little flour in them.

After a few years, Maria Renaldi struck a balance with her disease and her heritage. On Sunday she would have a little pasta and sauce; the rest of the week she would follow the diet carefully. She was able to maintain her weight and tolerated the three or four bowel movements per day that resulted.

One year ago, Mrs. Renaldi began to have significant pain in her legs, especially with walking, but even when she was just standing. The pain was not in her joints, but in her thigh and leg bones. Lying down provided prompt and almost complete relief. The pain was progressing so that she was unable to do much more than get to work and get home. She was unable to do housework or work in her garden.

She takes no medications and the remainder of her past history is unremarkable.

On physical examination she appeared tired and thin. Her blood pressure was 110/70, and her pulse was 80. Her general physical examination was unremarkable except for tenderness on the surface of both shins.

Laboratory Studies

Test	Maria Renaldi	Normal
Calcium	7.2 mg/dL	8.5–10.5 mg/dL
Phosphate	1.8 mg/dL	3–4.5 mg/dL
Albumin	4.3 g/dL	3.5–5.5 g/dL
BUN	7 mg/dL	8–22 mg/dL
Creatinine	0.7 mg/dL	0.3–1.5 mg/dL
Alkaline phosphatase	306 U/L	30–120 U/L
Liver function tests	Normal	Normal

Maria Renaldi's hypocalcemia is not explained by hypoalbuminemia. Her ionized calcium is almost certainly low. Although not yet measured, the PTH level should be elevated in response to the hypocalcemia, and the possible effects of an elevated PTH level are seen in the chemistry values presented. The increased bone turnover stimulated by the PTH results in elevation of the alkaline phosphatase. The low phosphate concentration probably is the result of PTH-mediated decrease in urinary phosphate reabsorption and the resultant increase in urinary phosphate excretion.

After reviewing these results, further studies were ordered:

Test	Maria Renaldi	Normal
Calcium	7.4 mg/dL	8.5–10.5 mg/dL
PTH	500 pg/mL	10–65 pg/mL
25-OH-vitamin D_3	6 ng/mL	Summer: 15–80 ng/mL Winter: 14–42 ng/mL

Nomogram: See Figure 6-7

Vitamin D deficiency occurs in many parts of the world. Even in areas where nutrition is generally adequate, some people, especially the elderly, may have mild vitamin D deficiency. Severe vitamin D deficiency, however, is relatively rare because many foods, especially dairy products, are supplemented with vitamin D. Intestinal malabsorption of fat can result in deficiencies of the fat-soluble vitamins A, D, E, and K. Ms Renaldi's weekend ''cheating'' led to some decrease in small bowel absorptive function, enough to interfere with vitamin D absorption. For patients with nontropical sprue, also known as gluten enteropathy, even small amounts of gluten result in small bowel mucosal damage that interferes with the absorption of many nutrients. Although she tolerated the malabsorption relatively well for a number of years, she did so at the expense of the calcium stored in her bones.

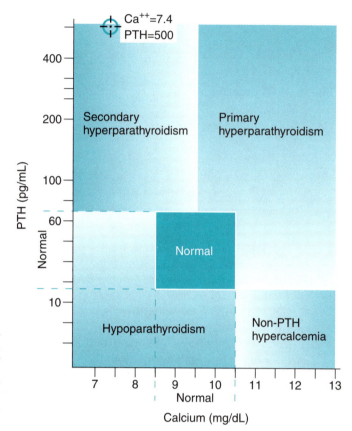

Figure 6-7. Nomogram for PTH versus calcium: Maria Renaldi. The elevated PTH level (secondary hyperparathyroidism) is appropriate for the low level of the serum calcium. A non-PTH mechanism is most likely responsible for her hypocalcemia, but inability to respond to parathyroid hormone also could be the explanation.

The secondary hyperparathyroidism that resulted from her inability to absorb vitamin D and calcium adequately has caused a significant increase in bone turnover. Over time, this has significantly decreased her skeletal calcium content. The PTH-stimulated bone turnover led to subperiosteal bone resorption. The resulting stretching of the periosteal membrane causes the intense, mechanically dependent bone pain.

Based on the evidence of vitamin D deficiency, Mrs. Renaldi was given a prescription for calcitriol—1,25-dihydroxyvitamin D$_3$. After 6 weeks of therapy with this potent form of vitamin D, Maria Renaldi was back working in her garden, and her leg pain was markedly improved. She had also given up her Sunday treats of pasta and sauce.

Her laboratory studies also improved:

Test	Maria Renaldi	Normal
Calcium	8.4 mg/dL	8.5–10.5 mg/dL
Phosphate	3.3 mg/dL	3–4.5 mg/dL
Alkaline phosphatase	188 U/L	30–120 U/L

Although not measured, her PTH level is probably much closer to normal, as indicated by the improvement in her pain, her alkaline phosphatase, and her serum calcium. Calcitriol is an extremely potent form of vitamin D. Because the molecule already has hydroxyl groups at the 1 and 25 positions, it does not require activation by hepatic or renal enzyme systems. The dose of this medication must be monitored carefully, because vitamin D intoxication can develop easily in patients treated with this unregulated form of vitamin D.

CASE PRESENTATION: CASE 5

Loss of height and back pain in a 70-year-old woman

Jane Johnson is 17, and although she had hoped to be 5′7″ tall, it was clear, because she hadn't grown in the past 2 years, that 5′6″ was as tall as she would get. It was curious, however, that she did indeed seem to be growing taller when she stood next to her grandmother, Wilma Larson.

Mrs. Larson has just turned 70 years old. Her general health has been excellent, but she does have occasional episodes of thoracic back pain. The pain radiates around to the front and usually gets gradually better over a period of 4 to 6 weeks. She has had 3 episodes of this pain. Although she hates to admit it, and would rather attribute the apparent increasing tallness of her granddaughter to normal adolescent growth, Mrs Larson is indeed getting shorter. She was 5′4″ when she got married at age 26 but is now barely 5′1″.

Mrs. Larson has been very careful not to gain weight and has only gained about 5 pounds over the past 20 years, but her clothes no longer fit. Her waist has increased by about 2 inches. She became more concerned when she was looking at recent pictures of herself. Why was she so stooped over? It was time for her checkup, and she put her shrinking height and expanding waist on the list of items to discuss with her doctor.

Mrs. Larson's past medical history was remarkable for an uncomplicated menopause at age 52. She had a few hot flashes but otherwise had very few symptoms and decided not to take any estrogen. Her diet has always been relatively healthy, although she avoids dairy products, since she thinks she gets some diarrhea and gas from them.

She is a nonsmoker and is on no medications.

Her mother died at age 76 of complications following a hip fracture.

Physical examination reveals a fair-skinned, small woman with a significant thoracic kyphosis—a dowager's hump. Her general physical examination was entirely unremarkable.

Laboratory Studies

Test	Wilma Larson	Normal
WBC	5900/mm^3	4300–10,800/mm^3
HCT	39%	37%–48% (female)
Calcium	9.8 mg/dL	8.5–10.5 mg/dL
Phosphate	3.4 mg/dL	3–4.5 mg/dL
Alkaline phosphatase	85 U/L	30–120 U/L
Albumin	4.1 g/dL	3.5–5.5 g/dL
Creatinine	1.1 mg/dL	0.3–1.5 mg/dL

X-rays of the thoracic and lumbar spine reveal marked kyphosis with multiple compression fractures (Figs. 6-8A and 6-9A).

Figures 6-8B and 6-9B shows a normal X-ray of the spine for comparison.

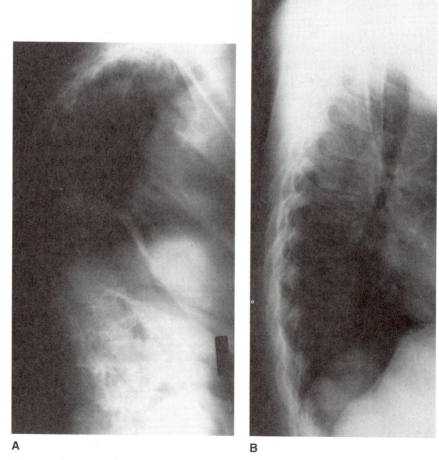

A

B

Figure 6-8. Lateral X-rays of the thoracic spine. (**A**) Wilma Larson's spine film shows diffuse osteopenia and multiple compression fractures, which result in a kyphosis. (**B**) Normal thoracic spine.

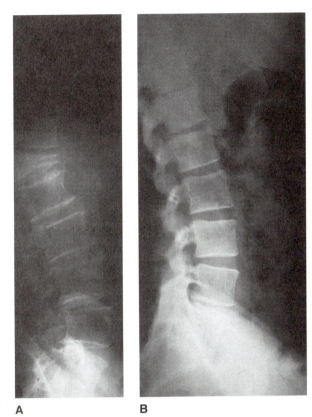

Figure 6-9. Lateral X-rays of the lumbar spine. (**A**) Wilma Larson's film shows a compression fracture and osteopenia compared with the normal film (**B**).

A   B

Mrs. Larson's loss of height is explained by the X-ray findings. The anterior wedging of the thoracic vertebrae results in the kyphosis and loss of height. The reason for these compression fractures most likely is postmenopausal osteoporosis. The normal calcium, phosphate, and alkaline phosphatase levels suggest that she does not have hyperparathyroidism or vitamin D deficiency as the cause of her bone weakness. Further evaluation clearly is indicated.

Additional Laboratory Studies

Test	Wilma Larson	Normal
TSH	1.1 mU/L	0.3–5.0 mU/L
Calcium	9.8 mg/dL	8.5–10.5 mg/dL
Immunoelectrophoresis	Normal	Normal
PTH	44 pg/mL	10–65 pg/mL

Nomogram: See Figure 6-10

Hyperthyroidism or overtreatment with thyroid hormone can increase bone turnover and lead to significant decreases in bone strength and increased risk for fractures. Multiple myeloma also can result in significant

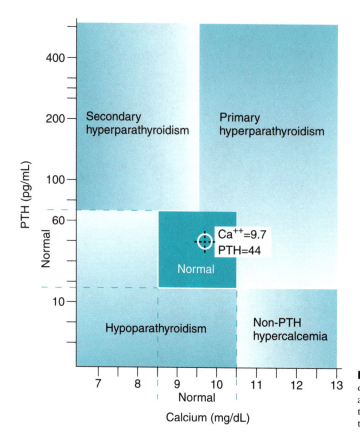

Figure 6-10. Nomogram of PTH versus calcium: Wilma Larson. Both the calcium and the PTH levels are normal, a finding that usually is the case in postmenopausal osteoporosis.

weakening of bone, but it is unlikely in Mrs. Larson's case because she has a normal immunoelectrophoresis. Other causes of loss of bone density (e.g., chronic obstructive pulmonary disease, diabetes mellitus, alcoholism, liver disease, rheumatoid arthritis, chemotherapy, or Cushing's syndrome) do not seem to be likely explanations for Mrs. Larson's problem.

Mrs. Larson has postmenopausal osteoporosis. It is a common, at times very painful, condition that affects many women—perhaps as many as 25 million in the United States—and is associated with a huge cost, both in health care expenditures and in pain and loss of function. Although osteoporosis can occur in men, it is much more common in women. A positive family history of osteoporosis, fair skin, relatively small size, and poor calcium intake are clear risk factors for the development of osteoporosis. Other risk factors include cigarette smoking, excessive alcohol intake, inactivity, and premature menopause.

Osteoporosis is a disease of low bone mass. There are decreases in both the protein and the mineral composition of bone. These deficiencies result in significant decreases in the density and strength of bone and in a significant increase in the risk for fracture. The underlying pathology is unclear. There are no clear, specific, and consistently found abnormalities in bone cells or in the function of the calciotrophic hormones—PTH, calcitonin, and vitamin D.

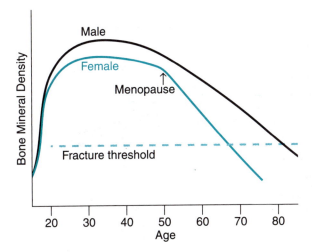

Figure 6-11. Bone mineral density for normal males and females as a function of age. Typical changes in bone mineral density are shown. Bone density rises rapidly during the teenage years and continues to rise gradually until about age 35. Men achieve higher bone density than women, and both begin to lose bone density after age 35. At the time of menopause, the loss of bone in women accelerates. As bone density falls, fracture risk increases; this risk is especially high after the fracture threshold is crossed. Because of lower bone density at peak and the increased rate of bone loss after menopause, women cross this line at a much earlier age than do men.

Bone mass increases rapidly during normal growth and development. In spite of the lack of linear growth after epiphyseal closure, bone density continues to increase in most individuals until about age 30 or 35 (Fig. 6-11). It remains relatively stable until the late 40s or early 50s, when bone density in both sexes begins to decline. The decline in bone density in women is markedly accelerated at the time of menopause. Some of this decline can be limited by the use of postmenopausal estrogen replacement. Because men do not experience the same, relatively sudden, decline in sex hormone levels seen in women at the time of menopause, a similar steepening of the curve of bone loss is not seen in men.

Mrs. Larson's bone density study confirms a significantly low bone density, and, although the study wasn't necessary diagnostically, reviewing it did help Mrs. Larson make the decision to take estrogen (Fig. 6-12). Her hip was studied because hip fractures are a common site of fractures in patients with osteoporosis. She had not wanted to take estrogen at the time of her menopause because she had so little in the way of symptoms and was worried about the potential risks. She is not enthusiastic about the possible return of menstrual bleeding, but Mrs. Larson agrees that estrogen replacement is a reasonable approach to her bone problem. The estrogen will be taken with a small daily dose of a progestational agent that will protect her from endometrial carcinoma, a risk of estrogen therapy. It is hoped that this regimen will minimize the amount of menstrual bleeding. She understands that estrogen therapy will not reclaim lost bone but hopes that it will stem further loss of bone. She also is taking some supplemental calcium and vitamin D, and although it is not clear how much of the calcium will be absorbed, it is hoped that calcium from her GI tract will supply her calcium needs and reduce the amount that is taken from bone. She also has started to walk for 20 minutes each day.

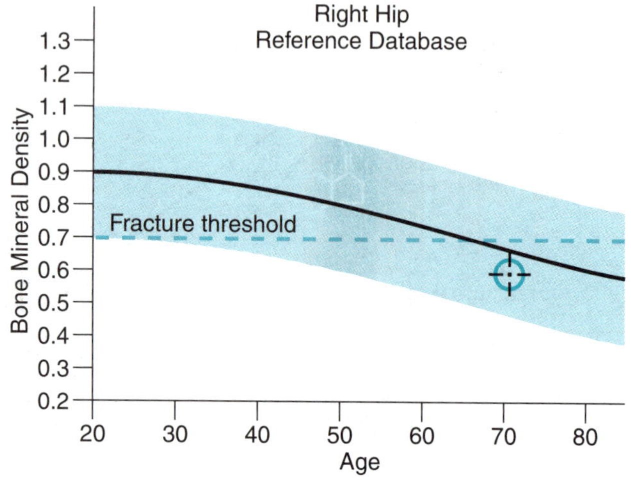

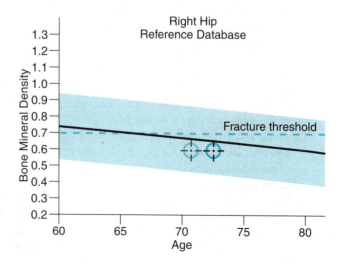

Figure 6-12. Bone mineral density study: Wilma Larson. The curve describes the average bone mineral density for a woman of Mrs. Larson's size and ethnic background; the shaded area includes two standard deviations around the mean. Mrs. Larson's bone mineral density is below average and significantly below peak bone density, a finding that puts her at increased risk of fracture.

Adequate calcium and vitamin D intake and sensible exercise are the foundation of osteoporosis management. Weight-bearing exercise decreases bone loss and helps improve strength and balance. Estrogen can be added to prevent further bone loss. Other agents that affect bone turnover and calcium metabolism also can be added to the regimen in addition to or in place of estrogen.

After a year of estrogen therapy, Mrs. Larson has not gotten any shorter and has had no further episodes of back pain. She is tolerating the estrogen therapy well and has not had significant vaginal bleeding. Her repeat bone density study is shown in Figure 6-13.

Figure 6-13. Bone mineral density study: Wilma Larson. This study was performed after 1 year of estrogen therapy. Although Mrs. Larson's bone mineral density is essentially unchanged, the lack of further loss of bone mineral density is encouraging. Without treatment, further loss of bone mineral density might have been expected.

Mrs. Larson's bone density is essentially unchanged. Her osteoporosis has not progressed further clinically or by bone density. Although she is not any worse, her condition is severe enough for consideration of other modalities of therapy. Antiresorptive therapy with either calcitonin or a bisphosphonate can decrease bone resorption and is especially helpful in patients who have evidence of increased bone turnover. Calcitonin administered either by injection or by nasal spray can be used to inhibit osteoclastic activity and to decrease bone resorption. Alendronate, a bisphosphonate, has a chemical structure similar to pyrophosphate, with a carbon atom connecting the two phosphorous atoms instead of an oxygen molecule. It binds tightly with calcium and, on the bone surface, inhibits the activity of osteoclast cells. This inhibition decreases bone turnover and can decrease further bone loss.

Mrs. Larson was pleased to see that she hasn't lost any more bone. She is not enthusiastic about taking another medication and will wait for another year and have another bone density before deciding about calcitonin or alendronate.

Mrs. Larson is concerned about her two daughters and her granddaughter, Jane. She has gotten some information from the Internet about calcium intake, postmenopausal estrogen replacement, exercise, and other factors to prevent osteoporosis. She has sent copies to her daughters and e-mailed some of the information to Jane, who is away at college. She hopes that increased calcium intake now, while bone is still being formed, will minimize the risk of osteoporosis in Jane's future.

KEY POINTS AND CONCEPTS

- The concentration of calcium in the blood and extracellular fluid space is very tightly controlled.
- Parathyroid hormone (PTH) is a short–half-life protein hormone, released in response to low calcium concentration that has the following effects:
  - Increases renal reabsorption of calcium, lessening urinary calcium losses.
  - Increases activation of vitamin D, resulting in increased GI calcium absorption.
  - Stimulates bone turnover, making calcium contained in bone available to increase extracellular calcium concentration.
- *Hypocalcemia*
  - Causes:
    - Vitamin D deficiency.
    - PTH deficiency or ineffectiveness.
    - Renal failure.
  - Treatment:
    - Calcium replacement—intravenous or oral.
    - Vitamin D.
    - Magnesium, when deficiency is present.

- *Hypercalcemia*
  - Causes:
    - Hyperparathyroidism.
    - Tumor production of a PTH-like molecule (PTHrP).
    - Vitamin D intoxication.
    - Metastatic bone disease.
  - Treatment:
    - Hydration to enhance renal excretion of calcium.
    - Antiresorptive agents such as calcitonin or bisphosphonates to decrease bone breakdown.
    - Surgery to correct hyperparathyroidism.
    - Cessation of vitamin D intake; in severe cases of vitamin D excess, glucocorticoids can be used to inhibit vitamin D effect.

SUGGESTED READING

Anderson JJB, Toverud SU. Diet and vitamin D: a review with an emphasis on human function. J Nutr Biochem 5:58, 1994.

Bilezikian JP. Primary hyperparathyroidism: another important metabolic bone disease of women. Journal of Women's Health 3:21, 1994.

Favus MJ, Christakos S, Goldrin SR. eds. Primer on the Metabolic Bone Diseases and Disorders of Mineral Metabolism, 3rd ed. New York: Raven Press, 1996.

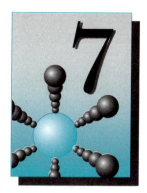

Glucose Regulation and the Endocrine Pancreas

In spite of wide variations in food intake and in physical activity, the circulating concentration of glucose in the blood is maintained within a relatively narrow range—60 to 120 mg/dL. This ensures that the tissues of the brain receive an adequate supply of glucose, the only metabolic fuel that these tissues can use under normal conditions. A complex series of hormonal factors controls this narrow range of glucose concentration. Each time a meal is ingested, glucose levels rise, and, in parallel, insulin levels increase. The insulin secreted leads to the intracellular distribution of glucose. This not only prevents a significant rise in glucose concentration but also provides glucose for intracellular metabolism. Glucagon, cortisol, catecholamines, and growth hormone, among other hormones, play a vital role in maintaining glucose concentration at times of fasting or increased demand for glucose. Figure 7-1 depicts the fluctuations in glucose, insulin, and glucagon over a 24-hour period in a normal subject ingesting a mixed meal. The minimal changes in glucose concentration reflect multiple feedback relationships among insulin secretion, gastrointestinal hormones, absorbed carbohydrates, stored carbohydrates, gluconeogenesis, and a number of other hormones that have an impact on glucose metabolism and regulation.

ANATOMY

Insulin and glucagon are produced by clusters of cells in the pancreas. More than 1 million groups of endocrine cells, referred to as the islets of Langerhans, are dispersed within the exocrine pancreas. These islets contain four cell types—*A, B, D,* and *F*—each of which produces a different hormone. The *A* cells produce glucagon, whereas the *B* cells are the site of insulin synthesis and secretion. *D* cells are the source of pancreatic somatostatin, and the *F* cells, which are more prevalent in the posterior lobe, produce pancreatic polypeptide. Although the islets of Langerhans make up only 2% to 3% of the mass of the pancreas, their blood

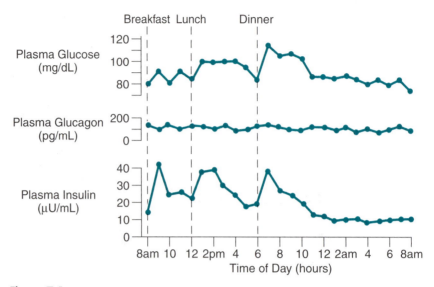

Figure 7-1. Changes in levels of glucose, insulin, and glucagon following the ingestion of mixed meals. In a normal, healthy person, moderate rises in plasma glucose are seen following the ingestion of mixed meals. Insulin levels rise sharply in response to food intake, but glucagon levels remain relatively stable.

supply is organized in such a way that they receive five to ten times the blood flow of comparable amounts of pancreatic exocrine tissue. The hormones produced by the islets of Langerhans are released into veins that drain into the portal vein. This presents a relatively high concentration of hormone to the liver, where many of the metabolic effects of these hormones occur.

CHEMISTRY

Insulin biosynthesis is controlled by a gene on the short arm of chromosome 11. The biosynthetic process originates in the rough endoplasmic reticulum of the B cells and results in the production of pre-proinsulin, a precursor molecule with a molecular weight of 11,500, which is cleaved by microsomal enzymes to proinsulin. Proinsulin is transported to the Golgi apparatus, where it is split into insulin and equimolar amounts of C peptide, also referred to as connecting peptide (Fig. 7-2). The 51-amino-acid insulin molecule consists of a 21-amino-acid A chain and a 30-amino-acid B chain. The A and B chains are connected by two disulfide bridges. The mature human secretory granule of the B cells contains both insulin and the 31-amino-acid C peptide, which has no known biologic activity but is released from the B cell in equimolar quantities with insulin. Human insulin differs from pork insulin by only one amino acid and from beef insulin by three amino acids. These similarities allow the use of animal insulins in patients who need insulin replacement. Currently, however, human insulin produced by genetic recombinant techniques accounts for most of the pharmaceutical insulin used.

Once secreted, insulin, like other protein hormones, is rapidly degraded and has a biologic half-life in the serum of 6 to 10 minutes. The duration of the biologic effects, however, may be much longer.

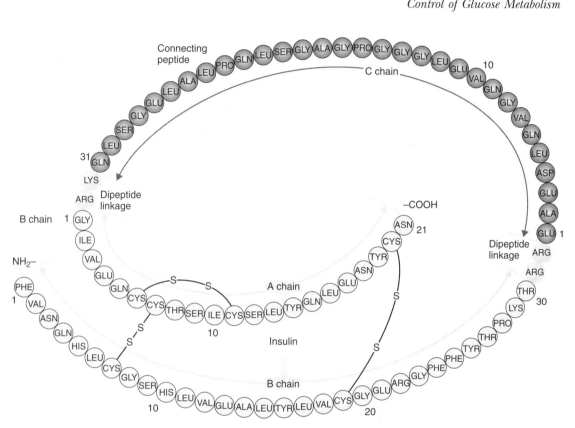

Figure 7-2. The proinsulin and insulin molecules. The amino acid sequence of the proinsulin molecule is shown. Within this molecule are the A and B chains of the active insulin molecule. Cleavage at the dipeptide linkages shown results in the production of the insulin molecule and the inactive C peptide.

CONTROL OF GLUCOSE METABOLISM

Glucose is the prime stimulator of insulin secretion, both in the fasting state and in the postprandial or fed state. Fasting insulin levels are in the range of 10 μU/mL (0.4 ng/mL or 69 pmol/L), and increase up to 100 μU/mL after a standard meal, with peak concentrations being reached 30 to 45 minutes after the meal. Amino acids, such as leucine, also are insulin secretagogues, and the effect of these nutrient stimulators is augmented by enteric hormones such as gastric inhibitory polypeptide and secretin. Pharmacologic agents such as phenytoin, colchicine, thiazides, and alpha-adrenergic agonists inhibit insulin secretion, whereas sulfonylureas, beta-adrenergic agonists, and pentamidine may stimulate the release of insulin.

There are three sources for the glucose that enters the circulation and is made available for the brain and other tissues. The source of glucose changes as an individual moves from the fed to the fasting state (Fig. 7-3). One source is exogenous, from ingested foods; the other two are endogenous and arise from the liver's capacity to break down glycogen (glycogenolysis) and to form new glucose (gluconeogenesis).

Most ingested carbohydrates are polysaccharides and consist mostly of starches; a small proportion consist of lactose (milk sugar) and sucrose. Digestion of starches begins in the mouth, aided by salivary ptyalin, which continues its

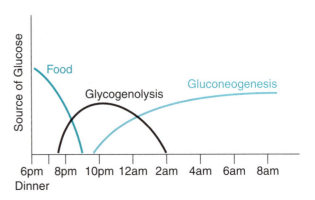

Figure 7-3. Sources of postprandial blood glucose. For 2 to 3 hours following a meal, ingested carbohydrates are the principal source of blood glucose. Between meals, glycogenolysis provides much of the circulating glucose. During periods of fasting, as glycogen is depleted, gluconeogenesis becomes the source of circulating glucose.

hydrolytic actions in the stomach until the pH becomes too low. In the small intestine, pancreatic amylase further breaks down starches to maltose and other small glucose polymers. The enzymes lactase, sucrase, and α-dextrinase are added from the epithelial cells along the brush borders of the small intestine to effect the splitting of all disaccharides to glucose, galactose, and fructose. Glucose represents more than 80% of the final product of carbohydrate ingestion and is absorbed immediately and passes into the portal circulation. Although the circulating concentration of glucose is the most important regulator of insulin secretion, the mechanism of glucose-stimulated insulin release is poorly understood. An old hypothesis assumed the presence of a membrane-bound glucose receptor in B cells, but none has ever been identified. It is more likely that the B cell recognizes glucose via its metabolic products; the metabolism of glucose within B cells results in an increase in cytosolic calcium that, in turn, sets off a series of events that lead to the secretion of insulin. Inositol metabolism, potassium channels, changes in cellular calcium flux, and G proteins all play a role in the process that links the initial metabolism of glucose to the release of insulin.

When glucose concentration increases rapidly, a short burst of insulin is released (early phase), and if the glucose level is maintained, insulin release falls off but then gradually rises again (the late phase). Sustained high levels of glucose result in a reversible desensitization of the B cell to glucose, but not to other insulin secretogogues. Cyclic adenosine monophosphate (cAMP) also is an important modulator of insulin release, but only in the presence of glucose. Glucose induces the formation of cAMP in the B cell.

For insulin to effect its multiple actions, the hormone must bind to specific, membrane-located, glycoprotein receptors that have a high affinity and specificity for the hormone. A schematic representation of the insulin receptor is shown in Figure 7-4. Most tissues have insulin receptors, but those in the liver, skeletal muscle, and fat account for the prime biologic actions of insulin. The brain and red blood cells do not require insulin. After insulin binds to its receptor, a number of insulin-receptor complexes are internalized into the cell, where they activate the processes of glucose transport, and intracellular protein, carbohydrate, and lipid synthesis.

Because the plasma membrane is impermeable to polar molecules such as glucose, the cellular uptake of this nutrient is accomplished by carrier proteins that are associated with the membrane. There are two classes of glucose carrier proteins—the Na^+ glucose transporter and the facilitative glucose transporters.

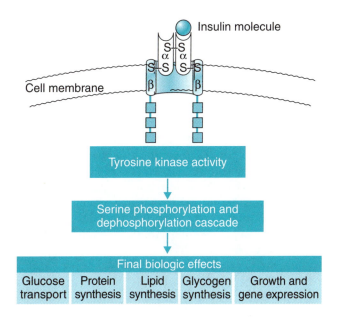

Figure 7-4. The insulin receptor. Located at the cell surface, the insulin receptor, when activated, induces a large number of events within the cell that lead eventually to the multiple effects of insulin.

The latter are present in almost all cells, and the various isoforms of these transporters have distinct tissue distributions that determine the disposal of glucose under differing physiologic conditions. The Glut 1 transporter (erythrocytes) and the Glut 3 transporter (brain) may be responsible for basal or constitutive uptake of glucose; the Glut 2 transporter (liver) mediates the bidirectional transport of glucose by hepatocytes. Glut 4 transporters in skeletal muscle and adipose tissue are responsive to insulin and mediate most of the insulin-stimulated uptake of glucose that occurs in these tissues. The Glut 5 transporter (small intestine) isoform may be involved with the transcellular transport of glucose by absorptive epithelial cells.

Insulin promotes anabolism and inhibits catabolism. Some of the actions of insulin are listed in Table 7-1. In the liver, glycogen, proteins (e.g., enzymes), and triglycerides are synthesized, whereas glycogenolysis, gluconeogenesis, and keto-

TABLE 7-1. *ACTIONS OF INSULIN*			
	LIVER	**ADIPOSE TISSUE**	**MUSCLE**
Anabolic Effects	Stimulation of glycogen synthesis	Stimulation of fatty acid uptake, synthesis, and esterification	Stimulation of amino acid uptake, protein synthesis, glycogen synthesis
Anticatabolic Effects	Inhibition of glycogenolysis, gluconeogenesis, ketogenesis	Inhibition of lipolysis	Inhibition of proteolysis, amino acid output

genesis are inhibited under the influence of insulin. In skeletal muscle, insulin stimulates active amino acid transport and ribosomal protein synthesis; insulin enhances glucose transporter activity and glycogen synthesis. In adipose tissue, insulin promotes triglyceride synthesis by increasing the availability of α-glycerol phosphate so that fatty acids are esterified while inhibiting lipolysis by restraining the activity of hormone-sensitive lipases.

The disposition of specific foodstuffs both after a meal and during fasting reflects the effects of hormones in addition to insulin. Glucagon, synthesized in the A cells of the islets of Langerhans under the regulation of a gene on chromosome 2, modulates the availability of substrates during the intervals between meals. By stimulating glycogenolysis, glucagon ensures an appropriate hepatic output of glucose in the early postprandial period; as hepatic glycogen stores are depleted, however, glucagon in collaboration with cortisol stimulates gluconeogenesis and ensures the maintenance of an adequate early morning (fasting) blood glucose concentration.

During an overnight fast, glucose is produced exclusively by the liver and is consumed for the most part by the brain. In the basal state, glucose turnover is approximately 2 mg/kg/min, so that individuals weighing 70 kg need between 95 and 105 g of glucose in the 12-hour period between dinner and the next morning's breakfast. Glycogenolysis accounts for about 75% of the liver's nocturnal output of glucose; gluconeogenesis is responsible for the remainder. Lactate, pyruvate, and amino acids, especially alanine, are the major substrates used for gluconeogenesis. The hormonal signal for the transition to the fasting state is the fall in circulating insulin. At basal levels of insulin, glucagon stimulates glycogenolysis and gluconeogenesis. When fasting is prolonged and insulin levels fall even further, gluconeogenesis becomes the liver's only means to maintain euglycemia because all glycogen stores are depleted. Simultaneously, fatty acids are mobilized from adipose stores to provide the energy source for muscle activity and preserve the available glucose for use by the central nervous system. In the liver, these fatty acids are oxidized, resulting in the production of ketone bodies—acetoacetate and beta-hydroxybutyrate.

If fasting is prolonged from days to weeks, other homeostatic mechanisms come into play. These mechanisms preserve body protein so that gluconeogenesis is slowed and the brain begins to utilize the ketone bodies acetoacetate and beta-hydroxybutyrate. The signal for the use of ketones by the brain appears to be the rise of these bodies in arterial blood. The extremely low levels of insulin present after extended starvation are similar to those seen in severe diabetes.

DISORDERS OF GLUCOSE METABOLISM

Diabetes mellitus is the major pathologic state related to glucose homeostasis. This disorder is characterized by elevations in both the basal and postprandial levels of glucose. Several forms of diabetes are recognized; they are listed in Table 7-2. Most patients with diabetes have either the insulin-dependent (IDDM) form, also referred to as type 1 diabetes, or the much more common non–insulin-dependent (NIDDM), or type 2 diabetes. Diabetes that is recognized during pregnancy, referred to as gestational diabetes, is a risk factor for the subsequent development of other forms of diabetes, and the detection and treatment of this form of abnormal glucose regulation are vital to the prevention of fetal mortality and morbidity. Diabetes also may appear in the setting of other diseases or as a consequence of pharmacologic or chemical agents.

TABLE 7-2.	*TYPES OF DIABETES MELLITUS*
CLINICAL CLASS	**CHARACTERISTICS**
Type 1 (Insulin-dependent[IDDM])	Onset before age 30 Insulinopenia Prone to ketonemia Dependent on insulin to prevent ketoacidosis and to sustain life
Type 2 (Non–insulin-dependent [NIDDM])	Onset usually after age 30 85%–90% of patients are obese Not prone to ketoacidosis Not dependent on insulin for survival, but may require it to control hyperglycemia
Gestational diabetes (GDM)	Onset during pregnancy
Secondary or other types of diabetes	Related to specific condition or agent: pancreatic disease, endocrinopathies, drugs, or chemical agents

Although the two common forms of diabetes have similar symptoms, similar abnormal glucose elevations, and similar complications, the mechanisms for the abnormal glucose regulation are strikingly different. Type 1, or insulin-dependent, diabetes (IDDM) is characterized by severe insulin deficiency. Insulin replacement therapy is absolutely required in the management of this condition. Type 2, or non–insulin-dependent, diabetes (NIDDM) usually occurs in the setting of significant or even elevated insulin levels in a state characterized by resistance to the effects of insulin. Although insulin is at times used in the management of type 2 diabetes, it often is not necessary because weight loss, exercise, dietary control, and, in some cases, oral hypoglycemic agents usually result in significant improvement.

Hypoglycemia can have disastrous effects on the function of the central nervous system and is defended against by a number of powerful, hormonally based, counterregulatory mechanisms. The secretion of cortisol, catecholamines, glucagon, and growth hormone is triggered by hypoglycemia and results in the normalization of blood sugar when liver function is normal and when substrates for glycogenolysis and gluconeogenesis are available.

THE PHYSIOLOGIC BASIS OF CLINICALLY USEFUL TESTS OF GLUCOSE METABOLISM

BLOOD GLUCOSE CONCENTRATION

The two common ways of determining the concentration of glucose in the blood are to measure the serum glucose or to obtain glucose values from a finger-stick blood sample.

Serum Glucose. The serum of blood drawn from a vein is analyzed for glucose concentration. Although also commonly called blood sugar and blood glucose, this reading really is a serum glucose concentration. The normal range in the fasting state is 60 to 110 mg/dL. Interpretation of the value requires knowledge of the time of sampling in relation to the time of the last ingestion of food and the content of that meal. Table 7-3 outlines the diagnostic criteria for various types of diabetes and gestational diabetes.

Finger-Stick Blood Sugar. In the finger-stick blood sugar test, used by many diabetic patients to monitor the control of their diabetes and in some screening programs, blood is obtained from the capillary bed of a fingertip or earlobe. The drop of blood obtained is analyzed as a whole blood sample on test strips that are read in a reflectance colorimeter or by a meter that monitors a glucose-dependent electrochemical reaction. Because whole blood is used, and because the glucose concentration inside red cells is lower than that seen in the serum, values for finger-stick blood glucose values are about 10% lower than venous serum glucose values obtained at the same time.

Glucose Tolerance Testing. Measuring the concentration of glucose in the serum in the fasting state and then at timed intervals after the ingestion of a given quantity of glucose has been a standard way to look for abnormalities of glucose metabolism. For most patients, such testing is neither necessary nor appropriate because the diagnosis and treatment of most glucose-related metabolic

---

TABLE 7-3. *CRITERIA FOR DIAGNOSIS OF DIABETES*

Diabetes in Nonpregnant Adults

Normal serum glucose values for nonpregnant adults after 75-g glucose load:

Time	Glucose
Fasting	<115 mg/dL (6.4 mM)
30 min	<200 mg/dL (11.1 mM)
60 min	<200 mg/dL (11.1 mM)
90 min	<200 mg/dL (11.1 mM)
120 min	<140 mg/dL (7.8 mM)

A fasting glucose >126 mg/dL (7.0 mM) or a 120-min value ≥200 mg/dL and one other level ≥200 mg/dL confirms the diagnosis of diabetes.

Gestational Diabetes

Screen all pregnant women at 24 to 28 weeks of gestation with a glucose concentration determined 1 hour after a 50-g glucose challenge:

If <126 mg/dL (7.0 mM), no further testing needed.

If >126 mg/dL (7.0 mM), administer 100 g of glucose.

100-g glucose tolerance test:

Time	Glucose
Fasting	<105 mg/dL
1 h	<190 mg/dL
2 h	<165 mg/dL
3 h	<145 mg/dL

If 2 or more values are abnormal, gestational diabetes is present.

problems can be based on the history, physical examination, and basic laboratory data. Abnormalities of glucose metabolism during pregnancy, however, often do require a modified glucose tolerance test for accurate assessment.

Ketones. Ketone bodies—acetone, acetoacetate, and beta-hydroxybutyrate—are the end products of fat metabolism. Ketones may be present normally in the urine of individuals who have been fasting for significant periods of time. Only small amounts of ketones are present in the serum, even during periods of fasting. Large urinary ketone excretion and significant serum levels of ketone bodies indicate that excessive fat catabolism is taking place and that ketoacidosis is developing. Ketones can be estimated by the use of nitroprusside-containing tablets or test strips. The intensity of the purple color that develops when a drop of urine is placed on a reagent tablet or strip provides a semiquantitative measure of the ketone concentration. Beta-hydroxybutyrate, the principal ketone body form found under conditions of acidosis, is not measured by the nitroprusside reaction but can be quantitated by other techniques in the laboratory. Serum ketones can be estimated using similar reagents. More accurate determination of ketone concentrations can be determined in the laboratory by enzymatic methods.

Hemoglobin A_{1C} (HbA_{1C}). Glucose is bound to the hemoglobin molecule in an irreversible fashion and in proportion to the height of the glucose concentration. The percentage of hemoglobin that is glycosylated is easily measured and can be used as an indicator of the average blood glucose level over the preceding 2 to 3 months, a time determined in large measure by the average lifespan of a red blood cell. Although it is not an established screening test for diabetes, it can be used as a report card for diabetic patients. The test can be affected by a number of factors, e.g., hemoglobinopathies, renal failure, and chronic alcohol ingestion. In addition, the normal range and the correlation of the value with the average glucose value may vary from laboratory to laboratory. The normal range for hemoglobin A_{1C} is 3.5% to 5.6%. Variations of this test include the glycated hemoglobin, glycohemoglobin, glycosylated hemoglobin, and HbA_1 tests.

Urinary Microalbumin Excretion. The earliest clinical sign of diabetic renal disease is the appearance of tiny amounts of protein in the urine. The amount of protein that indicates the presence of incipient nephropathy is too low to be detected during routine urinalysis and requires a more sensitive assay. The amount of protein can be quantified by a specific procedure to detect microscopic amounts of albumin (microalbuminuria). The test can be done on a 24-hour urine or other timed collection of urine (Table 7-4) or, more conveniently, on a random sample that is also analyzed for creatinine. The excretion of albumin can be expressed in terms of μg of albumin per mg of urinary creatinine.

TABLE 7-4. *URINARY ALBUMIN EXCRETION*

CATEGORY	24-hr COLLECTION	SPOT COLLECTION
Normal	<30 mg/24 hr	<30 μg/mg creatinine
Microalbuminuria	30–300 mg/24 hr	30–300 μg/mg creatinine
Clinical albuminuria	>300 mg/24 hr	>300 μg/mg creatinine

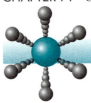

Polyuria, polydipsia, and weight loss in a 13-year-old girl

Robin Tyler was embarrassed—she had wet her bed. She did not want to tell her mother, but she had other concerns she needed to talk with her about. Robin was constantly thirsty and had been drinking several quarts of diet cola or water each day over the past several days. Robin's friends had started to tease her because no sooner had a class period ended than Robin would run to the rest room. In fact, before wetting the bed last night, she had been up to urinate at least five times. Last week, when she stepped on the scale before a soccer game, she noted her weight was 4 pounds less than it had been 3 weeks earlier, in spite of the fact that she recently had had a great appetite.

Yesterday when called upon in history class, Robin was terrified because she could not clearly see the blackboard on which her teacher had written the question. When Robin related all of these happenings to Sarah, her best friend, Sarah urged Robin to tell her mother. After wetting the bed, Robin decided to tell her mother all the things she had noticed over the past several days. Mrs. Tyler, an R.N. who works part-time as a school nurse, reassured her distraught daughter but immediately went to the drugstore and purchased a bottle of urine test strips. A random sample of Robin's urine tested positive for glucose and ketones. Mrs. Tyler arranged an appointment for Robin to see her pediatrician later that afternoon.

Past Medical History

Illnesses:	None
Operations:	None
Medications:	None
Habits:	Coffee: None
	Cigarettes: None
	Alcohol: None
	Drugs: None

Family History

Mother:	38 years old, healthy
Father:	40 years old, healthy
Brothers:	11 years old, healthy, and 9 years old, mild asthma
Maternal grandfather:	Type 2 diabetes

Review of Systems

Blurred vision, weight loss, polyuria, and polydipsia

Menstrual periods started at age 12 and have been relatively regular. She has noticed a cheesy vaginal discharge and some vaginal itching.

Physical Examination

A thin, worried young woman

Vital signs:	**Blood pressure 90/60; pulse 78, resting**
Height:	**5′6″**
Weight:	**118 pounds; 133 pounds at her checkup 4 months earlier**
Skin:	**Warm, normal**
HEENT:	**Normal**
Chest:	**Clear, normal breath sounds**
Heart:	**Normal**
Abdomen:	**Normal**
GYN:	**Normal breast and axillary and pubic hair development for her age; cheesy vaginal discharge noted**

Laboratory Studies

Test	Robin Tyler	Normal
WBC	5900/mm^3	4300–10,800/mm^3
HCT	39%	37%–48% (female)
Glucose	268 mg/dL	70–110 mg/dL, fasting
Serum ketones	Trace positive	Negative
Sodium	134 mEq/L	135–145 mEq/L
Potassium	3.0 mEq/L	3.5–5.0 mEq/L
Urinalysis:		
Color	Clear	Yellow, clear
Specific gravity	1.042	1.001–1.020
Blood	Negative	Negative
Glucose	4+	Negative
Ketones	2+	Negative
Protein	Negative	Negative
Nitrite	Negative	Negative
Leukocytes	Negative	<4 cells/high-power field
Red cells	Negative	<4 cells/high-power field
Vaginal discharge	Numerous hyphae on KOH prep—probable monilia	No hyphae

Polyuria, polydipsia, and polyphagia are the hallmarks of diabetes. Bed-wetting or enuresis may occur with severe polyuria and often is the first symptom of diabetes. When coupled with increased thirst and weight loss, diabetes mellitus is the first consideration. Robin's symptoms relate directly to hyperglycemia, which is a reflection of severe insulin deficiency. Her diabetes, appearing at age 13, is typical of the insulin-dependent, or type 1, form of diabetes. This disorder appears to be autoimmune in origin, with susceptibility related to certain HLA antigens located on the short arm of chromosome 6. The HLA antigens vary among racial groups: in Caucasians,

HLA-B8, HLA-B15, HLA-B18, HLA-CW3, HLA-DR3, and HLA-DR4 are most common, whereas only HLA-DR3 and HLA-DR4 are correlated with type 1 diabetes in Asians, Africans, and Latinos. HLA-DQ genes are more specific markers for the susceptibility because HLA-QW3.2 is commonly found in HLA-DR4 patients with diabetes, whereas a protective gene, HLA-DQ3.1, is found in nondiabetics who have an HLA-DR4 allele. Type 1 diabetes is primarily a disorder of the northern hemisphere, with the highest prevalences in Finland and the United States.

Both genetic and environmental factors contribute to the pathogenesis of type 1 diabetes (Table 7-5). The nature of the environmental component is unclear, although viral infections head the list of possibilities—coxsackievirus B4, rubella, and cytomegalovirus, among others, have been suggested—there remain questions about the interplay between environmental agents and the genetically determined susceptibility of affected individuals. Noninfectious agents such as bovine albumin found in cow's milk, environmental toxins, and ingestants also have been implicated. Whatever the initial antigenic stimulus, a series of defined reactions occur that are characterized by the following features:

1. An infiltration of lymphocytes in the islets of Langerhans (insulitis)
2. The presence of circulating antibodies directed against both cytoplasmic and cell-surface components of the B cell
3. Antibodies directed against insulin

These reactions culminate in the gradual destruction of the B cells, with preservation of the other cellular components of the pancreatic islets. The process usually requires months or years (Fig. 7-5) and can be delayed or inhibited by immunosuppressive treatment. Symptomatic diabetes does not manifest itself until 75% to 85% of the beta cells are destroyed.

Insulin deficiency immediately results in large increments in the output of glucose by the liver: both glycogenolysis and gluconeogenesis are unin-

TABLE 7-5.   *GENETIC AND ENVIRONMENTAL EVENTS IN THE PATHOGENESIS OF TYPE 1 DIABETES*

EVENT	CAUSE OR CONSEQUENCE
Genetic susceptibility	Determined by HLA-D on chromosome 6
Precipitating event: viral infection or external toxin or food (e.g., milk)	Currently no consensus on the exact precipitant
Insulitis	Islets are infiltrated by activated T cells
Autoimmunity phase	B-cell destruction implies transition to a non-self state
Antibody production: e.g., antibodies to insulin, GAD; >90% of B cells are destroyed	Type 1 diabetes: classic symptoms of polyuria, polydipsia, and polyphagia

GAD, glutamic acid decarboxylase

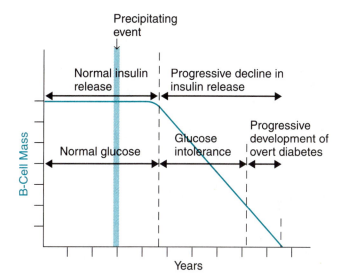

Precipitating event

Normal insulin release

Progressive decline in insulin release

Normal glucose

Glucose intolerance

Progressive development of overt diabetes

B-Cell Mass

Years

Figure 7-5. Stages in the onset of type 1 diabetes. Long before overt glucose intolerance and diabetes mellitus develop, there has been a significant decline in pancreatic B-cell mass. The large functional reserve of the pancreatic islet cells postpones the development of clinically apparent diabetes until the B-cell mass is significantly depleted.

hibited. The uptake of glucose by the two prime insulin-sensitive tissues—skeletal muscle and adipose tissue—is markedly diminished. The consequence of hepatic overproduction and peripheral underutilization of glucose is hyperglycemia. When the blood levels of glucose exceed the renal threshold (about 180 to 200 mg/dL), glucosuria occurs, with simultaneous loss of free water and large quantities of sodium, potassium, and other electrolytes. Dehydration and electrolyte depletion follow.

In addition to causing hyperglycemia, the absence of insulin leads to accelerated rates of lipolysis; the excess free fatty acids that result from this exaggerated breakdown of triglycerides are then available for hepatic ketogenesis. In the insulin-deficient state, glucagon increases the ketogenic capacity of the liver. The presence of excessive amounts of the ketones, acetoacetate and beta-hydroxybutyrate, in the basal state is a diagnostic criterion for type 1 diabetes, and differentiates it from type 2 diabetes. Enough insulin action is present in patients with type 2 diabetes to restrain lipolysis and prevent ketosis. If insulin deficiency is not corrected, unregulated gluconeogenesis and ketogenesis result in diabetic ketoacidosis. Ketone bodies are weak organic acids, but can cause significant acidosis if they accumulate, a condition that develops when production exceeds excretion. Ketoacidosis is the extreme state of insulin deficiency and can be prevented, as in Robin's case, by early detection of decompensated diabetes and the institution of insulin therapy. The pathogenesis of diabetic ketoacidosis is shown in Figure 7-6.

Monilial vaginitis is a common problem for women with diabetes. Increased glucose levels in vaginal secretions result in changes in vaginal flora that allow the uncomfortable overgrowth of monilial organisms.

Robin was both frightened and relieved. She was frightened because she knew diabetes was a significant problem and that she would have to learn to manage her disease. She was relieved because she knew that she would feel better soon, maybe even in time for next Saturday's soccer game.

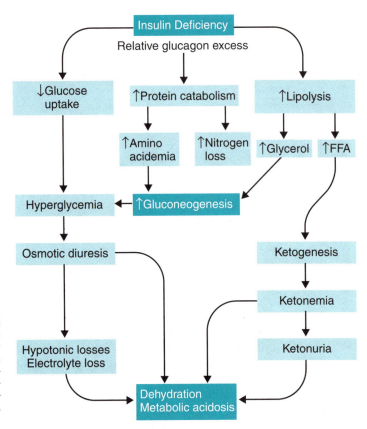

Figure 7-6. Pathogenesis of diabetic ketoacidosis (DKA). Diabetic ketoacidosis begins with a deficiency of insulin. The resulting rise in glucose levels, together with the increase in protein catabolism and lipolysis, lead to a dehydrating diuresis, electrolyte depletion, severe hyperglycemia, and marked acidosis. Correction requires replacement of insulin, electrolytes, and fluid.

During the visit to her pediatrician, Robin learned about insulin and was very surprised that she was able to give herself her first shot of insulin! She had dreaded it, but it really wasn't too bad. She also learned to do fingerstick blood sugars. In addition, she has homework! She has a booklet to read over the next few days that covers diet, exercise, insulin, and general care issues.

Robin had given herself 10 units of NPH insulin and planned to come back the next day for some more teaching and a check on her injection technique. That night, Robin had to get up only once and was relieved that her sheets were dry in the morning. Her blood sugar on arising was 198 mg/dL. She also felt less thirsty; her vision was still fuzzy, however. She hopes that tomorrow she will have time to pick up all the supplies she needs and the vaginal cream that was prescribed.

Insulin therapy and careful attention to the content and timing of meals and activity are the foundation of management for the type 1 diabetic. The goal is to replace insulin in a physiologic pattern. This means maintaining low levels of insulin at times of fasting or decreased food intake and higher levels at times of food intake and rising glucose concentrations. The low levels at times of fasting are required to restrain gluconeogenesis and lipolysis and to prevent ketoacid production and ketosis. The higher levels required after eating are necessary for appropriate intracellular distribution of glucose.

Because insulin is a protein molecule, it must be given parenterally. Orally administered insulin would be digested into its component amino acids and, therefore, would have no biologic effect. Subcutaneously injected insulin bypasses digestion and makes insulin available for its metabolic effects. An additional problem with insulin replacement is that the molecule has a very short half-life once it enters the circulation. Subcutaneous placement of insulin does provide some repository effect because it gradually enters the circulation from the injection site. Various preparations of insulin are available that provide a time-released effect from the subcutaneous injection site. The characteristics of the commonly available forms of insulin are shown in Table 7-6. Although insulin derived from animals, usually cows and pigs, has been used for years, most patients currently requiring insulin use human insulin produced by genetic recombinant techniques. Regular insulin is a buffered form of insulin that is gradually absorbed over a rela-

TABLE 7-6. *CHARACTERISTICS OF COMMONLY AVAILABLE INSULIN PREPARATIONS*

TYPE AND PREPARATION	COMPOSITION	ACTION PROFILE (hr)			COMMENTS
		Onset	Peak	Duration	
Short-acting					
Regular	Solution of zinc insulin	0.5–1	2–4	6–8	Usually given at mealtimes or to lower a markedly elevated glucose
Lispro	Reversed amino acids 28 and 29 on beta chain	0.2–0.5	0.5–2	3–4	Usually given 15 minutes before a meal as part of a multiple-dose regimen
Intermediate-acting					
NPH	Protamine zinc, phosphate buffer	1.5	4–12	18–24	Used to provide an insulin effect that lasts through the day or evening
Lente	Amorphous, acetate buffer	2.5	6–14	18–28	Similar to NPH insulin
Long-acting					
Ultralente	Amorphous and crystalline mix	4–6	18–24	36–40	Used to provide a background insulin effect, usually supplemented with frequent doses of a short-acting insulin
Mixtures					
NPH/Regular	70% NPH/30% regular	1–2	4–14	18–30	Biphasic action, not useful when frequent dose adjustments are needed

tively short period of time—2 to 6 hours. Lispro is a preparation of insulin that has a very rapid onset of action and a short duration of effect. NPH and Lente insulin are longer-acting preparations and have very similar characteristics. Ultralente insulin provides an even longer duration of insulin effect.

Insulin also can be administered by an external, motor-driven syringe pump that continuously injects regular or lispro insulin into the subcutaneous space. The pump system can be adjusted to provide a basal rate of infusion to maintain the necessary low levels of insulin. When activated by the patient, boluses of insulin can be administered, providing higher levels of insulin at times of increased glucose influx such as mealtime.

A similar re-creation of the physiologic pattern of insulin dynamics can be approached with the frequent—3 to 4 times a day—administration of a rapid-acting insulin against a background of longer-acting insulins. The Diabetes Control and Complications Trial (DCCT) provides evidence that excellent or tight control of glucose levels in patients with diabetes can significantly reduce the development of complications. Tight control, however, has some significant costs. Frequent testing, frequent adjustments of insulin doses, frequent injections, and, most importantly, the risk of hypoglycemia are all important aspects of what is required to maintain near-normal glucose levels. Multiple injection regimens or an infusion pump requires meticulous attention to a number of factors. Doses of insulin administered either by infusion pump boluses or by conventional subcutaneous injections are adjusted based on the blood glucose at the time of testing, the content of the meal to be ingested, and the activity planned. Because exercise has an insulin-like effect, lower doses of insulin are needed if vigorous exercise is planned.

After 3 weeks of education, practice, and adjustments of her insulin dose, Robin is feeling very well. Although her vision is better, it is still not back to normal, but she has no nocturia and the vaginal itch and discharge are gone. She is now on an insulin regimen of three shots a day, and she keeps a careful log of her finger-stick blood glucose results. A page from her logbook is shown in Figure 7-7.

Only a few of her friends know that she has diabetes, and she is not sure she wants anyone else to know. At a birthday party for her close friend, Sarah, last week, Robin had a piece of cake and some ice cream—the first time she has had sweets since she found out she had diabetes. Robin was worried about eating them. She knew that both the cake and the ice cream contain large amounts of sugar and that they would mess up her glucose values, but she really wanted to have some and was afraid that her friends would make a big deal of it if she didn't partake. Robin decided to have some, but to not finish her serving. As she predicted, her glucose that night before bed was 286 mg/dL—back to where she started! Robin took four units of regular insulin, and although she had to get up once during the night to urinate, her glucose was 145 mg/dL when she arose the next morning.

Two weeks later Robin's soccer team had made the regional finals, and everyone was very excited. The game was on Saturday morning at a school about 1 hour away by bus. The bus left her school at 11:30; the game was at

Date	Breakfast Glucose	Breakfast Insulin	Lunch Glucose	Lunch Insulin	Dinner Glucose	Dinner Insulin	Bedtime Glucose	Bedtime Insulin	Comments
Sun	overslept	18N/4R	122	—	92	4R	126	6N	Overslept, Took insulin @ 10:30
Mon	154	18N/4R	147	—	62	4R	162	6N	
Tue	194	18N/5R	FORGOT	—	118	4R	—	—	Fell Asleep! Forgot PM Dose
Wed	232	18N/6R	168	—	152	6R	110	6N	
Thu	137	18N/4R	—	—	164	6R	138	6N	
Fri	188	18N/5R	156	—	202	8R	140	6N	Pizza for lunch
Sat	166	18N/5R	118	—	110	4R	137	6N	

Figure 7-7. Robin's glucose log. Finger-stick glucose levels and insulin doses are recorded along with other information that can be used to help improve control in patients on intensive insulin regimens. N, NPH insulin; R, regular insulin.

2:30. The plan was for the team to have a light lunch on the bus and warm up on arrival at the tournament site. Robin has always gotten a little carsick, and the thought of eating on the bus was not a pleasant one. In addition, she was anxious about the game and had butterflies in her stomach. On the morning of the game her fasting sugar was 123 mg/dL. She took her usual dose of 4 units of regular insulin along with 18 units of NPH insulin and had a light breakfast. At 11:00 when she left for school to get the bus, her finger-stick glucose was 108 mg/dL, and she decided not to take any more insulin. Robin didn't feel like eating before going to school and wasn't going to try to eat on the bus. She also didn't want to eat too close to game time, so she decided not to eat at all.

Robin played goalie and was one of the best in the league. Each team scored once in the first period, and Robin made some great saves. Toward the end of the first period, however, Robin began to feel very strange. She was incredibly hungry and she was aware that her heart was beating very rapidly. Even though it was a chilly November day, she was sweating profusely. She also seemed to have trouble paying attention, and she missed an easy save. The coach was concerned about Robin's behavior and sent in a substitute goalie. On the sidelines it was clear to both the coach and Mrs. Tyler that something was radically wrong. Robin was confused, disoriented, and very irritable. Mrs. Tyler did a finger-stick blood sugar. The value was 12 mg/dL! Robin was getting more agitated. She refused to drink the orange juice she was offered, nor would she eat the candy that her mother had brought in case something like this happened. Although she had never done this before, Mrs. Tyler had been educated about the use of glucagon to reverse hypoglycemia and gave Robin a subcutaneous injection of glucagon. After about 15 minutes, Robin was back to herself, and a repeat finger-stick glucose was 147 mg/dL. She agreed to drink some orange juice and to eat several crackers. She was feeling much better, but very embarrassed, and very sorry that her team was down by one goal.

She convinced the coach and her mother that she was ready to play

again and returned to the game during the second period. No more goals were scored against Robin, and her team's offense really clicked during the last 10 minutes of the game. Robin's team won, 3 to 2.

The insulin-like effect of exercise, which lowers blood glucose, combined with decreased food intake during the day and the morning dose of NPH insulin, resulted in a significant hypoglycemic episode for Robin. Learning the signs and symptoms of impending hypoglycemia is vital for diabetics, their family, and their friends. Carrying glucose in tablet or gel form and having glucagon for injection available are strategies for dealing with the possible development of hypoglycemia. In addition, wearing a bracelet that identifies an individual as having diabetes often can speed the correct diagnosis and treatment.

The manifestations of hypoglycemia can be separated into neuroglycopenia and those signs and symptoms produced by the counterregulatory response to hypoglycemia (Table 7-7). Robin's confusion, lack of attention, and irritability probably were the result of neuroglycopenia. The hunger, the palpitations, and the sweating were produced by the autonomic response to hypoglycemia. The hormonal responses to hypoglycemia are presented in Table 7-8. Hypoglycemia triggers the release of catecholamines, which results in glycogenolysis and gluconeogenesis. The catecholamines also induce tachycardia and anxiety. Glucagon released from the pancreas also stimulates the release of glucose from the liver. Cortisol and growth hormone, in addition, are released and serve to counteract the effects of insulin. If Robin were not diabetic, she would have had a very low level of insulin during the game. Her morning dose of NPH insulin, however, gave her a significant level of circulating insulin. Her counterregulatory mechanisms were unable to counteract the effects of the insulin. Because the effect of the injected glucagon is short-lived, and because Robin's glycogen stores were significantly depleted by the counterregulation that did occur, it was very important that she eat some carbohydrate over the next few hours to replenish glycogen stores and prevent a return of hypoglycemia.

Other causes of hypoglycemia are usually related to medications or

TABLE 7-7. *SYMPTOMS OF HYPOGLYCEMIA*

ADRENERGIC SYMPTOMS	NEUROGLYCOPENIC SYMPTOMS
Palpitations	Headache
Anxiety	Inability to concentrate
Tremulousness	Fatigue
Hunger	Confusion
Sweating	Bizarre behavior
	Hallucinations
	Convulsions
	Coma

TABLE 7-8. *RESPONSE TO HYPOGLYCEMIA: THE ROLE OF THE COUNTER-REGULATORY HORMONES*

HORMONE	TIMING	EFFECTS
Epinephrine	Immediately, within minutes	Stimulates hepatic glucose production, limits glucose utilization, activates lipolysis, increases FFAs, limits insulin secretion by beta cells
Glucagon	Immediately, within minutes	Activates glycogenolysis and gluconeogenesis, increases hepatic glucose production, activates lipase in adipose tissue, increases FFAs, enhances hepatic capacity for ketogenesis
Cortisol	After 2–3 h	Stimulates hepatic gluconeogenesis, limits peripheral glucose utilization
Growth hormone	After several hours	Limits glucose utilization, may enhance lipolysis

substances that induce insulin secretion or interfere with gluconeogenesis, such as alcohol. Liver disease can result in inadequate hepatic glucose production and lead to hypoglycemia. Similarly, adrenal and pituitary insufficiency can lead to inadequate counterregulatory protection against hypoglycemia.

Robin is now 18 years old, has finished high school, and has started college. She loves her new friends and some of her classes, but the work is much harder and she doesn't have time to play soccer. The dining hall food isn't very good, and her day-to-day schedule is very chaotic. She is also getting fed up with testing her glucose and injecting insulin three or four times a day.

One Saturday morning she overslept and hurried to meet her friends for a football game. She forgot to take her insulin and didn't bother to test her glucose. During the game she was very thirsty and had two diet colas. At a fraternity party after the game, she had some punch that the brothers had concocted. She was too shy to ask the contents. She was thirsty and it tasted good, so she had several glasses. At 9 p.m. her friends could not arouse her, and she was taken to the local emergency room.

On arrival at the emergency room, Robin could not be aroused and was breathing very deeply and rapidly. Her breath smelled of alcohol. A finger-stick glucose in the ambulance on the way to the emergency room was over 400 mg/dL.

Physical Examination
Vital signs:	Blood pressure 90/40; pulse, 140 beats/min
	Respirations 32/minute, deep
Skin:	Warm and dry
HEENT:	Very dry tongue and mouth
Chest:	Clear

Heart:	Rapid, no murmurs
Abdomen:	Decreased bowel sounds, no masses
Extremities:	Unremarkable

Laboratory Studies

Test	Robin Tyler	Normal
WBC	12,900 with left shift	4300–10,800/mm³
Hct	51%	37%–48% (female)
Glucose	588 mg/dL	70–110 mg/dL, fasting
Sodium	138 mEq/L	135–145 mEq/L
Potassium	5.6 mEq/L	3.5–5.0 mEq/L
Chloride	90 mEq/L	98–106 mEq/L
Bicarbonate	6 mEq/L	21–30 mEq/L
BUN	30 mg/dL	8–22 mg/dL
Creatinine	3.4 mg/dL	0.3–1.5 mg/dL
Serum ketones	Strongly positive at 1:16 dilution	Negative
Arterial blood gases		
pO_2	114 mm Hg	80–100 mm Hg
pCO_2	18 mm Hg	35–45 mm Hg
pH	7.02	7.38–7.44
hCG (pregnancy test)	Negative	Negative, not pregnant Positive, pregnant
Alcohol	180 mg/dL	"Legal intoxication" = >80 mg/dL

An intravenous line had been started in the ambulance, and saline was started at 500 mL per hour. Shortly after arrival in the emergency room, Robin received an intravenous bolus of 10 units of regular insulin, and an intravenous insulin drip at 4 units per hour was started.

After 3 L of fluid, Robin was much more responsive and was surprised to find herself in the hospital—she had never been hospitalized before. By midnight her glucose was 184 mg/dL and her bicarbonate had risen to 12 mEq/L and her pH to 7.12. Her potassium level had fallen dramatically, to 3.4 mEq/L. In response to these changes, her IV fluids were changed to include glucose and potassium. Her insulin drip was continued at the same rate.

The next morning Robin was tired and achy but was feeling very much better. She was hungry and was able to take liquids without any problem. The laboratory tests drawn that morning showed marked improvement in her glucose (143 mg/dL) and in her electrolytes. Ketones were still present in her serum, but her BUN and creatinine were back to normal and alcohol was no longer detectable in her blood. She was started on 10 units of NPH insulin, slightly less than her usual morning dose, and a few hours later the insulin drip was discontinued. The next morning, Robin's glucose was 162 mg/dL, and her appetite and self-confidence were restored. She returned to her dorm room recommitted to monitoring her diabetes more carefully and resolved also to make sure she always knows what she is ingesting.

Although for many patients ketoacidosis is the initial presenting event of diabetes mellitus, Robin did not experience it until several years into the course of her diabetes. Adjustment to adolescent and adult life can, for some diabetics, lead to denial of their problem and experimentation with other, sometimes nontraditional ways of dealing with the problem. Alcohol, drugs, and changes in daily routine also can present challenges to good diabetic control. Most commonly, diabetic ketoacidosis is precipitated by some event that results in lack of adequate insulin effectiveness. Not taking insulin is clearly one way, but insulin effectiveness also can be severely limited in the face of several medical problems. Infections, especially of the urinary and gastrointestinal tract, myocardial infarction, and various inflammatory processes can stimulate the release of stress-responding hormones that antagonize the effects of insulin and lead to hyperglycemia and ketoacidosis in patients with insulin-dependent diabetes. One of the common complications of diabetes, neuropathy (discussed later in this chapter), can mask the usual symptoms of infection, inflammation, or infarction, and these conditions must be looked for carefully in all cases of ketoacidosis.

The key element in the precipitation of Robin's episode of ketoacidosis was that she did not take insulin on the morning of the football game. She had not taken any insulin during the day. This resulted in very low levels of insulin and started the process illustrated in Figure 7-6. Her insulin level fell below that needed to restrain lipolysis and ketogenesis. The alcohol ingested at the party further accelerated ketogenesis. The acidosis that resulted drives respiration and results in the development of Kussmaul's breathing (rapid deep breathing). The acidosis also drives potassium from the intracellular space into the extracellular space, resulting in a high serum potassium in the face of total body potassium depletion. As the acidosis is corrected and some potassium shifts back into the intracellular space, hypokalemia ensues and must be carefully corrected. The lack of insulin also leads to uncontrolled hepatic glucose production and decreased uptake and intracellular incorporation of glucose by insulin-sensitive cells. The resulting hyperglycemia leads to a dehydrating diuresis and the loss of both fluid volume and electrolytes—sodium, potassium, phosphate, and others. Hyperosmolality leads to altered mental status.

Management of ketoacidosis involves replacement of fluid, electrolytes, and insulin. Because the fluid losses may be deceptively large, fluid needs should be assessed carefully and continually. Hypoglycemia and hypokalemia must be avoided and usually are prevented by adding glucose and potassium to intravenous solutions once the initial hyperglycemia and hyperkalemia are corrected. Diabetic ketoacidosis is a fatal condition unless skillfully and promptly treated.

Ten years have passed since Robin's diagnosis, and she has adjusted well to her disease. She has had no further episodes of ketoacidosis and only

an occasional episode of mild hypoglycemia, which she responds to quickly. She takes 36 units of NPH insulin and 8 units of regular insulin before breakfast, 10 units of regular insulin before supper, and 12 units of NPH insulin at bedtime. Her hemoglobin A_{1C} measurements have ranged from 7.5% to 8.9% (normal—3.5% to 5.6%) during the last year.

Robin completed college last spring and was married in the fall. She and her husband would like to have a child, and her physician suggested that, before conceiving, Robin control her glucose a bit more tightly, because excellent regulation of glycemia not only improves the chances of conception, but greatly reduces the likelihood of congenital malformations.

Robin began to test her blood glucose four times daily and added a dose of regular insulin before lunch. Three months later, Robin reports that she has missed her period. An hCG beta-subunit test is positive, confirming pregnancy. On a number of occasions, Robin has noted a low glucose in the morning; she also has had some morning nausea.

During pregnancy, maternal metabolism adapts to provide the fetus with adequate supplies of nutrients needed for development. Some of the factors involved in this vital supply process are depicted in Figure 7-8. In normal pregnant women, basal or fasting levels of glucose tend to decrease slightly as the developing fetus requires increasing quantities of glucose. Pregnancy for nondiabetic women is "diabetogenic"; hormones produced by the placenta, especially human placental lactogen (HPL), and estrogens induce a degree of insulin resistance. This decrease in insulin effectiveness tends to make relatively more glucose available for the developing fetus. Women who cannot mobilize sufficient additional insulin to overcome the insulin resistance of pregnancy develop gestational diabetes. The diagnosis

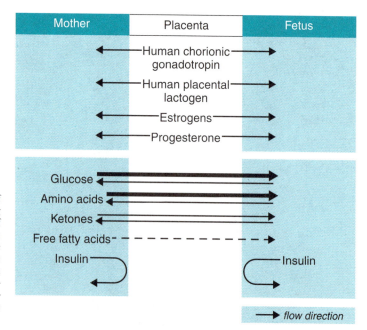

Figure 7-8. Source and distribution of hormones and metabolic fuels during pregnancy. The placenta is the source of a number of hormones that affect both maternal and fetal metabolism. Glucose and amino acids largely flow from the maternal side to the fetus. Ketones can be toxic to the developing fetus, and ketone levels should be minimized in pregnant women. Insulin does not cross the placenta significantly.

of gestational diabetes is based on different criteria than those used for other forms of diabetes (see Table 7-3).

Pregnancy in a patient with type 1 diabetes requires special attention to the regulation of glucose concentration. Ideally, efforts should be made to control glycemia close to physiologic levels before conception, but often this is not possible. When pregnancy occurs in a poorly controlled patient, efforts to regulate the glucose should be initiated as soon as the pregnancy is confirmed. Monitoring the blood glucose four to six times per day is advised. Insulin requirements actually may decrease early in the pregnancy. Later in the second and third trimesters, however, as insulin resistance induced by rising levels of human placental lactogen and other insulin-antagonist hormones becomes a dominant factor, insulin requirements rise progressively and usually are two to three times greater than prepregnant needs at the time of delivery. Some of the changes in responsiveness to insulin during pregnancy and the insulin resistance of late pregnancy are intracellular events that occur distal to the binding of insulin to its receptor. Early in the third trimester, insulin needs may rise 50% over a 4- to 6-week period.

Target blood glucose levels sought in the pregnant diabetic emulate those of the pregnant nondiabetic: pre-meal values should range from 60 to 105 mg/dL, and 2-hour postprandial levels should not exceed 120 mg/dL. Maintaining maternal glucose in this range is difficult but essential to avoid fetal demise, excessive fetal growth, and delayed pulmonary maturation—all unfortunate consequences of poor control of maternal glucose. Good glycemic control should be maintained throughout the pregnancy.

In the past, many women with type 1 diabetes were delivered before term to avoid the risk of intrauterine fetal death, especially from the respiratory distress syndrome. Now, with up-to-date, active prenatal care, most women with type 1 can be safely delivered at term. Spontaneous labor or labor induced once the cervix is favorable are the methods recommended.

Robin aggressively managed her glucose during her pregnancy and delivered a 7 lb 6 oz boy in the 38th week of her pregnancy. At one point her total insulin dosage was two times that of her pre-pregnancy requirement. Almost immediately after delivery, her insulin requirements returned to their previous levels. Two years later, Robin completed a second pregnancy without complications.

Robin is now 26 years old, and she and her husband are considering a third child. During her check-up she asks about getting ready for another pregnancy.

Her examination is remarkable for blood pressure of 120/84, mild background retinopathy, and absent ankle jerk reflexes and decreased vibratory sense in her feet.

Laboratory Studies

Test	Robin Tyler	Normal
Hemoglobin A_{1C}	7.8%	3.5%–5.6%
Creatinine	1.0 mg/dL	0.3–1.5 mg/dL
BUN	12 mg/dL	8–22 mg/dL
Urinalysis		
Color	Clear	Yellow, clear
Specific gravity	1.030	1.001–1.020
Blood	Negative	Negative
Glucose	1+	Negative
Ketones	Negative	Negative
Protein	Trace	Negative
Nitrite	Negative	Negative
Leukocytes	Negative	<4 cells/high-power field
Red blood cells	Negative	<4 cells/high-power field
Urine for microalbumin	110 μg/mg creatinine	<30 μg/mg creatinine

Robin now has three findings that indicate she is developing early complications of diabetes. She has small, but significant amounts of albumin in her urine and clinical evidence of both neuropathy and retinopathy. Although these complications can occur in any patient who has had diabetes for a number of years, the DCCT study indicates that they occur with less frequency in patients whose diabetes is under excellent control.

DIABETIC RETINOPATHY

Microaneurysms detected on the examination of the optic fundi indicate that an early lesion of diabetic retinopathy has developed. Retinopathy is categorized as either background (simple) or proliferative. In background retinopathy, the vessels may be dilated, constricted, or tortuous; in addition to microaneurysms, there may be dot, linear, or flame-shaped hemorrhages. Leakage of protein or lipid, or both, from hyperpermeable vessels produces hard exudates, whereas cotton-wool exudates result from microinfarctions of the retina.

Proliferative retinopathy reflects the most serious form of diabetic ophthalmopathy. Blindness occurs in many of these patients within 5 years of the appearance of proliferative changes. Proliferative retinopathy is characterized by the development of new blood vessels. The presence of these abnormal vessels may cause bleeding into the vitreoretinal space and lead to adhesions and proliferation of connective tissue and, ultimately, to retinal detachment. Photocoagulation with the xenon arc or argon laser is an effective treatment for proliferative retinopathy. The pathogenesis of retinopathy is thought to stem from ischemia, which is the result of focal occlusion of capillaries, and the formation of microaneurysms. Alterations in vascular permeability, blood viscosity, and clotting factors also are postulated to be culprits in the process. Hyperglycemia or other metabolic consequences of insulin deficiency or ineffectiveness probably are the proximate cause of diabetic retinopathy.

DIABETIC NEPHROPATHY

One of the major vascular complications of diabetes is the one that affects the kidney: diabetic nephropathy. In the past, 30% to 40% of all patients with type 1 diabetes developed diabetic nephropathy and progressed to end-stage renal failure that required dialysis or transplantation. Within the last decade, the development of a method to detect micro-quantities of albumin in the urine has provided an approach that permits early therapeutic intervention and, it is hoped, a marked reduction in the incidence of diabetic nephropathy.

The clinical course of diabetic nephropathy is presented in Table 7-9. Early in the course of type 1 diabetes, the glomerular filtration rate (GFR) and renal blood flow are elevated, and the kidneys actually increase in size and weight (see Table 7-9). The magnitude of the increase in GFR relates directly to the degree of hyperglycemia: good glycemic control reduces the GFR. Serum creatinine and the blood urea nitrogen (BUN) concentration often are reduced during this hyperfiltration phase. Usually after 2 to 3 years of type 1 diabetes, the histology of the kidney shows mesangial expansion, and the basement membranes thicken. Despite these changes, the GFR and blood flow remain elevated, but proteinuria is not present. In most patients who ultimately develop nephropathy, there is a latent period of 10 to 15 years during which laboratory tests are normal; the histologic changes are progressive, however, and small quantities of albumin may be detectable in the urine.

Three histologic changes characterize diabetic nephropathy: (1) glomerulosclerosis, in which the mesangial expansion and basement membrane thickening mentioned earlier progress to produce diffuse scarring of the whole glomerulus; (2) structural vascular changes in the small arterioles, which may be factors in the hypertension that often accompanies diabetic nephropathy; and (3) tubulointerstitial changes that ultimately lead to the disordered secretion of potassium and hydrogen ions that is a feature of end-stage diabetic nephropathy. The mechanism by which diabetes damages the

TABLE 7-9. *CLINICAL COURSE OF DIABETIC NEPHROPATHY*

CLINICAL PICTURE	YEARS AFTER ONSET
Kidneys enlarge; renal function supernormal	0–3
Mesangial expansion; basement membrane thickening begins	3–10
Silent period; no proteinuria, then microalbuminuria (30–300 μg/mg creatinine) develops	5–15
Proteinuria; intermittent, then persistent (>500 mg/24 hr)	>15
Azotemia begins; hypertension, edema, and renal failure ensue	15–20

kidneys remains undefined: it is not established whether glucose per se or a metabolic product resulting from hyperglycemia is the trigger. A genetic propensity for diabetic nephropathy contributes to its development. In some families in which multiple members have diabetes, nephropathy may affect 80% of the diabetic siblings. The pathogenic mechanisms probably include both the effects of hyperperfusion and the increase in the collagen-related components of the basement membrane. The altered permeability of the membrane may relate to the increased glycosylation of the membrane. In the end, mesangial expansion encroaches on the subendothelial space and the glomerular capillary lumen to cause a reduction in the GFR.

Microalbuminuria results when small amounts of albumin pass through the glomerular membrane and presages the development of nephropathy. Everyone with type 1 diabetes should be tested for microalbuminuria yearly after diabetes has been present for 5 years. Poor diabetes control, infection, exercise, and stress are other causes of microalbuminuria and must be excluded. When microalbuminuria is detected consistently, and other causes are excluded, and even if hypertension is not present, therapy with angiotensin-converting enzyme (ACE) inhibitors decreases and may eliminate the microalbuminuria. ACE inhibitors in patients with more advanced renal disease may induce hyperkalemia or, in some instances, may precipitate a decline in renal function, so serum potassium and creatinine should be measured frequently after treatment is started.

Hypertension typically accompanies the appearance of diabetic nephropathy. Patients with type 1 diabetes who are free of nephropathy rarely are hypertensive. Hypertension accelerates the nephropathy and warrants aggressive, immediate treatment. It is of paramount importance that patients with diabetes have blood pressures normalized (120/80 or less) to the extent possible without compromising cardiac or cerebral function. Restricted protein intake also may have a palliative effect on the progression of the nephropathy. End-stage renal disease remains a major cause of morbidity and mortality in type 1 diabetes patients. Preventive measures include excellent glycemic control, vigilant monitoring for microalbuminuria, and aggressive treatment of hypertension as soon as it is detected.

DIABETIC NEUROPATHY

Diabetes affects all parts of the nervous system. Peripheral nerves are the most commonly affected and account for the symptoms of numbness, paresthesias, hyperesthesias, and pain. Pain is often worst at night, may be deep-seated and lancinating (pseudotabes), and usually is self-limited. Abnormalities of gait and the deformity of joints (Charcot joints) connote the involvement of proprioceptive fibers. Mononeuropathies are less common than are polyneuropathies and may manifest themselves as a foot or wrist drop, or a paralysis of the third, fourth, or sixth cranial nerve. Radiculopathy is a sensory syndrome in which pain occurs through the distribution of one or more spinal nerves, usually in the chest wall or the abdomen. Autonomic neuropathy may affect the gastrointestinal and the genitourinary organs and may also be responsible for hypoglycemic unawareness or the blunting of the usual adrenergic response to hypoglycemia (Table 7-10). Amyotrophy is another form of diabetic neuropathy characterized by severe weakness and the loss of muscle mass in the proximal legs and pelvic girdle.

TABLE 7-10. *SYNDROMES OF AUTONOMIC NEUROPATHY*

Cardiovascular neuropathy
    Orthostatic hypotension
    Painless myocardial ischemia and infarction
    Resting sinus tachycardia (fixed heart rate)
    Sudden death

Gastrointestinal neuropathy
    Esophageal dysfunction
    Gastric paresis—delayed gastric emptying
    Diabetic diarrhea
    Gallbladder atony
    Fecal incontinence

Genitourinary neuropathy
    Erectile impotence
    Retrograde ejaculation with infertility
    Atonic bladder

Hypoglycemic unawareness
    Blunted adrenergic response to hypoglycemia
    (Contraindication to intensive glycemic therapy)

Diabetic neuropathy results from the loss of function of both large and small myelinated nerve fibers. The nerve damage seen in diabetic patients is associated with varying degrees of paranodal and segmental demyelination, proliferation of connective tissue, and the closure of capillaries resulting from thickening and reduplication of capillary basement membranes. The connection between diabetes and the neuropathies is not clear, but three hypotheses are under intense scrutiny: the metabolic, the vascular, and the axonal hypotheses.

The metabolic hypothesis centers around the lower levels of myoinositol and elevated levels of sorbitol in nerves exposed to hyperglycemia. These changes result in decreased Na^+-K^+ ATPase activity, which may lead to nerve dysfunction and structural damage. Ischemic disease secondary to vascular closure plays a role in the pathogenesis of mononeuropathies and perhaps in other forms of neuropathy. The axonal hypothesis is based on the presence of early functional changes in axonal transport followed by structural degeneration. Although there is no specific treatment for the diabetic neuropathies, it is important to identify the presence of neuropathy so appropriate compensatory and protective measures can be implemented.

Robin has decided not to have another pregnancy now. She is worried about her renal function and the potential development of nephropathy. She will redouble her efforts to keep her sugars in good control and would like to start an ACE inhibitor in hopes of decreasing the progression of nephropathy.

A visit with her ophthalmologist confirms that background retinopathy is developing. She will have further testing to see if laser therapy is indicated. Now she has even more reason to keep her glucose in good control.

Robin is in the silent period of the development of diabetic nephropathy. She hopes that careful attention to her diabetic control and blood pressure will prevent the progression of neuropathy and, in addition, will stem the progression of neuropathy and retinopathy.

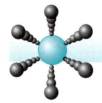

CASE PRESENTATION: CASE 2

Fatigue and hypertension in a 53-year-old man

Mr. James Howard, a 53-year-old real estate agent and father of three children, was seen for a routine checkup. Although his general health has not been a problem, he was noted to have an elevated blood pressure 18 months ago and was started on a diuretic (hydrochlorthiazide). His blood pressure was in the range of 120 to 130 over 86 to 90 when checked last month. He reports that tiredness and fatigue have been more notable lately, but he attributes these to pressures at work. He has been overweight ever since he left college. Like other members of his family, he has had a problem maintaining the weight loss he achieved after repeated diets. Currently, he weighs 212 lbs and is 5'9" tall.

Family History

Father died at age 63 of a myocardial infarction—he had his first coronary event at age 53. A 38-year-old brother was hospitalized 3 months ago with unstable angina and was found to have coronary artery disease.

Physical Examination

An overweight man with a protuberant abdomen and relatively thin legs and arms

Blood pressure: 142/94, pulse 88

The examination is negative except for the obesity noted above.

Laboratory Studies

Test	James Howard	Normal
Glucose (random)	284 mg/dL	70–110 mg/dL, fasting
Triglycerides (nonfasting)	364 mg/dL	<160 mg/dL, fasting
Cholesterol	244 mg/dL	<200 mg/dL
Sodium	142 mEq/L	135–145 mEq/L
Potassium	3.8 mEq/L	3.5–5.3 mEq/L
Chloride	103 mEq/L	98–106 mEq/L
Bicarbonate	25 mEq/L	21–30 mEq/L
BUN	12 mg/dL	8–22 mg/dL
Creatinine	1.1 mg/dL	0.3–1.5 mg/dL

After these laboratory results became available, Mr. Howard was asked to return to the lab in the morning, after an overnight fast, to obtain a fasting glucose and triglyceride measurement:

Test	James Howard	Normal
Fasting glucose	192 mg/dL	70–110 mg/dL
Fasting triglycerides	250 mg/dL	<160 mg/dL

Mr. Howard was instructed to set up an appointment to see the dietitian, and at the follow-up office visit later in the week, adult-onset diabetes was discussed.

Type 2 diabetes is a heterogenous disorder that accounts for over 90% of the diabetes in the United States. Both diminished tissue sensitivity and impaired B-cell function characterize the disorder. In fact, the defects in insulin secretion can lead to insulin resistance, and the presence of insulin resistance aggravates the B-cell defect. Early in their course, patients with type 2 diabetes usually have normal or elevated basal insulin levels with postprandial hyperinsulinemia that reflects insulin resistance. The insulin resistance of type 2 diabetes often is exaggerated by several other accompanying disorders that by themselves are associated with insulin resistance. Conditions associated with insulin resistance are listed in Table 7-11. As the disease progresses, as it does in most patients, the fasting glucose values increase and B-cell function is compromised. As the diabetic state progressively worsens and the hyperglycemia becomes more pronounced, the plasma insulin response to both oral and intravenous glucose diminishes progressively. The transition from normal to severe type 2 diabetes is depicted in Figure 7-9. The molecular basis of this impairment remains undefined.

The impairment of insulin secretion leads to continued output of glucose from the liver in the immediate postprandial period. This, when coupled with the decreased uptake of glucose by peripheral muscle, culminates

TABLE 7-11. *CONDITIONS ASSOCIATED WITH INSULIN RESISTANCE*

Obesity	Hormone excess states:
Hypertension	Glucocorticoids
Hyperlipidemia	Growth hormone
Hyperuricemia	Placental lactogen
Sedentary lifestyle	Catecholamines
	Thyroxine

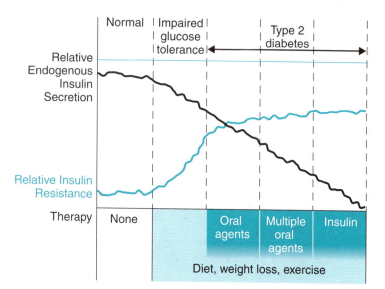

Figure 7-9. B-cell function and insulin resistance in type 2 diabetes. In type 2 diabetes, insulin resistance usually is combined with a decline in functional pancreatic B-cell mass. As this combination of abnormalities progresses, overt diabetes mellitus develops. Therapy at all stages is based on a combination of diet, weight loss, and exercise. As insulin deficiency and resistance progress, oral agents and insulin usually are added to the therapeutic regimen.

in severe hyperglycemia. In this setting, frank diabetes develops. Post-receptor abnormalities account for the insulin resistance in type 2 diabetes patients with fasting hyperglycemia. These defects cause a marked decrease in the transport of glucose into cells and an impairment at an unidentified intracellular step of insulin action. A defect at any given site of signal transduction could result in inappropriate insulin action or resistance.

For some patients, the presentation of clinical glucose intolerance may be precipitated by medications that affect glucose metabolism. Glucocorticoids and, as in Mr. Howard's case, diuretics may affect glucose metabolism in patients developing type 2 diabetes. By increasing hepatic glucose production and decreasing peripheral glucose uptake, glucocorticoids can increase glucose concentrations significantly. Thiazide diuretics decrease insulin secretion and may cause hyperglycemia in some patients. In others, an acute clinical condition (e.g., pneumonia, myocardial infarction, urinary tract infection, or gastroenteritis) can stimulate the secretion of stress-responding hormones that antagonize the effects of insulin and result in hyperglycemia.

By the time patients with type 2 diabetes, such as Mr. Howard, come to medical attention, fasting hyperglycemia is present, and the sequence outlined above has already progressed. Patients should be made aware of their diagnosis, instructed in the fundamental principles of management, and presented with a therapeutic plan. The vital elements of that plan are diet and exercise. For many patients with type 2 diabetes, an appropriate combination of nutrition and exercise is the only intervention needed to control the metabolic abnormalities associated with their disease. Approximately 80% to 90% of patients with type 2 diabetes are obese, and for these patients weight loss is the primary treatment goal. Caloric restriction that effects a reduction in weight of 5% to 10% reduces insulin resistance and improves glucose tolerance. Exercise enhances insulin sensitivity and increases skeletal muscle glucose uptake, not only during the activity but for several hours afterward.

Enhanced insulin sensitivity dissipates within 48 hours after exercise, so that repeated bouts of exercise at regular intervals help improve the condition. Exercise increases energy expenditure to create a greater caloric deficit than can be achieved with a hypocaloric diet alone. Aerobic exercise decreases abdominal or central obesity, the pattern of obesity associated with insulin resistance, hypertension, hypertriglyceridemia, and cardiovascular risks.

When patients with type 2 diabetes do not achieve near-normal glucose levels with nutritional therapy and an exercise program, pharmacologic treatment must be initiated. Oral hypoglycemic agents usually receive first consideration. The four classes of pharmacologic agents currently available are shown in Table 7-12. Sulfonylureas have been available for more than 40 years. They augment the secretion of insulin by B cells so that intact B cells are necessary for their effectiveness. Because sulfonylureas increase the amount of insulin that reaches the liver, these agents reduce the accelerated rate of hepatic glucose production and may reverse defects in the action of insulin. Metformin is a guanidine derivative that acts primarily to increase glucose utilization and does not stimulate insulin secretion. Another class of oral hypoglycemic agents, the α-glycosidase inhibitors, inhibit pancreatic alpha-amylase and membrane-bound intestinal alpha-glucoside hydrolase, thus preventing the hydrolysis of complex starches to oligosaccharides in the lumen of the small intestine and the hydrolysis of oligo-, tri-, and disaccharides to glucose and other monosaccharides at the brush border of the small intestines. In patients with diabetes, α-glucosidase inhibitors delay glucose absorption and lower postprandial hyperglycemia. The fourth class of oral hypoglycemic agents, the thiazolidinediones, affect glucose uptake peripherally and overcome insulin resistance. When oral hypoglycemic agents are ineffective, insulin therapy is initiated.

After several sessions of nutrition counseling, Mr. Howard begins to lose weight slowly. Moreover, he now follows an exercise program. Three months after his initial visit, Mr. Howard has lost 11 lbs, and his fasting glucose levels are all less than 120 mg/dL; most of his postprandial tests are under 200 mg/dL. His hemoglobin A_{1C} (normal = 3.5% to 5.6%) has fallen from 11.2% to 9.8%. He is no longer taking hydrochlorothiazide, and his blood pressure is 134/84.

TABLE 7-12.	*ORAL HYPOGLYCEMIC AGENTS*
CLASS	**MODE OF ACTION**
Sulfonylureas	Augment B-cell secretion of insulin; may decrease insulin resistance in target tissues
Biguanides	Primarily increase glucose utilization; do not stimulate insulin secretion
α-glucosidase inhibitor	Slows glucose absorption in the small intestine by inhibiting the splitting of disaccharides
Thiazolidinediones	Augment the effectiveness of insulin; reduce insulin resistance

For the next 6 months, Mr. Howard adheres to the nutrition and exercise program and feels better than ever. His weight is down to 196 lbs. His hemoglobin A_{1C} drops to 7.6%, and his triglycerides decrease to 212 mg/dL; his blood pressure is 132/82.

Four months later, Mr. Howard is promoted to an executive position that necessitates out-of-town travel. He finds it difficult to follow his treatment program. Within 5 months, he has not only regained all of the weight he lost, but now weighs 220 lbs. His glucose values are all above 200 mg/dL, and the Hgb A_{1C} is back over 11%. While traveling, about 1000 miles away from home, Mr. Howard became acutely short of breath and was taken by ambulance from his hotel room to the local hospital. Although he has never had any chest pain, his EKG shows evidence of a recent infarct, a finding confirmed by serial enzyme studies. Luckily, his course is uncomplicated and he is discharged after 5 days, committed to regain control over his diabetes.

Type 2 diabetes is accompanied by a high prevalence of premature cardiac, cerebral, and peripheral vascular disease. The risk for these macrovascular complications is magnified two- to seven-fold compared to age-matched nondiabetics. The relative risk for cardiovascular disease in women with diabetes is three to four times greater than that in nondiabetic women. Although diabetes is an independent risk factor, it often co-exists with other conditions such as hypertension, dyslipidemia, and obesity, all of which add to the risk potential. The accelerated atherosclerosis that accompanies diabetes is indistinguishable from that occurring in individuals without diabetes. Poor control of the diabetes aggravates the atherosclerotic process. When autonomic neuropathy also is present, the usual symptoms of coronary artery disease may not appear. The ischemia may, therefore, be silent and come to attention only when congestive heart failure or arrhythmias occur. Mr Howard's infarction was painless and was heralded only by the dyspnea of heart failure.

The cause of the accelerated atherosclerosis of diabetes is not completely understood, but multiple factors contribute to its pathogenesis. Abnormalities in lipid metabolism, hemostatic factors, and alterations in the endothelium and smooth muscle of blood vessels all play a role. Hyperglycemia directly and indirectly alters lipoprotein composition so that the lipid particles are more atherogenic. There is overproduction of very-low-density lipoprotein (VLDL) and low-density lipoprotein (LDL) particles and defective clearance of these particles. High-density lipoprotein (HDL) cholesterol, which is felt to protect against atherosclerosis, is reduced in such an environment. Increased platelet aggregation is another potential factor: platelets from diabetics have elevated von Willebrand factor and are more susceptible to aggregation. In addition, endothelial cells, which play an important role in arterial relaxation, may become dysfunctional in the presence of hyperglycemia. These and other undefined abnormalities related to hyperglycemia account for the excessive prevalence of myocardial infarctions, strokes, and gangrenous extremities that threatens every patient with diabetes.

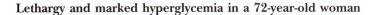

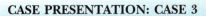

CASE PRESENTATION: CASE 3

Lethargy and marked hyperglycemia in a 72-year-old woman

Ms. Dorothy Lauer is a 72-year-old grandmother who recently lost her husband. She has always been in good health except for some arthritis in her knees and fingers. Six months ago, during a routine examination, a slight elevation of blood sugar was noted. Her fasting glucose concentration was 130 mg/dL, and she was advised to avoid sweets and to get her weight down by a few pounds. One month ago she developed some back pain, which was attributed to osteoporosis. Three weeks ago, she began to have a severe headache over her right temporal area that had a persistent, burning quality. Her scalp over that area became very tender. She had little relief from aspirin and acetaminophen. At the same time, she felt aching and stiffness in all her muscles, but especially those in the back of her neck, shoulders, and lower back. She was seen by her physician, who made a diagnosis of polymyalgia rheumatica. Her erythrocyte sedimentation rate was 130 mm/hr (normal: up to 25 mm/hr). A temporal artery biopsy showed arteritis, and prednisone (40 mg/day) was started with immediate results—both the headache and the muscle aches disappeared.

A week after the start of treatment, Ms. Lauer departed on a trip with friends to see the autumn foliage in northern New England. Her prednisone had been tapered to 30 mg/day. On the first day of the trip she noted increasing thirst, a constant dry mouth, and the need to urinate frequently. By the third day, she had a need to urinate hourly, and each trip to the bathroom also allowed her to satisfy an almost insatiable thirst. During the night she was up six to seven times to urinate. By the fifth day, she felt so tired and fatigued that she decided to stay in the inn while the others took a day trip. When they returned that evening, Ms. Lauer was worse: she was unable to get out of bed and appeared lethargic and confused. Her friends took her immediately to the local hospital.

Physical Examination

An elderly woman who appeared acutely ill and severely dehydrated. She was very sleepy and confused. She was not oriented to time and place, but, when aroused, recognized her friends.

Vital signs:	Blood pressure 100/62
	Pulse 108
	Respirations 12/min
	Body temperature 96.8°F
Skin:	Skin turgor is diminished
HEENT:	Lips and mucous membranes are very dry
Chest:	Clear
Heart:	Normal
Abdomen:	Decreased bowel sounds, no masses or apparent tenderness

Neurologic: **Mental status as above, little spontaneous movement but is able to move all extremities on command, deep tendon reflexes present and symmetrical but depressed, Babinski response negative**

Blood was drawn for laboratory tests, and an intravenous infusion of saline was started.

Laboratory Studies

Test	Dorothy Lauer	Normal
Glucose	1040 mg/dL	70–110 mg/dL, fasting
Ketones	Negative	Negative
Sodium	128 mEq/L	135–145 mEq/L
Potassium	4.0 mEq/L	3.5–5.0 mEq/L
Chloride	118 mEq/L	98–106 mEq/L
Bicarbonate	24 mEq/L	21–30 mEq/L
BUN	68 mg/dL	8–22 mg/dL
Creatinine	1.8 mg/dL	0.3–1.5 mg/dL
Hematocrit	56%	37–48% (female)
WBC	11,500/mm^3 with left shift	4300–18,800/mm^3

Because of persistent hypotension, the rate of intravenous fluid was increased and stress-dose glucocorticoids were administered. After 2 hours, Ms. Lauer had a minimal output of urine and a Foley catheter was placed.

Ms. Lauer's symptoms, clinical presentation, and laboratory data confirm a diagnosis of the nonketotic, hyperosmolar state. This life-threatening emergency can develop in patients with type 2 (non–insulin-dependent) diabetes and is analogous in some ways to the ketoacidosis of type 1 (insulin-dependent) diabetes. Ketonemia and acidosis usually are absent, however. Before the therapy with prednisone, Ms. Lauer's pancreas secreted adequate insulin to maintain her blood glucose levels below the renal threshold for glucose. Glucosuria and the resulting polyuria and polydipsia therefore did not occur, even though her blood glucose may have been elevated at times. The high doses of prednisone, administered for the temporal arteritis, aggravated her diabetes by increasing the rate of hepatic gluconeogenesis and simultaneously inhibiting glucose uptake and utilization by muscle and adipose tissue. Ms. Lauer's pancreatic secretory reserve for insulin was inadequate to offset the effects of the glucocorticoid (prednisone), and significant hyperglycemia developed. As blood glucose levels rose, the renal threshold for glucose was exceeded and glucosuria developed. A significant, volume-depleting, osmotic diuresis ensued.

The severe hyperglycemia seen in Ms. Lauer's case is a result not only of the overproduction of glucose and the underutilization of glucose, but also of a profound state of water depletion. In the days before her hospitalization, Ms. Lauer lost large quantities of free water, and her effective plasma volume became progressively depleted. In addition, an age-related decline in the effectiveness of the thirst mechanism may have resulted in inadequate fluid intake. Osmotic diuresis, in the face of poor fluid intake, quickly leads to volume depletion. Declining plasma volume results in decreased renal blood flow. Glomerular filtration is thereby reduced, and the ability to excrete glucose in the urine declines. The rising blood glucose concentration perpetuates the problem and allows a hyperosmolar state to develop.

This condition occurs most frequently in elderly people, many of whom have no previous knowledge of diabetes or who have had only mild glucose intolerance. This severe state of hyperglycemia often is precipitated by a stressful intercurrent illness, by prescribed medications, or by events such as vascular accidents, burns, or heat stroke. Some of the factors that can precipitate a nonketotic, hyperosmolar state are listed in Table 7-13. Patients become confused and lethargic as the hyperglycemia increases; profound weakness and coma follow. The neurologic picture may simulate a focal, acute cerebrovascular event or may be more generalized. Orthostatic hypotension, marked dehydration, and prerenal azotemia are additional clinical features.

Why ketogenesis and ketoacidosis are not present in the face of such severe hyperglycemia remains uncertain. Hyperosmolality by itself suppresses lipolysis, and levels of free fatty acids (the substrate for ketone production) in hyperosmolar coma usually are one-third of those seen in ketoacidosis. In most instances, small quantities of insulin are present, and the level of insulin may be sufficient to restrain ketogenesis. Glucagon levels in nonketotic, hyperosmolar coma are similar to those measured in diabetic ketoacidosis.

As her glucose levels rose, Ms. Lauer became progressively more lethargic and weak to the point that she was unable to drink. Severe dehydra-

TABLE 7-13. *PRECIPITATING FACTORS FOR THE HYPERGLYCEMIC, HYPEROSMOLAR, NONKETOTIC STATE*

Infections

Vascular accidents
  Cerebral
  Cardiac

Severe burns

Heatstroke

Acute pancreatitis

Medications:
  Thiazide diuretics
  Glucocorticoids
  Hydantoin
  Beta-blockers

Hyperalimentation

tion resulted, aggravating her mental confusion and disorientation. Maximal hepatic production of glucose rarely raises the plasma glucose above 500 mg/dL provided urinary output is maintained. Blood glucose values greater than 500 mg/dL indicate renal dysfunction, usually as a result of a reversible, prerenal mechanism—volume depletion.

After an hour, Ms. Lauer began to respond to the saline infusion; her glucose levels decreased to 754 mg/dL and her blood pressure rose to 100/74. As her urinary output increased, 10 mEq of potassium chloride was added to each liter of fluid. In addition, an infusion of regular insulin at the rate of 3.0 units per hour was started. Although the glucose values and osmolality continued to decline gradually, Ms. Lauer remained lethargic and was difficult to arouse during the first 24 hours in the hospital. After about 36 hours she became more alert and began to drink fluids and eat soft foods. Her blood glucose had declined to 234 mg/dL. On discharge she was given an injection of 20 units of NPH insulin and urged to see her primary physician the next day.

It is imperative that adequate fluid replacement be administered to correct hypotension and restore fluid volume. Usually, isotonic saline is the initial solution used, but in some patients, especially those with known cardiac disease, hypotonic saline may be a better choice. Careful monitoring for congestive heart failure is essential. Some clinicians advise measuring central venous or pulmonary arterial pressures when rapidly administering the large quantities of fluid needed for patients with nonketotic hyperosmolar coma. When hourly urine output exceeds 50 mL, or if serum potassium levels are falling, potassium should be added to the intravenous fluids. Although the plasma glucose values in the hyperglycemic, nonketotic, hyperosmolar state often are greater than 1000 mg/dL, relatively small amounts of insulin are needed to effect a rapid decline in glucose. The most important therapeutic factor is the restoration of an effective plasma volume and the subsequent reestablishment of normal renal function. Once renal blood flow is adequate, much of the excessive circulating glucose will be excreted. Insulin should be administered intravenously in hypotensive patients to ensure absorption and effectiveness.

Although Ms. Lauer was feeling very much better, she really did not like taking insulin shots and wondered if she would have to do this for the rest of her life. During a visit with her primary physician, the day after leaving the hospital, a random blood glucose was 218 mg/dL. Her prednisone dose was now 15 mg per day.

Six weeks later, both her prednisone dose and her insulin dose had been decreased to 10—10 mg of prednisone and 10 units of NPH insulin, and Ms. Lauer has been feeling well. A recent fasting blood glucose was 137 mg/dL. After 3 months and after a reduction of her prednisone dose to 7 mg per day, Mrs. Lauer was able to stop all insulin, and her blood sugars have remained in good range.

Ms. Lauer's hyperglycemia is now under control. The scenario described could easily be repeated, however, if levels of stress-responding hormones are again increased (endogenously or exogenously), but it is hoped it could be avoided by monitoring glucose levels carefully during times of stress or increased steroid dose. On a day-to-day basis, diet and exercise should control Ms. Lauer's diabetes.

KEY POINTS AND CONCEPTS

- The concentration of glucose in the blood is carefully controlled by a number of hormones and physiologic processes.
- Insulin, a protein hormone with a short half-life, is produced by the B cells in the pancreatic islets. Glucose stimulates the synthesis and release of insulin. The prime functions of insulin are to distribute glucose into cells and to promote the production of glycogen, protein, and lipids.
- Insulin and exercise are the principal factors in lowering blood glucose concentrations.
- A number of counterregulatory hormones (e.g., cortisol, glucagon, growth hormone, and catecholamines) work to maintain the blood glucose level in the face of decreased intake or increased utilization of glucose.
- Diabetes mellitus is the most common clinical abnormality of glucose metabolism and involves either the lack of insulin or the lack of insulin effect, or both:
  - When insulin is severely deficient (type 1 diabetes), it must be replaced to normalize metabolic function.
  - In states of decreased insulin effect or insulin resistance (type 2 diabetes), weight loss, dietary modification, exercise, and, for some patients, hypoglycemic agents usually return glucose metabolism to a more normal state.
- The complications of diabetes take many forms. Retinopathy, neuropathy, and atherosclerosis are among the most devastating. All can be decreased by good glucose control.
- Pregnancy is diabetogenic. Patients with preexisting diabetes require more insulin than usual when they are pregnant.

SUGGESTED READING

Atkinson MA, Maclaren NK. Mechanisms of disease: the pathogenesis of insulin-dependent diabetes mellitus. N Engl J Med 331:1428–1436, 1994.

The Diabetes Control and Complication Trial Research Group. The effects of intensive insulin treatment on the development and progression of long-term complications in insulin-dependent diabetes mellitus. N Engl J Med 329:977–986, 1993.

Franz MJ, Horten ES Sr, Bantle JP, et al. Technical review. Nutrition principles for the management of diabetes and related complications. Diabetes Care 17:490–518, 1994.

Lewis E, Hunsicker L, Bain R, Rhode R. The effect of angiotensin-converting enzyme inhibition on diabetic nephropathy. N Engl J Med 329:1456–1462, 1993.

Polonsky KS, Sturis J, Bell G. Non-insulin-dependent diabetes mellitus—a genetically programmed failure of the beta cell to compensate for insulin resistance. N Engl J Med 334:777–783, 1996.

Reaven GM. Role of insulin resistance in human disease. Banting Lecture. Diabetes 37:1595–1607, 1988.

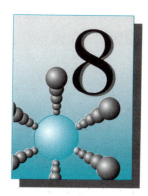

Lipid Metabolism

Lipids are fat-soluble molecules that are vital for normal cellular function but also are significant in the development of atherosclerosis, the leading cause of death in the United States. Lipid molecules, like cholesterol and fatty acids, provide a very efficient energy storage system, are essential for membrane function, and, in addition, provide the basic structure for steroid hormone synthesis. Lipids are ingested, synthesized, and metabolized by the body. A complex system of carrier proteins, apoproteins, transports these fat-soluble molecules in the aqueous circulatory system.

In addition to overingestion, abnormalities of lipid synthesis, transport, and metabolism are related to the development of atherosclerosis and a number of other abnormalities. Understanding, evaluating, and treating lipid abnormalities requires a clear understanding of the absorption, synthesis, transport, and degradation of these molecules.

ANATOMY AND BIOCHEMISTRY

The gastrointestinal tract is the site of fat and cholesterol digestion and absorption. The liver is responsible for multiple aspects of lipid metabolism, including the synthesis, degradation, and packaging of lipid molecules. Fat cells and capillary endothelium also are involved in lipid metabolism (Fig. 8-1).

Lipids are relatively insoluble in plasma and are transported in association with proteins. One example of the way in which lipids are transported in an aqueous environment is the binding of a free fatty acid, such as palmitic acid, to albumin. Cholesterol and triglycerides are transported as part of more complex lipoprotein particles. These particles are spherical and of varying size, with a hydrophobic core and a surface monolayer that is amphophilic, i.e., partly hydrophilic and partly hydrophobic, which promotes a stable oil–water interface. The core of these spheres contains cholesterol esters and triglycerides; the surface monolayer is composed of phospholipids, unesterified cholesterol, and apoproteins. Apoproteins are noncovalently bound to the lipids, and the resulting lipo-

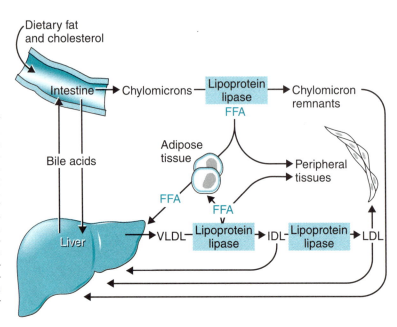

Figure 8-1. Overview of lipid metabolism. Dietary fat and cholesterol enter the circulation as chylomicrons. Under the action of lipoprotein lipase, free fatty acids (FFA) are released from the chylomicrons and become available for uptake by adipose cells, muscle, and the liver. The remaining chylomicron remnants are taken up by the liver. Very-low-density lipoproteins (VLDL) are produced by the liver. Lipoprotein lipase releases FFAs from the circulating VLDL, resulting in the production of intermediate-density lipoprotein (IDL) and low-density lipoprotein (LDL), which can be taken up by peripheral tissues or returned to the liver.

protein complexes vary in diameter from 10 to 500 nm. The characteristics of the major lipoproteins in human plasma are shown in Table 8-1. In addition to transporting lipid molecules, apoproteins play an important role in the distribution and metabolism of specific lipoproteins.

TRIGLYCERIDE METABOLISM

As much as 40% of the calories in Western diets come from triglycerides. During digestion, oral and pancreatic lipase hydrolyze dietary fat to monoglycerides and free fatty acids. These breakdown products of fat digestion are aggregated into micelles within the intestinal lumen and diffuse into the epithelial cells of

TABLE 8-1. LIPOPROTEINS IN HUMAN PLASMA

LIPOPROTEIN	PREDOMINANT CORE LIPID	DIAMETER	MAJOR APOPROTEINS, IN ORDER OF QUANTITY
Chylomicron	Triglyceride	80–500 nm	B-48, C, A-I, A-II, A-IV, proline-rich apoprotein
Very-low-density (VLDL)	Triglyceride	30–100 nm	B-100, C, E
Intermediate-density (IDL)	Cholesterol ester, triglyceride	25–30 nm	B-100, some C and E
Low-density (LDL)	Cholesterol ester	~21.5 nm	B-100, B-74, B-26
High-density (HDL)	Cholesterol ester	7.5–10.5 nm	A-I, A-II, C, E, D

the small intestine, where they are reconverted to triglycerides. These triglyceride molecules are coated with a monolayer envelope composed of five separate apoproteins—AI, AII, AIII, AIV, and apo B-48—all synthesized by the intestinal cells. The resulting structures, chylomicrons, may range from 80 to 500 nm in diameter and contain about 90% triglyceride, 1% cholesterol, 6% to 8% phospholipid, and 1% to 2% protein.

As chylomicrons pass through the mesenteric and thoracic duct lymph into the circulation, they lose phospholipids, apo AI, AII, and AIV, but take up apo CI, CII, CIII, and E. Apo CII is transferred from the high-density lipoprotein (HDL) particle, and its presence is essential for the activation of the enzyme lipoprotein lipase. This important enzyme is synthesized in parenchymal cells of various tissues but functions at the luminal surface of the vascular endothelium. Lipoprotein lipase hydrolyzes the triglycerides of chylomicrons immediately; the free fatty acids (FFA) liberated as a result are utilized differently in several peripheral tissues. In adipose tissue, they are re-esterified and stored, whereas in muscle they serve as sources of energy. The particle that remains after the hydrolysis of most of the triglyceride, the chylomicron remnant, contains cholesterol ester in the core and phospholipid, cholesterol, and apo B-48 and E in the surface monolayer.

Chylomicron remnants are removed from the circulation by the liver. The remnants bind to hepatocytes at apo E receptors and are taken up by absorptive endocytosis and hydrolyzed to yield amino acids, FFAs, and free cholesterol. As cholesterol from the chylomicron remnant accumulates in the hepatocyte, it suppresses the production of endogenous cholesterol by the inactivation of hydroxymethylglutaryl-CoA reductase (HMG-CoA), the rate-limiting enzyme involved in cholesterol synthesis. This is an example of negative feedback—the intracellular accumulation of a product (cholesterol) reduces the activity of the rate-limiting enzyme essential for its synthesis.

In hepatocytes, the carbon sources from a carbohydrate-containing meal provide building blocks for both synthesis of fatty acids and formation of glycerol. As a consequence, triglyceride synthesis is stimulated. These triglycerides are packaged by the liver as very-low-density lipoproteins (VLDL). The core of these VLDL particles is primarily triglyceride with a small amount of cholesterol ester; the surface membrane contains apo B-100, C, and E, as well as phospholipids and free cholesterol. VLDL particles are secreted by the liver and provide the majority of circulating triglycerides in the fasting state.

After they are secreted into the circulation by the liver, VLDL particles are cleared by the action of lipoprotein lipase (LPL) at the luminal surface of capillaries. The particles progressively lose triglyceride and become cholesterol-rich VLDL remnants, which, through further attrition of triglyceride, are converted into smaller, denser low-density lipoproteins (LDL). As with chylomicrons, the hydrolysis of VLDL is effected by lipoprotein lipase and requires the presence of apo CII; unlike the reaction with chylomicron remnants, the metabolism of VLDL remnants is slower and requires interactions with other proteins and enzymes. The conversion of VLDL to LDL usually requires about 12 hours.

CHOLESTEROL METABOLISM

Western diets provide up to 0.5 to 1.0 g of exogenous cholesterol per day, yet only 30% to 60% of the ingested cholesterol enters the cholesterol pool. Dietary cholesterol that is incorporated into chylomicrons ultimately is metabolized in the liver and is either converted to bile acids or secreted into bile. Most peripheral cells can synthesize cholesterol, but few cells can degrade it, so that special mechanisms are necessary to maintain cholesterol balance in these tissues. As noted, the LDL particles derived from VLDL deliver cholesterol to peripheral cells. Cells in such tissues as smooth muscle, the adrenal cortex, the luteal cells of the ovary, and fibroblasts have LDL receptors (apo B and apo E receptors) and use the delivered cholesterol in membrane formation or in steroidogenesis.

Among its many functions, the liver manufactures and secretes another lipoprotein—the disc-shaped, very dense, tiny particle, high-density lipoprotein. These particles contain phosphatidylcholine, free cholesterol, and apoproteins AI or E. After being secreted by the liver, HDL particles interact with the circulating enzyme lecithin-cholesterol acyltransferase (LCAT). This enzyme forms cholesterol esters by transferring fatty acids from HDL phosphatidylcholine to HDL free cholesterol. The cholesterol esters form the core of what now becomes the spherical HDL particle. The HDL particle contributes to reverse cholesterol transport, i.e., it carries cholesterol from peripheral tissues through the plasma to the liver, where the cholesterol can be removed from the body. This is the function that has given the HDL particle its reputation as the good cholesterol carrier. The liver plays a vital role in the regulation of cholesterol homeostasis. It secretes cholesterol into the circulation as a component of VLDL and into bile but removes cholesterol through its receptors for chylomicron remnants, LDL, and HDL. Genetic, hormonal, and dietary factors can alter these multiple hepatic functions and, consequently, also affect cholesterol balance in the body.

In summary, the plasma lipoproteins are soluble macromolecular complexes of triglycerides, cholesterol, and phospholipids and one or more specific proteins, referred to as apoproteins. These complexes are synthesized by the intestine or the liver. The apoproteins determine the fate of the several lipoproteins by targeting the delivery of lipids to specific tissues that possess specific receptors for the apoproteins. Plasma lipoproteins usually are divided into five major classes according to their density. They may be further classified on the basis of particle size, electrophoretic mobility, or apoprotein content (see Table 8-1).

DISORDERS OF LIPID METABOLISM

Lipid abnormalities contribute significantly to the development of atherosclerotic vascular disease. Lifestyle, diet, and genetic factors are the major contributors to lipid disorders. Obesity, lack of exercise, and excessive intake of cholesterol and saturated fat can, for many people, lead to the development of significant abnormalities of lipid metabolism. Other people, however, may have relatively low lipid levels in spite of obesity, lack of exercise, and high fat intake. Several clearly familial syndromes of hyperlipidemia have been described, and for some of these the metabolic abnormality has been well elucidated.

Excessive quantities of lipoprotein also can accumulate in disorders other than those that involve primarily the metabolism or defects in lipids or lipoprotein structure. These secondary forms of dyslipidemia may occur with endocrine diseases such as diabetes mellitus and hypothyroidism or may result as a consequence of other illnesses or drugs (Table 8-2).

TABLE 8-2. *SECONDARY HYPERLIPIDEMIC STATES*
Endocrine causes
Diabetes mellitus
Hypothyroidism
Acromegaly
Anorexia nervosa
Cushing's syndrome (endogenous or exogenous)
Glycogen storage disease
Non-endocrine causes
Renal disease
Alcohol
Dysglobulinemia
Antihypertensive therapy (e.g., thiazides, beta-blockers)
Estrogen or oral contraceptive therapy

Diet, weight loss, and exercise are the foundation of the treatment of lipid disorders. Lipid-lowering medications used adjunctively are helpful. They often are not very effective, however, unless combined with modifications in diet and lifestyle.

THE PHYSIOLOGIC BASIS OF CLINICALLY USEFUL TESTS OF LIPID METABOLISM

Inspection of Serum. If inspection of serum from a fasted individual reveals a milky opalescence, referred to as lactescence, triglycerides are likely to be elevated. The opalescence results because large, triglyceride-rich lipoproteins scatter light. If the serum appears hazy, that indicates a level of triglyceride above 200 mg/mL. Normally, chylomicrons are cleared from the serum during an overnight fast. The presence of chylomicrons is confirmed by a white supernatant layer that appears when the serum is permitted to stand for several hours in the refrigerator.

Cholesterol. Measurement of total cholesterol by standard techniques is essential in the evaluation of any lipoprotein disorder. The total cholesterol—both esterified and unesterified–is measured. This value includes the cholesterol in all the circulating forms of lipid. The level is not significantly affected acutely by food intake, and the patient need not be fasting. Although a range of statistically defined normal values usually is used in the interpretation of laboratory test results, recommended cholesterol values often are presented with an ideal rather than normal range. This reflects the fact that in many Western cultures the cholesterol levels observed in the population and the rates of vascular disease are significantly elevated.

HDL Cholesterol. HDL cholesterol can be measured by heparin-manganese techniques. The level is not much affected by recent food intake and can be measured accurately in the nonfasting state.

LDL Cholesterol. Although there are techniques that can measure LDL cholesterol directly, LDL usually is calculated based on total cholesterol, HDL cholesterol, and triglyceride concentrations. If the triglyceride level is <400 mg/dL, and if chylomicra are not present, the LDL cholesterol can be estimated by the following formula:

LDL cholesterol = total cholesterol − (HDL cholesterol + triglycerides/5)

Because the triglyceride concentration is affected significantly by recent food intake (see next section, Triglycerides), the level of LDL cholesterol should be calculated on the basis of the results generated on a fasting specimen. The National Cholesterol Education Program bases many of its treatment recommendations on the level of LDL cholesterol. A "desirable" LDL cholesterol is <130 mg/dL; a "high-risk" LDL cholesterol is 159 mg/dL or greater. In patients with existing coronary artery disease the treatment goal is an LDL cholesterol below 100 mg/dL.

Triglycerides. Triglycerides should be measured after a 12- to 14-hour fast and after 3 days with no alcohol intake. Triglyceride levels increase immediately after a meal and may take several hours to clear. Triglyceride clearance also is slowed by alcohol. In the fasting state, almost all triglyceride is carried by VLDL particles. Measurement of triglyceride levels is an important part of the evaluation of patients with obesity, diabetes, or possible early coronary disease.

Lipid Profile. Many laboratories offer a lipid profile, which usually includes total cholesterol, HDL cholesterol, triglycerides, and a calculated LDL cholesterol. Because triglycerides are part of most lipid profiles, the specimen should be drawn after a 12- to 14-hour fast and after 3 days without alcohol. If triglycerides are >400 mg/dL or if chylomicra are present, and in certain other clinical settings, it may be necessary to separate and quantitate lipoproteins on an agarose gel system.

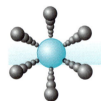

CASE PRESENTATION: CASE 1

Abdominal pain and lactescent serum in a 33-year-old man

William Leonard is a 33-year-old man who came to the emergency room with severe abdominal pain. The pain started about 4 hours before his arrival and was associated with nausea and vomiting. He described the pain as being "in the pit of my stomach." He tried antacids and a laxative, but nothing seemed to help. The pain radiated to his back and was slightly better when he sat up. The pain had started shortly after he left his brother's wedding reception. For the past several days he had been eating more and drinking more alcohol than usual.

Mr. Leonard works as a cook, and, although he has been overweight since high school, his general health has been good. Every day he walks to the luncheonette he owns with his brother, but he gets little additional exercise. Mr. Leonard's father and his father's brother both have diabetes and high cholesterol levels.

Examination in the emergency room showed an acutely ill, overweight man with a blood pressure of 100/66, pulse of 128, respiratory rate of 18/min, and temperature of 101°F. Basilar rales were present on the left side.

The abdominal examination showed diffuse tenderness on palpation, absent bowel sounds, and no palpable abdominal masses. On the dorsal surface of both forearms, pustule-like lesions with an erythematous border were present, consistent with eruptive xanthomata. A funduscopic examination of his eyes revealed lipemia retinalis.

Laboratory Studies

Test	William Leonard	Normal (Desirable)
WBC	16,500 with left shift	4300–10,800/mm^3
Hematocrit	52%	42%–52%
Glucose	254 mg/dL	70–110 mg/dL, fasting
Cholesterol	246 mg/dL	<200 mg/dL (ideal)
Triglycerides	18,500 mg/dL	<160 mg/dL (ideal)
Serum inspection	Grossly lactescent, white supernatant layer noted after overnight refrigeration	Clear, no supernatant layer after several hours of refrigeration
Amylase	1800 U/L	60–180 U/L

The presence of abdominal pain radiating to the back, with associated nausea, vomiting, relative hypotension, and significant abdominal tenderness, strongly suggests clinical evidence of pancreatitis. That diagnosis is supported by the markedly elevated amylase level. Although alcohol alone could be the cause of pancreatitis, Mr. Leonard's family history, the presence of eruptive xanthomata, and the extremely elevated triglyceride level point toward hypertriglyceridemia as the cause of his pancreatitis. Although the sample was not a fasting sample, the lactescent serum strongly suggests a severe hyperlipidemic state. From the family history of dyslipidemia, it can be assumed that Mr. Leonard previously has had elevated levels of triglyceride that were asymptomatic and undetected. At the reception, he consumed large quantities of fat in the form of cheese and red meat and drank alcohol-containing beverages. Each of these factors aggravated his hypertriglyceridemia, which, in turn, resulted in the development of pancreatitis.

Alcohol exaggerates the production of VLDL in individuals with primary hyperlipidemia. When metabolized, alcohol (ethanol) is converted to acetate. The acetate provided by ethanol metabolism leads to a reduction in the oxidation of fatty acids that usually would be required to supply acetate. These unmetabolized fatty acids are then incorporated into triglycerides. The added triglycerides increase the already expanded pool of triglycerides and overwhelm the available lipoprotein lipase. In addition, when Mr. Leonard ate fatty rich foods, chylomicron production by the intestine increased correspondingly. These chylomicrons were not cleared from the plasma because of the unavailability of sufficient lipoprotein lipase. Consequently, chylomicrons were deposited in the skin as eruptive xanthomas, were visualized circulating in the retinal veins (lipemia retinalis), and induced pancreatitis when free fatty acids were released in the capillary bed of the pancreas. When the concentrations of these lipids exceed the binding capacity of albumin, they lyse membranes and produce a chemical pancreatitis.

The elevated blood glucose, in this case, may be the result of acute pancreatic injury with decreased insulin secretion but also may represent early type 2 diabetes in this overweight man with a strong family history of diabetes.

Mr. Leonard was treated with intravenous fluids and nasogastric suction. He required large doses of narcotics to control his pain. After 48 hours his pain had decreased significantly, as had his amylase level. By 36 hours he was almost pain free and was able to tolerate clear liquids by mouth. His serum became less lactescent, and his triglyceride level fell to 852 mg/dL.

After 5 days of hospitalization, Mr. Leonard was discharged on a low-fat diet and was advised not to use alcohol. He also was made aware that weight loss, dietary changes, and exercise will be required to prevent this from happening again.

Although medications can be used to lower triglycerides, the foundation of effective therapy is weight loss, exercise, dietary modification, and avoidance of alcohol. In the treatment of patients with hyperchylomicronemia, saturated and polyunsaturated fat must be severely restricted because of the defect in clearing these fats. Once the acute pancreatitis subsides and the chylomicra are cleared from the serum, attention must be focused on the individual's total caloric intake. Mr. Leonard, like many obese individuals, most likely had an elevated level of VLDL triglycerides before the onset of pancreatitis. There is a positive correlation between levels of VLDL triglyceride and the degree of obesity, especially in people who gained weight during late childhood or adulthood and who are insulin-resistant.

When dietary management is ineffective and weight reduction fails to normalize the basal values of triglyceride, pharmacologic treatment can be

TABLE 8-3. *LIPID-LOWERING MEDICATIONS*

CLASS	MEDICATIONS	ACTION
Bile-binding resins	Cholestyramine, Colestipol	Interrupts enterohepatic cholesterol circulation, decreases LDL, increases VLDL synthesis
Nicotinic acid	Niacin	Decreases VLDL and LDL production, increases HDL production
HMG-CoA reductase inhibitors	"Statins," e.g., lovastatin, pravastatin, simvastatin	Inhibits the rate-limiting enzyme for cholesterol synthesis, decreases LDL
Fibric acids	Gemfibrozil, Clofibrate	Decreases triglycerides by increasing LPL (lipoprotein lipase) activity. Decreases secretion of VLDL, increases HDL

HDL, high-density lipoprotein; LDL, low-densiy lipoprotein; VLDL, very-low-density lipoprotein.

instituted. The commonly available lipid-lowering agents are listed in Table 8-3. Two classes of agents are used to lower triglyceride levels: niacin (nicotinic acid) and the fibric acid derivatives, clofibrate and gemfibrozil. Niacin acts by inhibiting lipolysis in adipose tissue and inhibits the secretion of VLDL by the liver. The fibric acid derivatives increase lipoprotein lipase activity and decrease VLDL production by the liver.

CASE PRESENTATION: CASE 2

Hypercholesterolemia in a 39-year-old man with a strong family history of heart disease

Walter Anderson, a 39-year-old insurance salesman and father of three children, had been in excellent health until 2 days ago. While playing tennis, he noted a tingling sensation in his left arm and transiently felt woozy. He decided to rest for a few minutes, and the tingling sensation and wooziness disappeared. Because of a strong positive family history of heart disease, Mr. Anderson sought medical attention the next day.

On further questioning, Mr. Anderson described other occasions when he had experienced left shoulder and arm discomfort during physical activity. A detailed review of symptoms was unremarkable.

Mr. Anderson's family history revealed that his father experienced his first myocardial infarction when he was 36 and died of coronary heart disease (CAD) at 43. Mr. Anderson's older brother, now 47, has had angina for more than 5 years and takes several medications for hypertension, in addition to nitroglycerin tablets for acute attacks of chest pain. Although he is not certain, Mr. Anderson thinks that other members of his family have high cholesterol levels.

Physical Examination

Height:	5'10"
Weight:	190 pounds
Blood pressure:	150/90
HEENT:	Normal
Chest:	Normal
Heart:	Normal
Abdomen:	Normal
Extremities:	3-cm soft protuberant nodule (xanthoma) of left elbow
EKG:	Normal

Laboratory Studies

Test	Walter Anderson	Normal (Desirable)
Cholesterol	310 mg/dL	<200 mg/dL
Triglycerides	120 mg/dL	<160 mg/dL
HDL cholesterol	30 mg/dL	>60 mg/dL
LDL cholesterol	240 mg/dL	<130 mg/dL (primary prevention) <100 mg/dL (secondary prevention)
Inspection of serum/plasma	Clear, no supernatant	Clear, no supernatant

The strong family history and the elevated total and LDL cholesterol levels suggest a diagnosis of the heterozygous form of familial hypercholesterolemia, an autosomal dominant disorder that is characterized by absence, deficiency, or defective internalization of LDL (B-100) receptors on the cell membranes of all tissues. Skin fibroblasts from the rare homozygous form of familial hypercholesterolemia have absent or defective LDL or B-100 receptors, so that affected individuals cannot normally bind, internalize, or catabolize LDL. The prevalence of the heterozygotic form of this disorder in the population is 1 : 500. Homozygotes with the disorder have higher cholesterol levels, usually above 600 mg/dL, and develop xanthomas in the Achilles and patellar tendons and extensor tendons of the hands in early childhood. These xanthomas appear as a fusiform mass in the tendon, often are painful, and represent infiltration of cholesterol esters into the tendon.

Eighty-five percent of men with the heterozygous form of familial hypercholesterolemia experience a myocardial infarction before the age of 60. CAD is especially prominent in individuals with low levels of HDL, probably representing a coincidental inheritance of the two traits. Homozygotes often develop fatal coronary disease as teenagers. Smoking and hypertension exacerbate the appearance of CAD. Levels of LDL cholesterol increase during childhood and adolescence, and the average level in heterozygotes at the time of diagnosis is 350 mg/dL. Triglycerides usually are normal.

Secondary causes for an elevated cholesterol must be considered even when the family history points to a primary cause. Among the disease states that are accompanied by elevated LDL cholesterol are hypothyroidism, nephrosis, monoclonal gammopathies, cholestasis, and anorexia nervosa. Hypothyroidism impairs the biliary excretion of cholesterol to a greater degree than it slows the biosynthesis of this lipid. Atherogenesis can be accelerated in myxedema. The metabolism of the LDL particle also is slowed in nephrosis because the surface content of the phospholipids is altered. Increased hepatic secretion of VLDL also may be a factor in the lipemia of nephrosis. Cholestasis is accompanied by the production of abnormal lipoproteins, which may account for the high LDL cholesterol noted in this condition. The elevated cholesterol of anorexia probably is a consequence of diminished biliary excretion. Patients who are found to have elevated cholesterol levels but do not have a strong family history must be evaluated for causes other than familial hypercholesterolemia.

A stress test showed fair exercise tolerance, but was stopped because of left arm pain and light-headedness. The EKG tracing showed evidence of active ischemia. Ten days later, cardiac catheterization showed three significant coronary artery stenoses, which were successfully opened with angioplasty. A follow-up exercise tolerance test showed marked improvement.

Six months later Mr. Anderson has been exercising for 30 minutes each day, has lost 15 pounds, and knows the cholesterol and fat content of most foods. He is making a major effort to lower his cholesterol and fat intake.

Laboratory Studies

Test	Walter Anderson	Normal (Desirable)
Cholesterol	265 mg/dL	<200 mg/dL
Triglycerides	105 mg/dL	<160 mg/dL
HDL cholesterol	28 mg/dL	>60 mg/dL
LDL cholesterol	216 mg/dL	<130 mg/dL (primary prevention) <100 mg/dL (secondary prevention)

Cholesterol intake should be reduced to less than 300 mg per day, and saturated fat intake should be less than 10% of the total caloric intake, because saturated fats decrease the clearance of LDL cholesterol. Lowering LDL cholesterol even further should prevent recurrence of significant coronary stenosis and may even reverse existing atherosclerosis. Although diet, weight loss, and exercise are the vital foundation for management of hypercholesterolemia, they often are not adequate to achieve significant reductions (>20%) in cholesterol levels. Further reductions often can be made with drugs that inhibit HMG-CoA reductase or with agents that bind bile acids and thereby reduce the cholesterol pool and increase hepatic LDL cholesterol clearance. The commonly available lipid-lowering agents are listed in Table 8-3. Inhibition of hepatic cholesterol synthesis and increasing cholesterol excretion often, when combined with diet, weight loss, and exercise, result in significant reduction in serum cholesterol levels.

Four weeks after adding pravastatin, 20 mg per day, to this diet and exercise regimen the following lipid studies were obtained:

Test	Walter Anderson	Normal (Desirable)
Cholesterol	176 mg/dL	<200 mg/dL
Triglycerides	125 mg/dL	<160 mg/dL
HDL cholesterol	27 mg/dL	>60 mg/dL
LDL cholesterol	124 mg/dL	<130 mg/dL (primary prevention) <100 mg/dL (secondary prevention)

After reviewing these results, Mr. Anderson has decided to become a vegetarian, thereby completely eradicating both cholesterol and saturated fat intake. In addition, although his brother warned him that it causes gas and constipation, Mr. Anderson has agreed to add cholestyramine to his regimen. He hopes that the changes in diet and lifestyle, along with these medications, will arrest or even reverse the progression of his coronary artery disease.

Mr. Anderson's children are having their cholesterol levels checked. Early intervention may prevent or delay the development of vascular disease in them.

The cases presented represent examples of lipid disorders in which great progress has been made in understanding the pathogenesis. Most lipid abnormalities are not as well defined, however, and probably are the result of a complex combination of heredity and lifestyle. The goal is prevention of vascular disease. Management of lipid abnormalities should be coordinated with reduction of other risk factors in an overall program of vascular disease risk reduction.

KEY POINTS AND CONCEPTS

- Lipids are transported in the circulation, associated with proteins in soluble lipoprotein complexes.
- Lipoproteins are spherical and vary greatly in size. Lipids, cholesterol esters, and triglycerides occupy the core, whereas the proteins compose the surface.
- The mucosal cells of the small intestine and the liver are the main sites of lipoprotein synthesis.
- The individual lipoproteins attach to tissues through their protein components, which are specific for receptors located on the surface of those tissues.
- Cholesterol and triglycerides are the two major lipid forms that are related to common clinical disorders. These disorders may have a familial basis or may be secondary to other diseases or medication, and are made worse by obesity, high-fat diet, and lack of exercise.

- Hypercholesterolemia predisposes individuals to vascular disease of the coronary, cerebral, and peripheral arteries. Hypertriglyceridemia predisposes to pancreatitis.
- Dietary and pharmacologic approaches, in addition to lifestyle modifications, are prescribed to correct dyslipidemic problems.

SUGGESTED READING

Eckel R. Lipoprotein lipase. N Engl J Med 320:1060–1068, 1989.

Shepard J, et al. Prevention of coronary heart disease with pravastatin in men with hypercholesterolemia. N Engl J Med 333:1301–1307, 1995.

Summary of the Second Report of the National Cholesterol Education Program (NCEP) Expert Panel on Detection, Evaluation, and Treatment of High Blood Cholesterol in Adults (Adult Treatment Panel II). JAMA 269:3015–3023, 1993.

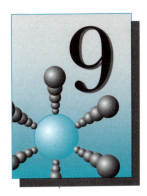

Reproductive Function in the Male and Female

From an endocrinologic point of view, the human reproductive system is a four-tiered system that includes (1) the central nervous system; (2) the pituitary; (3) the gonad; and (4) organs and peripheral tissues that are affected by sex hormones.

Central nervous system input is processed through the hypothalamus, where gonadotropin-releasing hormone (GnRH) is produced and released (see Chapter 2). GnRH stimulates the release from the pituitary of the gonadotropins, luteinizing hormone (LH), and follicle-stimulating hormone (FSH). These hormones, in turn, stimulate the production of sex steroid hormones and gametes by the ovary in the female and the testis in the male. An overview of the reproductive axis is shown in Figure 9-1. Gonadal sex hormone production results in the development of primary sexual characteristics in the male and in the development of secondary sexual characteristics in both sexes. Although there are clear and significant differences between the reproductive systems of males and females, there also are many similarities. GnRH and the gonadotropins, LH and FSH, are the same molecules in males and females, and both males and females have circulating androgens and estrogens. The relative amounts of these sex steroid hormones, however, differ markedly between the genders, as do the patterns of secretion. The hormonal differences between males and females are both quantitative and qualitative.

ANATOMY

Neurons in the arcuate nucleus of the hypothalamus are the source of the peptide hormone GnRH in both males and females. GnRH is the signal that activates the gonadal axis. The neurons that secrete GnRH are influenced by a number of neurotransmitters and hormones, including dopamine, prolactin, catecholamines, endorphins, and sex steroid hormones. The GnRH-secret-

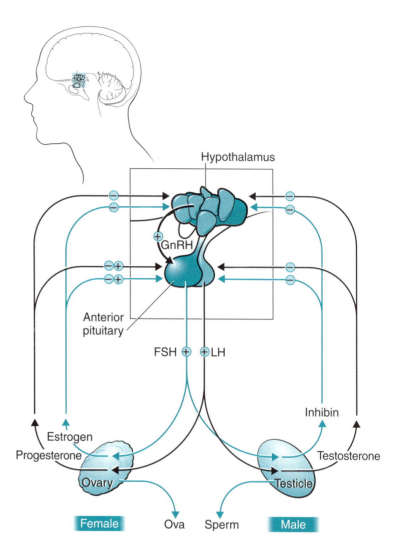

Figure 9-1. Overview of the gonadal axis. The release of LH and FSH begins at puberty and continues through adulthood. In the male, classic negative feedback loops control the production of testosterone and sperm. In the female, a more complex system, which involves both positive and negative feedback loops, controls ovarian function until the time of menopause, when ovarian function ceases.

ing neurons originate embryologically in the olfactory region of the brain and migrate to the arcuate nucleus. This neuronal relocation occurs in response to a specific protein, which must be present for normal development to occur. Once released, GnRH is carried by the hypothalamic–pituitary portal system to the anterior pituitary, where it stimulates gonadotrophs to synthesize and release the gonadotropins, LH and FSH (see Chapter 2). The gonadotropins, in turn, stimulate the gonads to make sex steroid hormones and to make gametes available for reproduction.

THE FEMALE GONAD: THE OVARY

The mature ovary is about $5 \times 2 \times 1$ cm and weighs between 4 and 8 g. The size and weight of the ovary vary during the menstrual cycle and decrease after menopause. The ovaries are covered by a reflection of the peritoneum called the mesovarium and are attached posteriorly to the broad ligament of the uterus

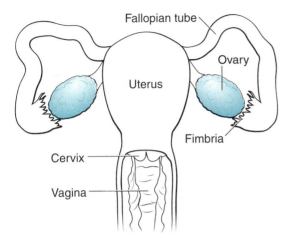

Figure 9-2. Gross anatomy of the ovary, uterus, and female duct system.

(Fig. 9-2). In addition to protection, the mesovarium also provides a conduit for the vascular and neural supply of the ovary. Vascular, lymphatic, and neural supply enter the ovary at an area referred to as the hilum. The arterial supply is derived from branches of the ovarian and uterine arteries. Venous drainage is into the ovarian vein. The ovaries are attached to the uterus by the ovarian ligaments and are adjacent to the ipsilateral Fallopian tube and fimbria (see Fig. 9-2).

An outer layer of columnar cells, the germinal epithelium, covers each ovary. Immediately below this cover is a layer of fibrous tissue referred to as the tunica albuginea. The bulk of the mature ovary is made up of follicles in various stages of development (Fig. 9-3). The innermost portion of the ovary, the medulla, consists of fibrous tissue, blood vessels, nerves, and lymphatic vessels.

The basic functional unit of the ovary is the follicle. A large, but finite, number of follicles are present at birth. These undeveloped groups of cells are referred to as primordial follicles and consist of an oocyte, arrested in the diplotene stage of meiotic prophase, surrounded by a layer or cluster of granulosa cells.

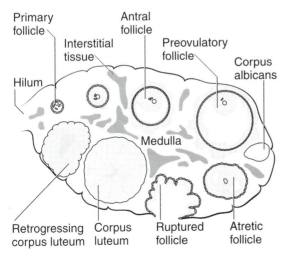

Figure 9-3. The anatomy of the ovary. Ovarian follicles in various stages of development are seen, including a ruptured follicle and a corpus luteum.

A basement membrane covers the granulosa cells and separates the follicle from other follicles and the surrounding ovarian tissue. A continuous process of frustrated follicular development results in the involution of many follicles, so that by the time of puberty, only about 400,000 follicles remain. Approximately 400 of these reach full development and release an oocyte during a woman's menstrual life.

The progression of follicular development is shown in Figure 9-4. As follicles develop, they enlarge with the formation of the zona pellucida, a membrane-like layer produced by the granulosa cells that surround the oocyte. When further development of a follicle is stimulated by the presence of gonadotropins, there is marked proliferation of the surrounding granulosa cells. Outside the basement membrane of each follicle is a layer of steroid hormone–producing theca cells. The thecal cells, in concert with the granulosa cells, produce estrogen. Inside the developing follicle, a fluid-filled space develops within the proliferating granulosa cells. As this space, the atrium or antrum, enlarges, the follicle reaches 2 to 2.5 cm in diameter. This is the preovulatory stage of follicular development. Eventually, ovulation occurs with rupture of the follicle and release of the oocyte. After ovulation, the atrial space is filled with blood, and the residual structure is referred to as a corpus hemorrhagicum. Blood vessels from the thecal layer invade the previously avascular granulosa layer. The color and function of the granulosa cells change after ovulation. The now yellow-colored structure, the corpus luteum, produces both estrogen and progesterone. If the egg is fertilized and a pregnancy results, hCG stimulation of the corpus luteum provides estrogen and progesterone to support the developing pregnancy. If no pregnancy results after about 14 days, the follicle becomes hormonally inactive and is replaced by fibrous tissue.

FEMALE DUCT STRUCTURES

In most species, a duct system provides a route for a gamete to be delivered to the outside world. In mammals, the role of this duct system in the female has been expanded and specialized to provide a site for the fertilization of ova and for the nurturing of embryos. The duct system, derived from mullerian ducts, includes the oviducts or Fallopian tubes, the uterus and its lining, the endometrium, and the vagina (see Fig. 9-2). Although these structures develop without hormonal stimulation, they are very sensitive to the effects of the female steroid sex hormones, estrogen and progesterone. The bulk of the uterus consists of muscular tissue, the myometrium, which is arranged around a central space, the uterine cavity. At the caudal end, the uterus constricts to a narrow cylinder, the uterine cervix, which is lined with mucus-producing cells and connects the uterine cavity with the vagina. The epithelial lining of the uterus, the endometrium, varies in thickness and in secretory activity during the menstrual cycle. The endometrium is very thin and inactive in the prepubescent and postmenopausal female. During pregnancy, the uterus expands significantly by a combination of passive stretching and cell growth. At the time of delivery the cervix dilates, and contraction of the myometrium results in delivery of the developed baby.

THE MALE GONAD: THE TESTICLE

The adult testicle is an ovoid mass with a volume of approximately 20 mL, an average length of 4.6 cm, and an average width of 2.6 cm. During embryologic

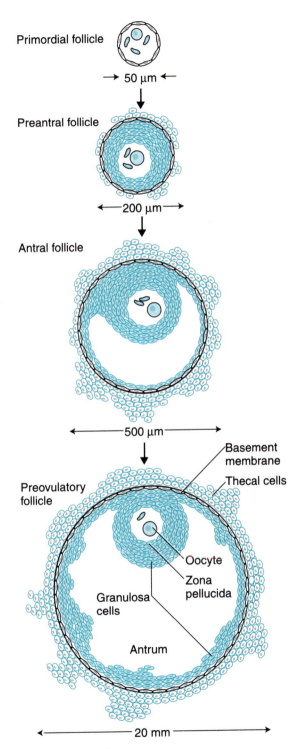

Primordial follicle

→ 50 µm ←

Preantral follicle

←—200 µm—→

Antral follicle

←———500 µm———→

Preovulatory
follicle

Basement
membrane

Thecal cells

Oocyte

Zona
pellucida

Granulosa
cells

Antrum

←————— 20 mm —————→

Figure 9-4. The sequence of development of the ovarian
follicle. Increases in cellularity and size characterize the
development of an ovarian follicle. Most follicles do not
progress to full development. Thecal cells in concert with
granulosa cells produce estrogen. Eventually, ovulation occurs, with rupture of the follicle and release of the oocyte.

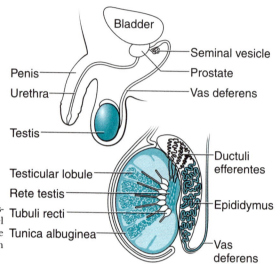

Figure 9-5. Anatomy of the male reproductive duct system and the testicle. Sperm produced by the testicles travel through the epididymis to the vas deferens. Fluids are added by the seminal vesicles and the prostate to form semen.

development, the testes descend from the abdominal cavity into the scrotum. The scrotum provides protection and keeps the testicles approximately 2°C cooler than the intra-abdominal temperature. The anatomy of the testicle and the associated duct structures is shown in Figure 9-5.

The bulk of the testicle is made up of seminiferous tubules, which are the sites of sperm production (Fig. 9-6). Sertoli cells line the basement membrane of these tubular structures, and the tight junctions between Sertoli cells form a barrier that provides a protected environment for sperm production. The Sertoli cells also provide a supportive environment in which sperm can mature. These cells also are the source of an androgen-binding protein that provides a high intratubular concentration of testosterone. This paracrine effect (i.e., a hormone having

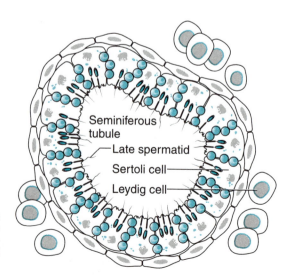

Figure 9-6. Cellular anatomy of the testicle. Sertoli cells line the seminiferous tubules. Spermatids mature in the protected and enriched space provided between the Sertoli cells. Leydig cells are interspersed near the Sertoli cells.

a special effect in the gland that produces it) is vital for spermatic development. The Sertoli cells also are the source of inhibin, a hormone that completes the feedback loop that controls spermatogenesis by inhibiting FSH secretion by the anterior pituitary.

MALE DUCT STRUCTURES

The path taken by sperm from the site of formation to the outside world and potentially to the duct system of a female starts with the seminiferous tubules. These tubules are highly convoluted loops that start and end at another duct structure, the rete testis. The seminiferous tubules are arranged in lobules and supported by fibrous tissue. Sperm move from the rete testis on to the epididymis through multiple ductuli efferentes, where ciliated epithelium facilitates their passage. The tortuous epididymis provides a storage and nurturing function for the sperm. During sexual arousal and with ejaculation sperm are expelled into the vas deferens and, eventually, through the urethra. The seminal vesicles and the prostate also are part of the male duct structure. These exocrine glands provide citrate and fructose that nourish and support the sperm. The final product of the testicles and the male duct system is semen, of which sperm constitutes about 10%.

THE HORMONES OF THE REPRODUCTIVE AXIS

HYPOTHALAMIC-RELEASING HORMONE: GnRH

GnRH is a polypeptide that is secreted in bursts into the hypothalamic–pituitary portal system. This manner of secretion allows a relatively high concentration of this releasing hormone to be delivered in pulses to the gonadotrophs of the anterior pituitary. The release of GnRH from the hypothalamus is controlled by a number of factors, including the neurotransmitters norepinephrine, which stimulates, and dopamine, which inhibits, release. Endorphins also decrease release. GnRH stimulates the secretion of both FSH and LH. The secretion of LH is consistently stimulated by pulsatile bursts of GnRH. FSH secretion also is under the influence of other hormones, including estrogen and inhibin, which inhibit FSH secretion. Because of these modulating factors, FSH secretion does not always occur in significant amounts when GnRH is present. GnRH has a very short half-life and is not found in significant amounts in the systemic circulation. For gonadotropin secretion to be stimulated, GnRH must be presented to the gonadotrophs in a pulsatile fashion, a process facilitated by its very short half-life. Continuous infusion of GnRH or administration of a long–half-life analogue results, after an initial episode of stimulation, in down-regulation that essentially shuts off gonadotropin secretion.

GONADOTROPINS: LUTEINIZING HORMONE AND FOLLICLE-STIMULATING HORMONE

Both LH and FSH are glycoprotein hormones that resemble TSH and hCG. These four very similar hormones share a common alpha subunit, but each has a unique beta chain that confers a distinct identity and function. Like other protein hormones, these glycoprotein hormones have relatively short half-lives. Although the names follicle-stimulating hormone and luteinizing hormone are taken from their effects on the female, the same hormones are present in the male. In the male, LH stimulates production of testosterone and FSH stimulates production of sperm.

ANDROGENS

Androgens are steroid hormones. In the male, testosterone and its reduced dihydro form are the principal androgens. In females, in addition to small amounts of testosterone and dihydrotestosterone produced by the ovary, weaker adrenal androgens and ovarian precursor molecules such as androstenedione and dihydroepiandrosterone (DHEA) and its sulfate may, if present in large enough amounts, have significant androgen effects.

The effects of androgens are seen in a number of different tissues. Skin appendages, e.g., sebaceous glands and hair follicles, are affected by androgens. At low levels, in both males and females, androgens stimulate the growth and maintenance of axillary and pubic hair and change the chemistry of sebum production, which may result in the development of acne. At higher levels, androgens stimulate growth of body hair and beard, while at the same time they inhibit scalp hair growth in many men. Muscle growth, laryngeal growth, and red cell production also are stimulated by androgens. In addition, these hormones may have important behavioral effects.

In males, testosterone is produced by the Leydig or interstitial cells of the testis. Testosterone also can be produced by the ovary or by the interconversion of various steroid molecules in body fat and other tissues. A series of enzymatically controlled reactions within the Leydig cells produces testosterone from cholesterol, the primary raw material. The cascade of androgen synthesis shares many of the components of the adrenal cortical biosynthetic pathway of steroid hormone production. Some testosterone produced by the Leydig cells is secreted into the seminiferous tubules, where it is bound to a protein made by the Sertoli cells. This reservoir of protein-bound testosterone provides the high local level of androgen effect required for normal spermatogenesis.

Once secreted into the bloodstream, testosterone circulates in both free and protein-bound forms. About 60% is bound to sex hormone–binding globulin (SHBG), a hepatically produced binding globulin. Some additional testosterone is bound to albumin. About 2% of the circulating testosterone is unbound and free to enter cells and bind to intracytoplasmic receptors. The testosterone-receptor complex—in a fashion similar to that seen with other steroid hormones, thyroid hormone, and vitamin D—enters the nucleus, precipitating changes in gene transcription. The corresponding changes in protein synthesis eventually result in the biologic effects of testosterone.

In most androgen-sensitive tissues, testosterone is converted to dihydrotestosterone (DHT), a more potent form of the androgen. Testosterone and dihydrotestosterone bind to the same receptor, but testosterone has significantly less affinity for that receptor than does its reduced counterpart. The prostate, scalp, and beard effects appear to occur only with DHT.

ESTROGENS

Although not required for the development of primary sexual characteristics in the female, estrogen is required for maturation of the female reproductive duct structures—the vagina, uterus, and Fallopian tubes. Estrogen also stimulates both the ductal and stromal development of the breast and leads to the distribution of body fat typically seen in females. In both sexes, estrogen mediates the closure of epiphyses that ends linear growth. Estrogen also stimulates the growth of the endometrial lining of the uterus and increases the production of vaginal secretions and cervical mucus. In addition, estrogen plays a role in lipid metabolism, calcium metabolism, and blood coagulation.

Estradiol (E_2) is the principal estrogen produced by the ovary. Like testosterone, it is transported in the bloodstream by the binding protein SHBG. LH and FSH stimulate production of estradiol by the coordinated actions of the thecal and granulosa cells. Levels of estradiol vary widely during the menstrual cycle.

PROGESTERONE

Progesterone is produced relatively early in the synthesis of all steroid hormones. Significant circulating levels are found only in the female, however, and only following ovulation, when ovarian steroid production is modified and a relative enzyme block results in the production and secretion of significant amounts of progesterone. Progesterone and similar synthetic compounds, referred to as progestins, stimulate glandular development of the breast and also induce secretory changes in the endometrial lining of the uterus. High levels, which continue to rise, are seen in pregnancy, and progesterone is vital to the establishment and maintenance of a pregnancy. Progesterone increases body temperature slightly and increases the ventilatory response to CO_2.

OTHER HORMONES

Inhibins are glycoprotein hormone products of gonadal function that regulate FSH production and secretion. Mullerian inhibitory substance (MIS) is a product of the Sertoli cell in the testicle that inhibits the development of the mullerian duct structures in the developing male embryo.

THE ANATOMY AND PHYSIOLOGY OF SEXUAL DEVELOPMENT

The developing mammalian embryo has the potential to differentiate into either the male or the female form of the species. The anatomic primordia for the development of the internal duct structures and the external genitalia of either sex are present in all embryos, regardless of genetic sex.

FEMALE EMBRYOLOGIC DEVELOPMENT

Female embryologic development is the default process because it is preprogrammed and does not require any hormonal signaling. The internal duct structures of the female, the uterus and fallopian tubes, are formed from the mullerian ducts (Fig. 9-7). Fusion of the lower aspects of the mullerian ducts results in the formation of the upper two-thirds of the vagina. This structure merges with the urogenital sinus, which provides the lower one-third of the vagina. The process of female internal duct development does not require the presence of a stimulating hormone signal and occurs unless inhibited by testicular production of MIS.

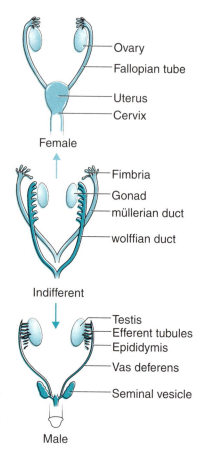

Figure 9-7. Progression of mullerian and wolffian ducts into the primary duct structures of the female and male. The female reproductive duct system from the fimbriae at the end of the fallopian tubes up to the lower one-third of the vagina is derived from the mullerian ducts. In the male, the wolffian ducts provide the epididymis, the vas deferens, and the seminal vesicles.

During the first few months of life, there is a low level of function of the hypothalamic pituitary ovarian axis in the female infant. Gonadotropin secretion is insufficient to induce ovulation and falls to very low levels by the end of the first year. Gonadotropin levels remain low until puberty.

MALE EMBRYOLOGIC DEVELOPMENT

The embryologic development of a male fetus, on the other hand, requires hormonal signaling provided by testosterone and MIS, both produced by the fetal testis. The differentiation of the bipotent fetal gonad into a testis is determined by the SRY (*S*ex-determining *R*egion of the *Y* chromosome) gene, which is located on the Y chromosome. The placental gonadotropin, hCG—a glycoprotein hormone that is very similar to the pituitary gonadotropins, LH and FSH—stimulates the fetal testis to function and to produce testosterone and MIS.

Testosterone produced by the fetal testis promotes the development of the wolffian ducts into the internal duct system of the normal male. The epididymis, the vas deferens, and the seminal vesicles are all derived from the wolffian ducts in response to the signaling provided by the presence of testosterone (see Fig. 9-7). Testosterone also results in the external virilization of the developing male fetus. External virilization, however, is only accomplished when testosterone is present in the reduced, more active form, dihydrotestosterone. 5-alpha reductase, an enzyme present in many androgen-sensitive tissues, converts testosterone into dihydrotestosterone. The presence of testosterone and its conversion to the dihydro form also are required for the normal development of the scrotum, prostate, and penis.

The fetal testis also produces MIS, a glycoprotein growth factor that inhibits development of the mullerian ducts and prevents the preprogrammed (default) development of female internal ductal structures—the uterus, fallopian tubes, and upper two-thirds of the vagina.

For the first few months following birth, the testes continue to produce some testosterone, stimulated by pituitary gonadotropins in response to hypothalamic GnRH release. After about 6 months, GnRH secretion stops and gonadotropin and testosterone levels fall to very low levels, where they remain until puberty.

PUBERTY

The mechanism for the dampening and essential inactivity of the gonadal axis from shortly after birth until the time of puberty is unclear. The pubertal process occurs over a 4- to 5-year period and is associated with several other events, among them hormonal, anatomic, and social changes. Early in the process of puberty, CNS inhibition of GnRH release declines, and the gonadal axis begins to function. In addition to the resumption of gonadal axis function that occurs at puberty, the pubertal process also involves increased androgen production by the adrenal cortex and a marked increase in the production of the growth factor IGF-1. The mechanism for the waking of the dormant gonadal axis and the increasing production of adrenal androgens at the time of puberty is not well understood. Age, body weight, nutrition, social setting, and genetics have been identified as factors related to the onset of puberty.

In both boys and girls, the first measurable indication of sexual maturation is a rise in DHEA-sulfate, a weak adrenal androgen. This change in adrenal cortical function occurs independently of the commencement of gonadal axis function. The axillary and pubic hair development seen in both sexes in early puberty is the result of adrenal androgen production. Later in the process of sexual development, gonadal androgens play a larger role, especially in males. The initiation and maintenance of axillary and pubic hair require relatively low levels of androgen. Much higher levels are needed for the development of male pattern beard and body hair growth. Increased axillary apocrine sweating and increased sebaceous gland function also are common androgen-mediated events that occur during puberty in both males and females.

As puberty progresses, GnRH secretion, as measured by gonadotropin levels, begins in nocturnal pulses that become more frequent and eventually occur throughout the day. The gonadotropins, in turn, stimulate gonadal maturation, the production of sex steroid hormones, and, eventually, the production of ova and sperm.

The growth spurt that is seen in both boys and girls at the time of puberty depends on the presence of sex steroid hormones. Sex hormones stimulate the production of IGF-1. Normal bone mineralization and epiphyseal closure in both males and females require the presence of estrogen. In individuals who lack either the aromatization enzyme necessary for estrogen production or a functional estrogen receptor, bone mineralization is deficient and, as a result of failure of epiphyseal closure, linear growth continues into adulthood. The importance of estrogen in bone development in males is underscored by the finding of bony abnormalities (e.g., decreased mineralization and failure of epiphyseal closure) in an otherwise normal male with a mutation in the estrogen receptor gene.

Female Puberty

Although an increase in growth rate—a growth spurt—usually is the first physical manifestation of the gonadal axis wakening of puberty in the female, breast budding, which occurs in the United States at a mean age of 9.5 years, is, for most girls, the first physical sign of the changes that are occurring. Estrogen produced by the ovary in response to FSH stimulation results in the initiation of breast development. At about the same time, development of pubic and axillary hair usually begins. During the next year of pubertal development in the female, there is an even greater rise in linear growth velocity. This growth spurt peaks before menarche, the onset of menstruation, which occurs, on average, at 12.5 years of age in the United States. The stages of female puberty are outlined in Table 9-1.

Although a small amount of linear growth and some additional breast development may occur after menarche, the process of female puberty is, from a hormonal and anatomic point of view, essentially completed by the first episode of menstrual bleeding. During the first year or so after menarche, menstrual periods typically are irregular and small in volume. Ovulatory cycles with regular episodes of bleeding usually begin after about 1 year, although menstrual patterns during adolescence can vary widely.

Male Puberty

The onset of puberty in the male is heralded by enlargement of the testicle. This is the first physical sign that the gonadal axis has again begun to function and that the process of puberty has started. As the testicles enlarge, testosterone production and secretion increase significantly, and, eventually, sperm production begins. The androgen-dominated changes of male puberty bring about an increase in muscle mass, male pattern hair growth, and laryngeal enlargement that results

TABLE 9-1. *THE EVENTS OF FEMALE PUBERTY*

EVENT	MEAN AGE (yr)	RANGE (yr)
Breast budding	11.2	8–13
Onset of pubic hair growth	11.5	8–13
Maximal growth rate	12.0	9.5–14.5
Menarche	12.5	10–16.5
Adult breast development	15.3	13–18
Adult pubic hair development	14.4	13–18
Regular menses	13.8	12–18

TABLE 9-2.	THE EVENTS OF MALE PUBERTY	
EVENT	**MEAN AGE (yr)**	**RANGE (yr)**
Testicular enlargement	11.6	9.5–13.5
Onset of pubic hair growth	12.0	10–14
Onset of penile enlargement	12.5	10.5–14.5
First ejaculation	13.5	12–16
Adult genital development	14.9	12.5–16.5
Adult pubic hair development	15.2	13.5–17

in voice change. An impressive growth spurt usually is also part of the process. Spontaneous or easily produced erections and nocturnal emissions of semen are common events in male puberty. The high levels of testosterone also lead to increased estrogen levels, which explain the gynecomastia that is commonly seen in early male puberty. The small nubbins of subareolar breast development usually resolve after a few months but can be an upsetting development that occurs in the face of a number of other significant changes. The events of male puberty are listed in Table 9-2.

ADULT GONADAL AXIS FUNCTION

In both the adult female and the adult male, feedback loops control gonadal function. The male system functions in a fashion that is similar to the hypothalamic–pituitary–adrenal axis or the hypothalamic–pituitary–thyroid axis. End products of the system, testosterone and inhibin, exert a tonic, negative feedback control over their own production. The female axis differs in at least three ways: (1) a complex interrelationship with both positive and negative feedback loops results in the creation of a menstrual cycle; (2) placental gonadotropin production, during the course of a pregnancy, takes over control of gonadal function; and (3) a preprogrammed failure of the end organ, the ovary, results in menopause and a syndrome of hormonal deficiency.

Steroid hormones of all classes—glucocorticoids, mineralocorticoids, androgens, estrogens, and progestins—are each produced by a series of enzymatically controlled, cytoplasmic reactions. Starting with either cholesterol, or, in some cases, acetate, the basic steroid molecule is formed. A number of different molecular modifications—side chain cleavage, hydroxylation, dehydrogenation, and aromatization—result in production of the various steroid hormones. Steroid hormone molecule production occurs exclusively in gonadal, adrenal cortical, or placental tissue, and these tissues share many of the same enzyme systems. The basic steroid hormone biosynthetic cascade has been expanded to include the paths of testosterone and estrogen production (Fig. 9-8). Minor, but important, modifications of steroid hormones can occur in peripheral tissues, especially the liver and adipose tissue. These peripheral modifications can result in relatively uncontrolled increases in androgen and estrogen levels in some individuals.

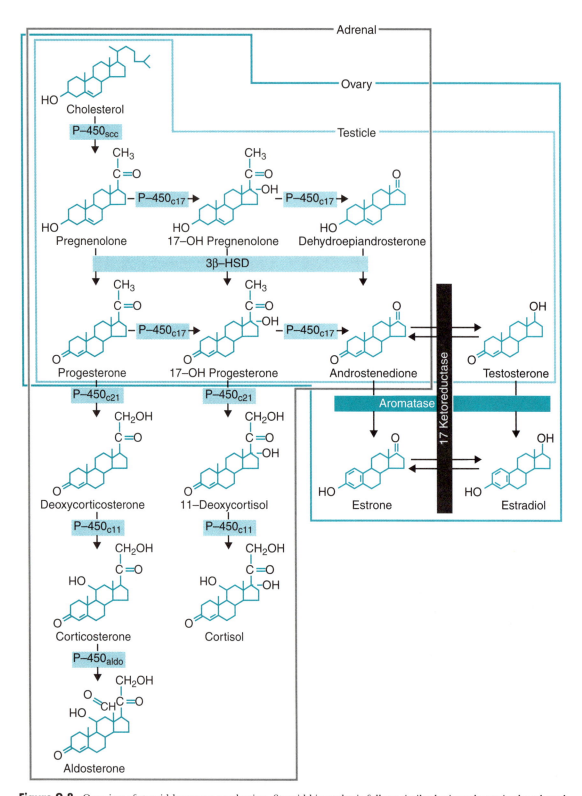

Figure 9-8. Overview of steroid hormone production. Steroid biosynthesis follows similar basic pathways in the adrenal cortex and in the gonads. The adrenal cortex lacks the aromatase and 17-ketoreductase enzymes needed to make sex hormones. The gonads lack the 21-hydroxylase and 11-hydroxylase enzymes required for production of glucocorticoids and mineralocorticoids.

FEMALE GONADAL AXIS FUNCTION

The Menstrual Cycle

The ovulatory menstrual cycle is the result of a complex series of endocrine gland and target tissue events. Although in some ways the time of menstrual bleeding is part of the previous cycle, it is associated hormonally with the beginning of a new cycle, and the dating of the menstrual cycle is based on the onset of menstrual bleeding, a clear-cut clinical event. The first day of bleeding is the first day of the menstrual cycle.

A number of significant events occur during the menstrual cycle (Fig. 9-9). LH and FSH enhance the development of a cohort of ovarian follicles. In a process that is ongoing from infancy until the time of menopause, groups of ovarian follicles are continually beginning to develop. The process that controls these attempts at follicular maturation is unclear. Most of these developing ovarian follicles do not survive and undergo atresia or involution. A few are rescued from involution by having matured to a certain level at a time when sufficient FSH and LH are present to foster further growth. In the process of being rescued from atresia, one or two follicles become dominant. Follicular domination is the result of a complex set of events within the follicle and the gonadal axis. When the LH receptors on the surface of the ovarian thecal cells are activated, steroid hormone production is stimulated (Fig. 9-10). Thecal cells cannot themselves produce estrogen, but they do provide the androgen precursors, androstenedione and testosterone, necessary for estrogen production. These androgens are converted into estrone and estradiol in the adjacent granulosa cells in a process that is enchained in the presence of FSH. In addition, FSH stimulation of the granulosa cell results in an increase in FSH receptors on the surface of these cells. The estrogen production that occurs in the developing follicles decreases pituitary FSH secretion by negative feedback. The follicle or follicles in which this process of estrogen production and FSH receptor induction is most successful survive and are able to maintain function in the face of falling FSH levels. Those follicles without a sufficient number of induced FSH receptors involute and atrophy in the face of falling FSH levels. This process usually results in the selection of one or two dominant follicles. The developing follicles are the source of the estrogen rise that is seen during the first half, or follicular phase, of the menstrual cycle. The length of this phase of the menstrual cycle can vary, but it usually is about 14 days.

The estrogen produced by the developing dominant follicle has a significant effect on production and release of LH by the pituitary. During the follicular phase of the menstrual cycle, estradiol stimulates the synthesis of LH by the gonadotrophs, but, at the same time, the presence of estrogen inhibits the release of LH. This simultaneous stimulation of production and inhibition of release leads to a significant storage pool of LH in the gonadotrophs of the anterior pituitary. Eventually, the storage sites become full and overflow with a massive release of LH, which occurs over a 24- to 36-hour period. This LH surge usually occurs at the middle of the menstrual cycle, around day 14, and triggers ovulation. At the same time there is a smaller surge in FSH release. Ovulation marks the end of the follicular phase and the beginning of the luteal phase, or last half, of the menstrual cycle.

The LH surge causes ovulation by the induction of prostaglandins, proteases, collagenases, and tissue plasminogen activators, which digest the capsule of the

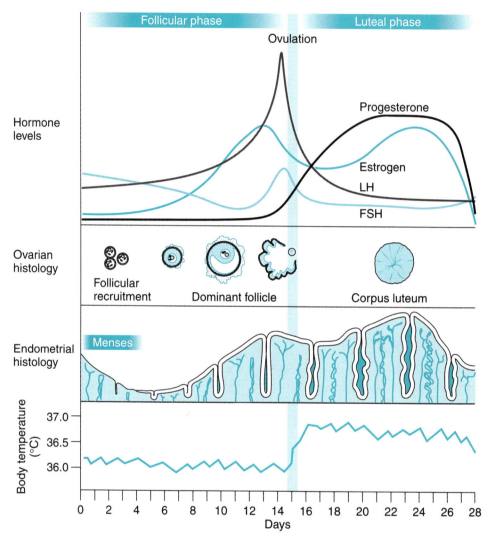

Figure 9-9. The menstrual cycle. Day 0 is the first day of menstruation. During the first half, or follicular phase, of the cycle, ovarian follicles are recruited and a dominant, estrogen-producing follicle develops. The rising estrogen levels stimulate thickening of the endometrium. At about day 14, a surge of LH triggered by the rising estrogen level results in ovulation. After ovulation, the remaining follicle becomes the progesterone- and estrogen-secreting corpus luteum. In the last half, or luteal phase, of the cycle, progesterone is produced together with estrogen. The endometrial lining becomes more vascular and secretory, ready for the implantation of a fertilized egg. Unless maintained by placental hCG, the corpus luteum fails, estrogen and progesterone levels fall, and menstruation results. The rise in basal body temperature at the time of ovulation is caused by the rise in progesterone.

ovary and allow extrusion of the oocyte. A surrounding group of granulosa cells provides support and protection for the oocyte. In the oocyte, meiotic division proceeds to metaphase II, where it is arrested until fertilization occurs. In addition to causing ovulation, the LH surge affects ovarian steroid hormone production. LH produces a partial 17-hydroxylase block. This enzyme block, relatively early in the biosynthetic pathway of steroid hormone production (see Fig. 9-10), shunts some steroid hormone production away from estrogen toward progesterone.

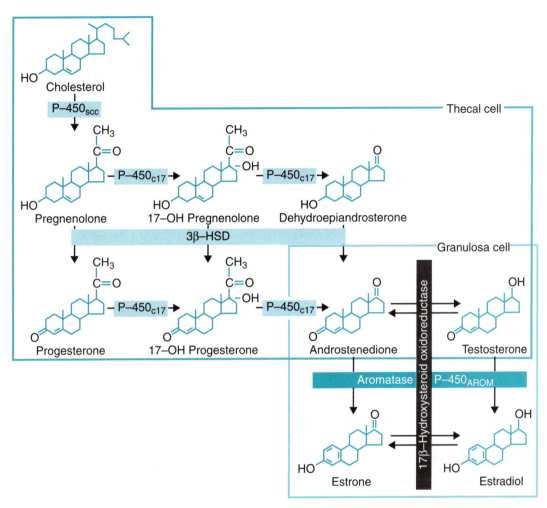

Figure 9-10. Ovarian steroid hormone production. The thecal and granulosa cells of the ovarian follicle work in concert to produce estrogen. Progesterone is produced after ovulation, when a relative 17-hydroxylase deficiency develops.

Whereas estrogen is the dominant sex steroid hormone in the first, or follicular, phase of the menstrual cycle, both estrogen and progesterone are found in abundance in the second, or luteal, phase. The presence of progesterone also induces a slight rise in body temperature that is maintained until the end of the menstrual cycle.

After ovulation, the dominant follicle becomes a corpus luteum, or "yellow body." The follicle becomes yellow as a result of the changes in steroid biosynthesis that occur after ovulation and result in increased progesterone production. The corpus luteum has a limited lifespan, and during the last 7 days of the cycle, it becomes less responsive to LH, resulting in a decline in production and secretion of estrogen and progesterone. If a pregnancy occurs, however, hCG, the placental gonadotropin, can stimulate the corpus luteum to continue to function, maintaining the hormonal and endometrial environment required for development of the embryo. In the absence of a pregnancy, the corpus luteum atrophies, estrogen and progesterone levels fall below those needed to support the endometrium, and menses occur. The low level of estrogen also signals a rise in FSH that begins a new cycle.

During the menstrual cycle, a number of changes occur at the endometrial level (see Fig. 9-9). Estrogen stimulates thickening and proliferation of the endometrial lining during the follicular phase. After being primed with estrogen, further changes in the endometrial lining occur with the addition of progesterone in the luteal, postovulatory phase of the menstrual cycle. Progesterone causes the endometrium to enter a secretory phase marked by further development of blood vessels and glandular formation. Once developed, the endometrium requires the continued presence of adequate amounts of both estrogen and progesterone. A reduction in the level of these hormones precipitates shedding of the endometrial lining, which is the onset of menstruation. When placental hCG production is adequate to maintain the corpus luteum, the continued production of estrogen and progesterone maintains an endometrial environment suitable for implantation of an embryo and for support of a pregnancy.

Menopause

Once the ovaries have been formed, the number of ovarian follicles is established—new follicles are not created. Only a few ripen to ovulation, and even fewer are supported for an extended period of time by a progressing pregnancy. Most follicles involute. The net effect, over time, of this process is menopause, the cessation of menstruation. The average age of menopause in the United States is 51 years, but the menopausal process for most women is heralded by a change in menstrual pattern in the 3 to 5 years before menstruation ceases completely. During this perimenopausal period, many cycles are anovulatory. Estrogen production usually is maintained, but the decreased frequency of ovulation reduces fertility and also results in the erratic production of progesterone. The change in progesterone secretion seen in perimenopausal women can have variable effects on menstrual pattern—for some women, the unopposed presence of estrogen results in endometrial hyperplasia with heavy, irregular bleeding, whereas for others menstrual bleeding may be scant and unpredictable. During this perimenopausal period, ovulatory cycles do occur on occasion.

Later in the approach to menopause, estrogen levels fall. Hot flashes—fleeting episodes of sudden warmth and, often, sweating—are indicative of falling estrogen levels. These episodes, in which body surface temperature rises by $2°$ to $4°C$ and core temperature falls by $0.2°$ to $0.3°C$, are an estrogen withdrawal phenomenon. Hot flashes are caused not by estrogen deficiency alone but by declining estrogen levels.

Hot flashes can be controlled by the administration of exogenous estrogen, but they will disappear after several weeks or months without any therapy. There are other, more permanent, changes induced by the lack of estrogen that occur at the time of menopause. The vaginal mucosa gradually atrophies, making intercourse uncomfortable and urinary tract infections more common. During the first 5 years following menopause, there is an accelerated loss of bone mineral content that increases the risk of osteoporosis and associated hip and spinal fractures. In addition, the relative freedom menstruating women have from atherosclerotic cardiovascular disease ends with menopause. The beneficial effects of estrogen on lipid metabolism and blood vessel function are no longer present. Estrogen replacement therapy, for many women, provides relief of hot flashes, reverses the development of vaginal atrophy, stems the loss of bone mineral, and decreases cardiovascular risk. Clearly, however, the risks of estrogen replacement therapy must be carefully considered. The risks and benefits of ERT must be weighed thoughtfully by each individual patient. The decision is often not easy.

MALE GONADAL AXIS FUNCTION

The function of the male reproductive axis is relatively straightforward compared to the events in the female. Testosterone production is under tonic feedback control by the hypothalamic–pituitary–gonadal axis. Although levels of testosterone vary moderately during a 24-hour period, usually reaching higher levels in the morning, the feedback control mechanism is similar to that seen in other glandular systems. Falling levels of free testosterone stimulate an increase in the synthesis and release of LH in response to GnRH stimulation. The resulting increased levels of LH stimulate Leydig cells to produce and secrete more testosterone, completing the loop.

When LH binds to the cell surface receptor of the Leydig cell, it triggers an increase in intracytoplasmic cAMP, which, in turn, activates the biosynthetic pathway for testosterone production. The series of reactions that result in the production of testosterone are shown in Figure 9-11. Some of the testosterone has local, paracrine effects in the testicle, providing the high local concentration of testosterone necessary for sperm production. The remaining testosterone is released into the circulation.

Sperm production is a continuous, self-sustaining process that is not limited by a finite supply of primordial substrate, as is the case in female oocyte production. Sperm production occurs over a 74-day period and requires several specific conditions, including spermatogonia, the support of Sertoli cells, a tubular structure in which to grow, a high local testosterone concentration, and a low temperature, $2°C$ cooler than the man's core temperature. Sperm production is stimulated by FSH (Fig. 9-12). FSH stimulation induces changes via receptors on the Sertoli cells that result in the development of the supportive environment necessary for sperm production. In the process of FSH stimulation and successful Sertoli cell function, a glycoprotein hormone, inhibin, which inhibits pituitary FSH secretion and completes the feedback loop that controls sperm production, is secreted.

Although there is some decline in testosterone levels and sperm count as men age, there is no dramatic cessation of gonadal function in men comparable to menopause.

OVERVIEW OF PATHOLOGY

Abnormalities in gonadal axis function can be divided into those conditions that reflect failure of normal development (*primary* failure) and those malfunctions that develop after the establishment of normal reproductive axis function (*secondary* failure). Primary gonadal failure can be caused by a large number of genetic, developmental, or anatomic defects, and the evaluation of patients with primary dysfunction requires a thorough understanding of the molecular biology, anatomy, and physiology of normal sexual development and function.

Secondary reproductive axis dysfunction can be caused by a failure of function at any one of the four tiers of the reproductive axis. Alterations in central

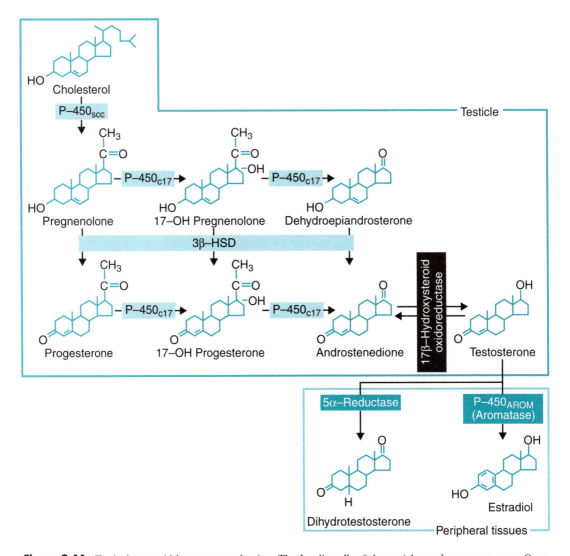

Figure 9-11. Testicular steroid hormone production. The Leydig cells of the testicle produce testosterone. Once secreted, testosterone can be activated in some target tissues to dihydrotestosterone. This more potent form of testosterone is required for many aspects of male sexual development and virilization. In both sexes, androgen precursors are converted to estrogens in peripheral tissues. The physiologic effects of testosterone are the result of the combined effects of the hormone itself and its androgen and estrogen metabolites.

nervous system input, either pathologic or adaptive, may result in failure of GnRH secretion and subsequent axis dysfunction. A hypothalamic tumor or drug-induced neurotransmitter imbalance can result in dysfunction. Adaptive shutdown of the axis occurs at times of stress, both emotional and physical, and is seen most clearly in states of malnutrition.

At the pituitary level, gonadotropin secretion often is the first function of the anterior pituitary to be clinically affected by an expanding lesion. Other functions of the pituitary often are preserved. Excessive prolactin secretion, the most common of the pituitary overproduction syndromes, often is the cause of shutdown of reproductive axis function. Dysfunction at the gonadal level may occur

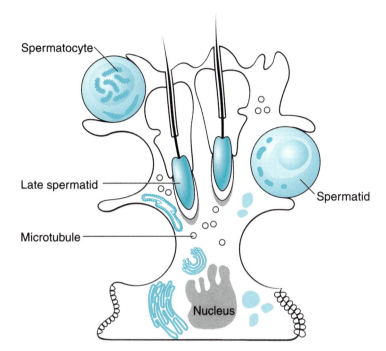

Spermatocyte

Late spermatid

Microtubule

Spermatid

Nucleus

Figure 9-12. The Sertoli cell. The Sertoli cells surround developing spermatids and provide a protected environment rich in testosterone, which is necessary for germ cell development. Sertoli cells line the seminiferous tubules, and tight junctions between Sertoli cells provide a blood–germ cell barrier.

as a result of trauma, infection, chemotherapy, or poorly understood changes in function. Reproductive duct function also can be disturbed by trauma, inflammation, or infectious processes resulting in abnormal menstrual bleeding in the female and in infertility in both sexes.

Syndromes of hyperfunction of the reproductive axis are relatively rare. Excessive pituitary gonadotropin secretion is very uncommon. Hyperfunction of the ovary or testicle is more common, but still very much less common than are syndromes of hypofunction. Premature puberty also can occur.

THE PHYSIOLOGIC BASIS OF CLINICALLY USEFUL TESTS OF REPRODUCTIVE FUNCTION

BOTH SEXES

Sexual History

A history of sexual development, behavior, and experience is extremely important in the evaluation of disorders of the reproductive axis. Awareness of concerns about sexual identity and adequacy, fertility, and contraception are important aspects of the evaluation and treatment of patients with reproductive axis dysfunction. A history of sexual abuse may make the evaluation of some patients very difficult.

Chromosomal Evaluation

A karyotype may be helpful in the evaluation of patients with primary disorders of the reproductive axis. A less definitive, but inexpensive and rapidly available, test can be done by counting the Barr bodies, nuclear clumps of inactivated sex chromatin, in a scraping of buccal or vaginal cells. When a large number of Barr bodies are present, an inactivated X chromosome is likely to be present. When no or few Barr bodies are seen, an inactivated X chromosome usually is not present.

FEMALE

Menstrual Calendar

A record of dates and descriptions of the pattern of menstrual bleeding and perimenstrual symptoms can provide helpful information in the evaluation of reproductive dysfunction. Breast tenderness and the character of vaginal discharge, when present, also provide important clues.

Basal Body Temperatures

In addition to a simple menstrual calender, measurement of body temperature on arising, before any activity, with an accurate and sensitive thermometer can be useful in charting ovulation and in helping couples effectively time intercourse. At the time of ovulation, there is a progesterone-mediated rise of about $\frac{1}{2}°F$ in basal body temperature that is maintained during the luteal phase of the menstrual cycle.

Pregnancy Tests

Based on identification of the unique beta subunit of hCG, samples of blood or urine can be easily evaluated to determine pregnancy. Kits that can provide a result within a few minutes are available for use at home, in the doctor's office or clinic, or in the laboratory. Pregnancy testing is a vital part of the evaluation of any woman with amenorrhea.

Follicle-Stimulating Hormone

Serum FSH levels are readily available. Low values are seen in prepubertal females, whereas high levels are seen after menopause. Because the concentration of FSH varies widely during the menstrual cycle, it is important, when possible, to correlate the level reported with the phase of the menstrual cycle.

Luteinizing Hormone

LH levels also are readily available and, like FSH, can vary widely, depending on the developmental stage of the patient and the phase of her menstrual cycle. In the evaluation of some patients, especially those with possible polycystic ovary syndrome (PCO), simultaneous LH and FSH levels can be helpful.

Prolactin

Prolactin, when present at higher than normal levels, inhibits gonadal axis function and should be tested early in the evaluation of menstrual abnormalities or infertility. Elevated values, unrelated to a medication or a pregnancy, should lead to further evaluation with MR imaging or CT scanning of the pituitary and functional evaluation of the anterior pituitary.

Estrogen Evaluation

Progesterone Challenge. Progesterone challenge is a test of functional estrogen level that can provide extremely helpful information at a very modest cost.

The testing strategy is based on the fact that exposure to, and then withdrawal from, a medication that mimics the effects of progesterone results in menstrual bleeding if the endometrium has been prepared by the presence of estrogen. Bleeding occurs in this test only if the following conditions are met:

1. The patient is not pregnant. A pregnancy test should be done before performing this test because there are potential teratogenic effects of progestin exposure.
2. The uterine cervix and the vagina are patent, allowing menstrual flow to be appreciated.
3. The endometrium has been exposed to enough estrogen to allow the administered progestational agent to cause the development of secretory endometrium.

A 5-day course of medroxyprogesterone, an orally administered progestational agent, 10 mg per day, is given. Two days after the last pill, bleeding is expected. When withdrawal bleeding does occur, it indicates that all the above conditions have been met. Lack of withdrawal may indicate pregnancy, blockage in uterine outflow, or estrogen deficiency.

Vaginal Cytology. The presence of estrogen results in changes in vaginal epithelium that can be noticed both by the patient and by cytologic examination. A history of vaginal dryness or dyspareunia and vaginal mucosal atrophy on examination indicate estrogen deficiency. A scraping of vaginal cells, prepared in the same fashion as a Pap smear, is an easy and inexpensive means of assessing estrogen levels. A cytologist can classify the vaginal cells and provide a functional assessment of estrogen effect. The more superficial cells are seen on the smear, the greater the estrogen effect.

Estradiol. Levels of estradiol and other estrogens can be measured. Although these tests are expensive and the values can vary widely, in selected clinical situations they can be helpful.

Progesterone

Because progesterone is produced by the ovary only during the last half, or luteal phase, of the menstrual cycle, measurement of progesterone levels following ovulation can provide evidence of ovulation and corpus luteum function.

Androgen Evaluation

In some cases of amenorrhea or infertility, and when hirsutism, or virilization, is present, an assessment of androgen levels is necessary. Because levels of SHBG are decreased in states of androgen excess, testosterone should be measured in both its bound and free forms. DHEA-sulfate is a relatively weak adrenal androgen that can be measured to explore a possible adrenal cortical origin of excess androgens. When hirsutism or virilization is evaluated, analysis of a 24-hour urine collection for 17-ketosteroids is an effective way to look for the possible presence of an adrenal cortical carcinoma as the source of increased androgen levels.

Pelvic Ultrasound

As an adjunct to a pelvic examination, a pelvic ultrasound study can provide important anatomic information. Uterine size and abnormalities can be assessed.

The width of the endometrium, the endometrial stripe, also sometimes can be determined, and the size and character of the ovaries can be assessed.

MALE

Testosterone

Testosterone circulates in both a bound and a free form. Accurate assessment of testosterone function may require assessing or estimating the effective or free concentration of hormone. The normal range of total testosterone concentration in the adult male is very wide (300 to 1000 ng/dL), and testosterone values in a single patient can vary somewhat over a 24-hour period. Borderline abnormalities should be evaluated with repeat samples. The total testosterone level usually is adequate in males, but, in some cases, measurement of the free testosterone concentration is vital in the elucidation of a clinical problem.

Luteinizing Hormone

Because LH stimulates the production and secretion of testosterone, LH levels are particularly helpful in evaluating hypogonadism. When paired with testosterone values, the level of LH can separate primary (testicular) from secondary (pituitary) or tertiary (hypothalamic) hypofunction.

Follicle-Stimulating Hormone

FSH stimulates spermatogenesis in males. Levels are elevated in cases of testicular failure or decreased sperm production resulting from a testicular-based defect.

Prolactin

Elevated prolactin levels can result in gonadal axis dysfunction and should be measured in cases of infertility and impotence.

Semen Analysis

In the assessment of the male reproductive axis, semen analysis can provide very useful data. A specimen, provided by masturbation into a clean, sterile vessel, should be produced at or near the laboratory so that it can be processed immediately. The specimen should be provided after 3 days without an ejaculation. The sample is evaluated for volume, pH, and number, motility, and appearance of the sperm.

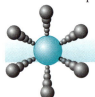

CASE PRESENTATION: CASE 1

Amenorrhea and dyspareunia in a 34-year-old woman

Eleanor O'Reardon hadn't had a menstrual period in over 6 months, but she was sure that she wasn't pregnant. She did not have the nausea and breast tenderness that had come with each of her three pregnancies. She has also had hot flashes that were very uncomfortable. She would suddenly feel incredibly hot and become very sweaty. Luckily, the episodes were short-

lived, but they were dramatic. She was not sleeping well, possibly because of hot flashes during the night. Intercourse had become very uncomfortable because of vaginal dryness. At age 34, she didn't think that menopause could be the explanation.

Ms. O'Reardon has three healthy children ranging from 4 to 10 years of age. Her menses started when she was 11 years old, and, after a year of irregular periods, she had regular periods until she became pregnant at age 23. Her general health has been excellent, and she is on no medications. She is a nonsmoker and uses only small amounts of alcohol and caffeine. She exercises three times a week for 45 minutes.

Her mother, aged 72, became menopausal at age 49 and recently was hospitalized for surgery to repair a hip she fractured when she tripped over a throw rug. Ms. O'Reardon's 38-year-old sister is still having regular menstrual periods.

A detailed review of systems is unremarkable. Her weight has been stable.

Physical Examination

Ms. O'Reardon is a healthy-appearing woman.

Height:	66″
Weight:	140 lb
Vital signs:	Blood pressure 110/70; pulse 88
HEENT:	Normal
Neck:	Normal, no goiter
Chest:	Clear
Breasts:	No masses, no galactorrhea
Heart:	Normal
Abdomen:	Normal
Pelvic:	Normal external genitalia, mild vaginal atrophy, healthy-appearing cervix
	Bimanual pelvic examination: unremarkable, ovaries not palpable, uterus normal size

Laboratory Studies

Test	Eleanor O'Reardon	Normal
Urine pregnancy test (hCG)	Negative	Negative, not pregnant Positive, pregnant

During the office visit, the results of the pregnancy test became available, confirming that Ms. O'Reardon was not pregnant. Ms. O'Reardon was given a prescription for five 10-mg tablets of medroxyprogesterone, a progesterone-like drug that can be administered orally. She was told that she might have a menstrual period 2 days after taking the last pill.

The facts that Ms. O'Reardon had clearly developed normally and that she has had three normal pregnancies significantly limit the diagnostic explanations for her amenorrhea. Ms. O'Reardon has *secondary amenorrhea,*

amenorrhea that develops after the establishment of a menstrual pattern. *Primary amenorrhea* is the term used to describe the lack of menstrual periods in a woman who has never menstruated. Pregnancy and menopause are the most likely causes of secondary amenorrhea for women in Ms. O'Reardon's age group. Pregnancy, in Ms. O'Reardon's case, seems highly unlikely, especially in view of her history and symptoms. She has none of the symptoms associated with her previous pregnancies and, unless fertilization occurred very recently or there is a laboratory error, the urine test effectively rules out pregnancy. A pregnancy test should be part of the initial evaluation of any woman with amenorrhea.

Ms. O'Reardon's amenorrhea is accompanied by classic symptoms of estrogen deficiency—hot flashes, sleep disorder, and vaginal dryness. Estrogen deficiency can be assessed in a number of ways. Estrogen levels can be measured, but, clinically, the easiest, and often the most helpful, method of assessing functional estrogen level is to use a progestational agent such as medroxyprogesterone. When withdrawal bleeding occurs in response to an exogenous progestin such as medroxyprogesterone, several important conclusions can be drawn:

1. Estrogen is present. The endometrial lining has been prepared adequately, by the presence of estrogen, for an episode of withdrawal bleeding to occur. Enough hypothalamic–pituitary–ovarian function is present to provide the estrogen needed.
2. Endometrium is present and the outflow path is patent. Menstrual flow is not blocked by cervical or vaginal stenosis.
3. A pregnancy is not present.

If withdrawal bleeding does not occur, estrogen deficiency is likely, unless, of course, one of the uterine conditions noted above is present.

Ten days after her initial visit for this problem, Ms. O'Reardon returned for a follow-up visit. She had had no bleeding in response to the progestin challenge. The following laboratory studies were reported:

Test	Eleanor O'Reardon	Normal
FSH	88 mU/mL	*Female:* Prepubertal: <5 mU/mL Pre- or postovulatory: 5–20 mU/mL Ovulatory surge: 12–40 mU/mL Postmenopausal: >30 mU/mL
Prolactin	10 ng/mL	5–25 ng/mL

The history, the physical examination, the lack of response to medroxyprogesterone, and the laboratory results indicate that Ms. O'Reardon has end-organ ovarian failure. Menopause, the cessation of menstruation, is a natural event in the life of a woman that occurs in the United States at an average age of 51 years. The finite number of oocytes present at birth are depleted, and new ones are not created. In Ms. O'Reardon's case, menopause is occurring at a very early age. Autoimmune oophoritis probably is the cause of Ms. O'Reardon's ovarian failure. As with the auto-immune destruction of other glands such as the thyroid and the endocrine pancreas, the ovary also can be destroyed. This form of premature men-opause usually is seen in women who already have exhibited autoimmune failure of another gland, such as the thyroid, the adrenal cortex, or the pancreas. Antiovarian antibodies can be measured, but the result would have no significant effect on the management of Ms. O'Reardon's case. Estrogen and progesterone can easily be replaced from exogenous sources. Another pregnancy, if desired, would require a major intervention and would probably involve the use of a donor egg.

Although the O'Reardons had decided several years ago not to have any more children, the loss of reproductive potential was, nonetheless, up-setting. In addition to the discomforts related to estrogen deficiency, Ms. O'Reardon was very concerned about her risk of developing osteoporosis. Worried that her mother's recent hip fracture meant that she, herself, would be plagued by brittle bones as she aged, Ms. O'Reardon came prepared to discuss the possibility of estrogen replacement therapy.

Although some basic concepts and guidelines regarding estrogen re-placement therapy (ERT) do exist, the decision process must address the individual needs, risks, and concerns of each woman. A careful risk–benefit assessment should be done when ERT is initially considered and must be reviewed periodically. Some aspects of the risk–benefit analysis are listed in Table 9-3.

Women with significant risk factors for heart disease or osteoporosis probably benefit more from ERT than those without such risk factors. Sim-ilarly, the risks of ERT itself must be individually assessed. A history of hy-pertension, venous thrombosis, gallstones, or migraine headaches might lessen the desirability of ERT for some women. A history of breast cancer is also, for most women, a reason not to embark on ERT. ERT appears to pose an increased risk of breast cancer for all women, but especially for those with a family history of breast cancer. The hope that routine examinations and mammograms will find malignancies at an early stage supports the need for increased vigilance on the part of the woman and her caregivers. For women who have not had a hysterectomy, the risk of endometrial carcinoma posed by ERT can be essentially eliminated with the concurrent administration of a progestational agent.

After reviewing the risks, Ms. O'Reardon decided to start ERT. She will continue to do monthly breast self-examinations and have regular mammo-grams. Because she has no family history of breast cancer, Ms. O'Reardon is comfortable with the small increase in breast cancer risk that is seen in women undergoing ERT. Frankly, it is the risk of osteoporosis and heart disease that worries her most. She has been to the health club once but plans to start aerobics four times a week later this month. Calcium supplements and a multivitamin are now part of her daily routine.

Three months after starting a continuous regimen of estrogen and med-roxyprogesterone, Ms. O'Reardon returned for a follow-up visit. The initial breast tenderness stopped after a couple of weeks. She had some vaginal

TABLE 9-3. *THE RISKS AND BENEFITS OF ESTROGEN REPLACEMENT THERAPY (ERT)*

BENEFITS	RISKS
Decreased hot flashes—improved sleeping	**Common, But Mild**
Less vaginal dryness—more comfortable intercourse, fewer urethral symptoms and urinary tract infections	Weight gain
	Breast tenderness
	Nausea
Improved cholesterol levels—increased HDL cholesterol, lower LDL cholesterol	**Intermediate**
Decreased vascular disease	Hypertension
Decreased risk of osteoporosis	Migraine exacerbation
? Decreased risk of dementia	Gallstones
	Endometrial cancer (not a problem if the patient has had a hysterectomy or if a progestational agent is used)
	Breast cancer—increased incidence
	Rare, But Disastrous
	Myocardial infarction
	Stroke
	Pulmonary embolus

spotting early in the treatment but has not had any bleeding for the past several weeks. The hot flashes have stopped, she is sleeping much better, and, for the first time in many months, intercourse is comfortable and more enjoyable.

On physical examination, her blood pressure is 130/80 and her breast examination is normal.

Ms. O'Reardon plans to revisit her decision regarding ERT each year, but for now, it seems to be the right decision for her.

ERT is an important option to consider in women with premature ovarian failure, at least until the normal age of menopause. The decision and the regimen should be reviewed each year, along with careful attention to risk factor modification. Patients with premature ovarian failure also are at risk for other glandular failure syndromes (see Chapter 11) and should be monitored for the development of other endocrine deficiencies.

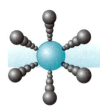

CASE PRESENTATION: CASE 2

Primary amenorrhea in an 18-year-old woman

Theresa Fleming has grown up and developed normally in almost every way. She is 18 years old and in her senior year of high school. She is captain of the swim team and had the lead role in the spring musical production.

Theresa seemed to go through puberty normally—she had normal breast development and was the second tallest girl in her class. She was a little concerned that she had never had a menstrual period, but her mother was even more concerned. Her mother had menarche at age 14, and her 13-year-old sister just started to have periods. Theresa has a steady boyfriend but has not had intercourse.

Past Medical History

Medical:	No significant illnesses
Surgical:	No operations
Allergies:	None
Habits:	No cigarettes
	Rare alcohol
	One caffeinated beverage per day
Medications:	None
Family history:	Unremarkable
Review of systems:	Noncontributory

Physical Examination

General:	Tall, healthy-appearing young woman
Vital signs:	Blood pressure 110/70; pulse 62
Height:	71″
Weight:	145 pounds
Skin:	Normal
Hair:	Normal scalp hair, absent axillary and pubic hair, very little arm and leg hair
HEENT:	Normal—full visual fields
Chest:	Clear lungs
Breasts:	Normal adult breast development; no galactorrhea
Heart:	Normal
Abdomen:	Normal
GYN:	Normal-appearing external genitalia, short vagina, no cervix visible
	Bimanual examination: No palpable uterus

Laboratory Studies

Test	Theresa Fleming	Normal
CBC	Normal	Normal
Glucose	88 mg/dL	70–110 mg/dL, fasting
T$_4$	8.8 μg/dL	5–12 μg/dL
TSH	1.1 mU/L	0.3–5.0 mU/L
Prolactin	24 ng/mL	5–25 ng/mL
Electrolytes	Normal	Normal
8 a.m. cortisol	24 μg/dL	15–25 μg/dL

Theresa Fleming has *primary amenorrhea;* she has never had a menstrual period. The differential diagnosis of primary amenorrhea includes all the possibilities that cause secondary amenorrhea, but a number of developmental and fundamental metabolic conditions also must be considered. Although Theresa looks quite normal to her family and schoolmates, the lack of sexual hair and the lack of a visible—not seen on examination—cervix or palpable uterus are the keys to understanding her clinical condition and planning further evaluation. A pregnancy test should be done because pregnancy is common in this age group and would explain the amenorrhea. The test is inexpensive and noninvasive, but it is highly unlikely to be positive, given Theresa's history and physical findings. A progesterone challenge is not indicated because it is not clear whether she has a uterus. Evaluation of pituitary function is always an appropriate consideration in the evaluation of primary amenorrhea (see Chapter 2, Case 1), but Theresa's normal growth and development, her normal tests of thyroid function and prolactin, and her normal 8 a.m. cortisol make a pituitary lesion less likely.

The lack of sexual hair indicates either a lack of androgen or an inability to respond normally to androgens. Further evaluation must include an exploration of her androgen status.

Additional Laboratory Studies

Test	Theresa Fleming	Normal

Testosterone	1232 ng/dL	*Male:*
		    Prepubertal: <100 ng/dL
		    Adult: 300–1000 ng/dL
		Female: 20–90 ng/dL

LH	22 mU/mL	*Female:*
		    Prepubertal: <5 mU/mL
		    Pre- or postovulatory: 3–35 mU/mL
		    Ovulatory surge: 40–150 mU/mL
		    Postmenopausal: >30 mU/mL
		Male:
		    Prepubertal: <5 mU/mL
		    Adult: 3–18 mU/mL

Buccal smear	<6% Barr bodies	Male: <20% Barr bodies Female: >50% Barr bodies
Karyotype	46,XY	Male: 46,XY Female: 46,XX

Theresa has normal male testosterone levels. The low number of Barr bodies suggests that she has only one X chromosome. The karyotype confirms a normal male genotype.

Often referred to as the hairless woman syndrome, Theresa has *testicular feminization,* a syndrome that is based on a lack of sensitivity to androgens. Individuals with this condition are genetically male but phenotypically and socially female. Target tissue resistance to androgens can explain all of the findings seen in women with this syndrome.

The presence of the SRY gene on the Y chromosome leads to the differentiation of the fetal gonad into a testis. During embryologic development, hCG stimulation of the fetal testis results in the production of both testosterone and MIS. MIS inhibits the development of the mullerian ducts and thereby prevents the preprogrammed development of female internal duct structures—the uterus, fallopian tubes, and upper two-thirds of the vagina. The testosterone needed to bring about wolffian duct development and external virilization is present, but in patients with testicular feminization, the receptors for testosterone are either absent or nonfunctional. Because of this lack of functional testosterone receptors, neither the internal nor the external male genital tract structures develop, and the preprogrammed development of a fetus with female external genitalia proceeds.

At the time of puberty, the testicles, which remain in an intra-abdominal location, begin producing testosterone. The levels of testosterone usually are at the high end of the normal male range and are, on occasion, even higher than normal. There is, however, no testosterone effect because of the receptor defect. The receptor defect itself, at the level of the hypothalamus and pituitary, results in increased testosterone production as a result of the lack of negative feedback. Some of the testosterone is aromatized in fat cells and in the liver to estrogen at levels that result in normal female breast development and body fat distribution. The estrogen also provides the sex hormone necessary for normal bone growth and epiphyseal closure during puberty.

Although patients with this syndrome are genetically male, their general and external genital appearance is clearly female. Their breast development and body fat distribution are also those of a normal female. Although they are infertile, such individuals appear to be normal females.

Because intra-abdominal testes have a significant potential for malignancy, they should be removed. This removal results in testosterone depletion, and adrenal androgens are not able to supply enough estrogen precursors to maintain adequate estrogenization; therefore, estrogen replacement therapy should follow gonad removal. Because the lower third of the vagina may not be adequate for intercourse, vaginoplasty or, for some patients, vaginal dilators can be used to elongate the vagina. Age-appropriate counseling and education also are a vital part of the management of this condition, both at the time of diagnosis and through the course of the patient's management. Infertility and questions of sexual identity and function are major issues that usually need to be addressed.

Theresa's spring vacation wasn't much fun. She underwent exploratory surgery with the removal of her gonads and at the same time had a vaginoplasty procedure. She tolerated the procedures well and is now on estrogen replacement therapy.

She is excited about starting college in the fall. During her winter break Theresa will return for a checkup and more discussion.

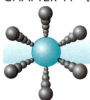

A 17-year-old male who has not yet gone through puberty

Charlie Goddard's visit to the medical center was prompted by his need for a pre-college physical. In addition to his immunization records and past medical history, the school form called for a physical examination. Charlie is 17 years old and, although he feels well, there are a few things he wanted to discuss with his doctor.

He could not help noticing in the shower room after basketball practice that his body was different from those of his classmates. Charlie had some axillary and pubic hair, but it was clearly less than his peers. His penis and scrotum also appeared smaller. Of greatest concern to Charlie were the nubbins of breast tissue that had developed when he was about 13 years old. Charlie has not been active sexually and has not had erections or nocturnal emissions.

Charlie had grown up and developed normally, but he never really had an adolescent growth spurt—he just seemed to keep on growing slowly. His pants and sport coat sleeves had to be lengthened every 4 to 6 months.

Past Medical History

Illnesses:	None of significance
Surgery:	None
Allergies:	None
Medications:	None
Habits:	Caffeine: None
	Alcohol: None
	Nicotine: None
	Recreational drugs: None
Family history:	Negative
Review of systems:	Negative

Physical Examination
Tall, thin, young man

Height:	73 inches
Arm span:	74 inches
Weight:	148 pounds
Vital signs:	Blood pressure 110/70; pulse 68
Skin:	Normal
Hair:	Scant axillary and pubic hair
HEENT:	Normal
Chest:	Normal
Breasts:	Moderate gynecomastia—nubbins of firm tissue, 3 cm in diameter, beneath each nipple
Heart:	Normal
Abdomen:	Normal
Genitals:	Small penis—4.5 cm in length
	Testes—1.5 × 1 × 1 cm, bilaterally and very firm
Extremities:	Long, thin arms and legs

Laboratory Studies

Test	Charles Goddard	Normal
CBC	Normal	Normal
Testosterone (total)	115 ng/dL	Adult male: 300–1000 ng/dL
LH	42 mU/mL	*Male:* Prepubertal: <5 mU/mL Adult: 3–18 mU/mL

Even though he is 17 years old, Charlie appears to have completed only the very first stages of puberty. His small, firm testes are the clinical clue to his problem. Normally, increasing testicular volume is the first physical manifestation of puberty in males. The low testosterone level provides laboratory confirmation of his clinical androgen deficiency. The elevated LH value points to testicular failure as the etiology.

Many of the clinical features of Kleinfelter's syndrome are present in this case—limited pubertal development, small firm testes, gynecomastia, and continued slow growth without a clear adolescent growth spurt.

When Charlie returned to the office to pick up his college health form, he was told that additional tests were necessary. A buccal smear—a scraping of the buccal mucosa with a tongue blade—was done, and blood for a karyotype was drawn. Charlie made a follow-up appointment to discuss the results of all the testing the following week.

Test	Charles Goddard	Normal
Buccal smear	59% Barr bodies	Female: >50% Barr bodies Male: <20% Barr bodies
Karyotype	47,XXY	Male: 46,XY Female: 46,XX

Results

The buccal smear shows Charlie to have a level of Barr bodies consistent with a normal female, indicating that Charlie has an extra X chromosome. The karyotype confirmed the diagnosis, showing a 47,XXY pattern. Charles Goddard's clinical presentation and the laboratory results generated so far are diagnostic of Kleinfelter's syndrome.

Maternal meiotic nondisjunction, which results in an egg with two X chromosomes, is the most common cause of this syndrome. The presence of a Y chromosome provides the SRY gene necessary for gonadal differentiation into a testis. Enough fetal testicular function is present to provide the MIS and testosterone necessary for regression of internal female reproductive ducts and for external masculinization. The testicle in a patient with Kleinfelter's syndrome is not able to support normal adult male function, however. When testicular biopsy is done, it shows fibrosis and hyalinization, with obliteration of seminiferous tubules. Leydig cells are present and may appear hyperplastic but usually are hypofunctional. Testosterone levels in men with Kleinfelter's syndrome can vary widely, with some even extending into the lower limits of the normal male range. The Leydig cells of men with Kleinfelter's syndrome are known to produce estrogenic compounds. These estrogens contribute to the development of gynecomastia.

Charlie was relieved to hear that something could be done to address his concerns. Hormonal therapy would give him a more masculine appearance, with increased muscle mass, increased body hair, and some enlargement of his penis. Silicone testicular prostheses could be implanted to give his scrotum a more normal appearance. The gynecomastia might improve with hormonal therapy, but, if it does not, surgical removal of the extra tissue is possible.

Charlie is going to start on relatively low doses of testosterone by injection. Because an injection of testosterone is given every 3 to 4 weeks, he will be able to have four shots before he leaves for college. The plan is to increase the dose gradually over the first 6 to 12 months of therapy. Follow-up care can be arranged with his college health service, and, eventually, Charlie can decide whether to continue the shots. He may opt to learn to administer the shots himself, or try a skin-patch preparation for hormone delivery.

Puberty is a complex process of physical, emotional, and social change. Androgen levels suddenly increasing into the normal adult male range can precipitate a number of dramatic developments, including acne, spontaneous erections, and changes in voice and personality. It is hoped that the initiation of puberty for Charlie will be a gentle process. Replacement testosterone therapy usually is continued indefinitely in patients with Kleinfelter's syndrome. In addition to bringing testosterone levels into the normal male range, this therapy lowers LH secretion and thereby decreases Leydig cell stimulation, which should decrease estrogen production and relieve some of the gynecomastia. Cosmetic procedures to decrease residual gynecomastia and to increase scrotal volume can be very helpful for some patients.

Orally administered testosterone is rapidly degraded by the liver. Modification of the molecule—methylation—decreases this rapid metabolism, but the modified testosterone molecule has been associated with hepatic abnormalities and hepatomas. Two transdermal systems for administration of testosterone are available. One version, which must be worn on the scrotum, may be difficult to use for men whose hypogonadism is associated with a small scrotal area. The other patch may be worn anywhere on the skin, and, aside from some problems with skin irritation at the site of the patch, works well for some men. The traditional method of testosterone replacement has been to place an ester of testosterone—ciprionate or enanthate—in an oil and inject the suspension intramuscularly. The testosterone diffuses from the oil over 2 to 4 weeks. Because the injection is intramuscular, it is more difficult to self-administer than is a subcutaneous injection such as insulin, and many patients rely on a second person for administration. Most patients with Kleinfelter's syndrome are infertile. Mosaic forms of Kleinfelter's syndrome do exist (e.g., 46,XY and 47,XXY); individuals with these mosaic forms may have only a few of the clinical manifestations of Kleinfelter's syndrome. Some may even be fertile. For most patients with Kleinfelter's syndrome, all the manifestations, except for infertility, can be adequately managed with a combination of hormonal therapy and plastic surgery.

CASE PRESENTATION: CASE 4

Steroid use in a 27-year-old body builder

J. J. Edmunds and his wife, Loretta, had been trying unsuccessfully to have a second child for the past 9 months. They are both 27 years old and are in excellent health. Their first child, Alexa, is now 2 years old and healthy. Mrs. Edmunds' pregnancy occurred about 2 months after stopping contraceptives. The pregnancy was uncomplicated and ended with a normal vaginal delivery. Loretta Edmunds breast-fed Alexa for 3 months and then weaned her daughter when she returned to work. Her menstrual periods resumed about 6 months postpartum and have been regular, about every 28 days, since then. Mrs. Edmunds has some mid-cycle lower abdominal pain, notes breast tenderness during the last half of her cycle, and has cramps during menstruation.

The Edmunds have intercourse three or four times a week and have not had any problems with the mechanics of intercourse. Loretta Edmunds' past medical history, review of systems, and physical examination are all unremarkable. J. J. Edmunds has been in excellent health. He eats a balanced diet that is high in protein and does not use alcohol or tobacco. He works out daily at the local gym, which is down the street from the market where he is an assistant produce manager.

A year ago Mr. Edmunds' body building program seemed to have reached a plateau. He was not adding any further muscle bulk. A friend at the gym suggested that he try some injections used by body builders in Europe. Although expensive—$25 apiece—they seemed to work well, increasing both his strength and his muscle bulk. He did note some acne and some tenderness of his nipples, but otherwise he did not note any significant side effects.

Physical examination of J. J. Edmunds revealed a large man with prominent muscle development. His general physical examination was remarkable for small soft testicles that measured approximately 2 cm in their longest diameter.

Laboratory Studies

Test	J. J. Edmunds	Normal
Testosterone	1610 ng/dL	*Male:* Prepubertal: <100 ng/dL Adult: 300–1000 ng/dL
LH	<2 mU/mL	*Male:* Prepubertal: <5 mU/mL Adult: 3–18 mU/mL
Semen analysis:		
Volume	4 mL	2–6 mL
Count	0.8×10^6/mL	$>20 \times 10^6$/mL
Motility	20% motile	>60% motile
Morphology	70% normal	>60% normal

A repeat semen analysis 2 weeks later yielded similar results.

The fact that Mr. and Mrs. Edmunds have had one child together is an important piece of information, ruling out developmental abnormalities in either that might cause infertility. Loretta Edmunds' menstrual pattern and the associated breast tenderness and cramps suggest that she is having ovulatory periods. Although a tubular or uterine abnormality could have developed since her last pregnancy, there is no history to support this possibility, and it would seem an unlikely cause of this couple's infertility.

J. J. Edmunds' low sperm count, on the other hand, is clearly a significant finding. Barring any questions of Alexa's paternity, Mr. Edmunds' sperm count must have been more normal 3 years ago when their first child was conceived.

When the Edmunds returned to discuss the results, the discussion centered on what might have altered Mr. Edmunds' sperm count. He had no history of testicular trauma and no pain or discomfort in his genitals. At first, he was reluctant to discuss the performance-enhancing injections that he was taking, but he did eventually tell his wife and physician about his drug use.

Exogenous androgens in supraphysiologic doses increase muscle mass and strength. In addition, they have significant effects on the endogenous androgen economy of the individuals who take them. By satisfying the sex hormone feedback loop, exogenous androgens shut off the hypothalamic–pituitary–gonadal axis in both males and females. In J. J. Edmunds' case, the resultant decrease in LH led to testicular atrophy and a significant decrease in the local testicular production of testosterone, which is vital for normal sperm production.

Six months after J. J. Edmunds stopped using exogenous steroids, Loretta Edmunds was pregnant. J. J. had lost some of the strength and bulk that

he had developed with hormone injections, but the Edmunds were pleased that they would have another child.

Endogenous androgens are available and useful for syndromes of androgen deficiency. In some cases of wasting syndromes, end-stage HIV infection, for example, they may improve well-being and increase weight and muscle mass. In normal individuals, the use of exogenous androgens in supraphysiologic doses can result in behavioral changes, including the precipitation of psychosis. Acne, prostatic enlargement, aggravation of preexisting prostate cancer, and gynecomastia can result. In addition, as in J. J. Edmunds' case, infertility and testicular atrophy may occur. Most of the effects of exogenous androgens are reversible, although it takes several months for the testicular atrophy to resolve and sperm production and semen analysis to return to normal.

In females, exogenous androgens in supraphysiologic doses often cause hirsutism and also can lead to acne and amenorrhea. Discontinuation of androgen use usually clears up the acne and brings about the return of menses, but once hair follicles are stimulated to develop, hair can continue to grow, leaving hirsutism as a permanent sequela of androgen use in females.

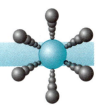

CASE PRESENTATION: CASE 5

Hypogonadism and anosmia in a 24-year-old man

All Jason Fernandez thought he needed when he made the appointment was a new prescription for his hay fever medication. His previous physician had retired, and a new physician was now taking care of Mr. Fernandez. During the visit, Jason's records were reviewed. Although Jason is now 24 years old, he looks more like a 13- or 14-year-old. Interestingly, since his visit 2 years before, his height had increased by about 1 inch. During this brief visit, his prescription was renewed and an appointment was made for a follow-up.

Jason Fernandez's past medical history is unremarkable. He has never had surgery. He is a nonsmoker and uses no alcohol. Jason works as a technician in a chemistry laboratory at a nearby university. He is not currently on any medications, except for the antihistamine he uses during the hay fever season. At times, even outside the hay fever season, Jason does experience difficulty recognizing odors. This diminished sense of smell has turned out to be an advantage in the laboratory where he works. He can easily handle certain chemicals that many of his coworkers find quite unpleasant.

A detailed review of systems reveals that he is continuing to grow slowly. Every year his pants need to be adjusted to account for another half inch or so of growth. Jason has not had much in the way of pubertal development. He has not been active sexually. He does not have erections or nocturnal emissions.

Physical Examination

A healthy, eunuchoid man who looks much younger than his age

Height:	72 inches
Weight:	180 pounds
Arm span:	75 inches
Blood pressure:	130/82
Skin:	Normal
Hair:	Sparse facial, axillary, and pubic hair
HEENT:	Normal
Neck:	Normal
Chest:	Normal
Heart:	Normal
Abdomen:	Normal
Genitals:	Small penis, 3.1 cm in length
	Small, soft testes, approximately $1 \times 1.5 \times 1.5$ cm
Extremities:	Normal

Laboratory Studies

Test	Jason Fernandez	Normal
Testosterone, total	157 ng/dL	*Male:* Prepubertal: <100 ng/dL Adult: 300–1000 ng/dL
LH	<2 mU/mL	*Male:* Prepubertal: <5 mU/mL Adult: 3–18 mU/mL
Prolactin	6 ng/mL	5–25 ng/mL
TSH	1.2 mU/L	0.3–5.0 mU/L

Jason Fernandez has not gone through puberty. His childlike appearance is caused by the preservation of prepubertal body fat distribution and the lack of facial hair. He has continued to grow. Continued growth without normal pubertal development has resulted in the production of eunuchoid proportions—i.e., an arm span greater than his height. The lack of epiphyseal closure allows long bones to continue to grow. Jason's arm span—the sum of four long-bone segments—is greater than his height—a measurement including only two long-bone segments that constitute about 50% of an individual's height.

The low testosterone and LH values would be normal for a prepubertal youngster, but clearly are abnormal for a 24-year-old man. Jason has hypogonadotrophic hypogonadism, a finding also supported by his lack of testicular development. Although the laboratory data available do not allow differentiation between a hypothalamic and a pituitary etiology for the hypogonadotrophic hypogonadism, when these findings are combined with anosmia—an inability to smell—it is referred to as Kallman's syndrome. In Kallman's syndrome, the hypothalamus does not produce GnRH, although other hypothalamic functions usually are normal.

Kallman's syndrome can be hereditary or sporadic. One form involves a genetic defect, which leads to variable deletions in KAL, a 680-amino-acid peptide that appears to play a role in neuronal migration. The absence of a normal form of this protein prevents the migration of GnRH-producing neurons from the olfactory area to their appropriate location in the hypothalamus. The absence of a normal form of this protein also impairs olfaction.

Further evaluation of Jason's condition led to additional testing. During an hour-long GnRH stimulation test, Jason had blood drawn to establish a baseline LH level. He then received an intravenous bolus of 100 μg of GnRH. His blood LH level was measured four more times at 15-minute intervals.

GnRH Stimulation Test (#1)

Time (min)	LH	Normal
0	<2 mU/mL	*Male:* Prepubertal: <5 mU/mL Adult: 3–18 mU/mL
15	<2 mU/mL	
30	3 mU/mL	LH should rise to a value at least 2.5
45	<2 mU/mL	times baseline at some point during
60	3 mU/mL	the 1-hour test.

After daily injections of GnRH for 7 days, Jason had another GnRH stimulation test

GnRH Stimulation Test (#2)

Time (min)	LH	Normal
0	<2 mU/mL	*Male:* Prepubertal: <5 mU/mL Adult: 3–18 mU/mL
15	10 mU/mL	
30	12 mU/mL	LH should rise to a value at least 2.5
45	16 mU/mL	times baseline at some point during
60	12 mU/mL	the 1-hour test.

The lack of an initial response to the administration of GnRH followed by a normal response after several exposures to GnRH is consistent with a hypothalamic deficiency of GnRH. During the first test, the gonadotroph cells of the anterior pituitary had not been exposed to GnRH for a sufficient length of time to promote LH and FSH synthesis and release. After repeated exposures, a response can be recruited. In addition to providing important diagnostic information, the results of GnRH testing offer helpful information about possible therapeutic approaches to this condition.

The options for treating patients with hypothalamic-based hypogonadotrophic hypogonadism can, most simply, include replacement of the end-organ sex hormone—testosterone for a male and estrogen and progesterone for a female. When fertility is desired, gonadal stimulation must be involved so that sperm or eggs can be produced. In this situation, gonadotropins can be administered parenterally. Another option, one that is especially useful for patients with hypothalamic hypogonadotrophism, is the use of pulsatile GnRH. Continuous administration of GnRH, or long-acting analogues, results in down-regulation and decreased production of gonadotropin. Pulsatile administration of the native short–half-life hormone, GnRH, however, recruits gonadotropin responses and can, in many cases, result in enough gonadal function to provide fertility.

Jason returned to discuss the results. Although the nature of the problem was clear to Jason and his parents, the next step was not so clear. In many ways, Jason did not want to do anything. Although he did not like looking so young, and wondered if his arms would keep on getting longer, he was basically happy the way he was. Jason was very apprehensive about going through puberty at 24 years of age. Fertility was not a concern, and all those shots could be a real hassle. Jason eventually decided to start a "go low, go slow" approach, using testosterone to put him through puberty slowly.

After 6 months of testosterone use, Jason had essentially stopped growing. He had developed enough facial hair to require shaving every day or every other day. His muscle bulk had increased, and he was beginning to look older. He did have some mild nipple swelling and irritation and a moderate degree of acne on his face and upper back. Overall, the changes have been gradual and he has accommodated well to them. His penis has enlarged significantly, and he is beginning to have erections and nocturnal emissions of semen.

Four years later, Jason Fernandez returned with another agenda. He and his wife wanted to have a child. They came in to discuss other options for managing his gonadotropin deficiency. The testosterone patches that he has been using have worked well, and he has been able to function normally sexually. He has normal erections and can ejaculate without difficulty. Analysis of his semen, however, shows no sperm.

After reviewing the options, Jason Fernandez began pulsatile GnRH treatments with a small infusion pump. He wears the pump on his belt next to his beeper, and it provides pulses of GnRH throughout the day. After 4 months of therapy, Jason's sperm count was approaching normal. His wife became pregnant a month later.

In addition to sporadic cases, both X-linked and autosomal modes of inheritance of Kallman's syndrome have been described. Jason's children will need to be followed carefully for the possibility of Kallman's syndrome.

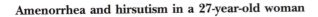

CASE PRESENTATION: CASE 6

Amenorrhea and hirsutism in a 27-year-old woman

Florence Jackson had not had a menstrual period in over 6 months. In addition, she had noted increasing facial and body hair. Ms. Jackson is 27 years old. Her menstrual periods started when she was 11 and have never been regular. The interval between menses can range from 3 weeks to 3 months or more. The bleeding pattern varies from 2 days to 7 days, and her periods usually are not associated with cramps. Ms. Jackson has never been pregnant, and she and her partner use condoms for contraception. Ms. Jackson's general health has been excellent. She is not on any medications and does not use any drugs. In spite of exercising for half an hour two to three times a week, and trying to control her caloric intake, Ms. Jackson is about 20 to 30 pounds heavier than she would like to be. A detailed review of systems is otherwise unremarkable.

Physical Examination

General:	An overweight woman with above average amounts of facial hair
Height:	64 inches
Weight:	210 pounds
Blood pressure:	110/70
Skin:	Moderately increased facial hair in the area of her sideburns, beneath her chin, and above her upper lip. Moderate amounts of periareolar and presternal hair and a male escutcheon. No striae.
Neck:	Normal, no thyroid enlargement
Chest:	Clear
Heart:	Normal
Breasts:	Normal, no galactorrhea
Abdomen:	Obese, no organomegaly
Pelvic exam:	Normal external genitalia. Clitoris, normal size. Vaginal mucosa and cervix appear normal. Bimanual exam unremarkable, but limited by her weight.
Extremities:	Normal

Laboratory Studies

Test	Florence Jackson	Normal
hCG—beta subunit	Negative	Negative, not pregnant
		Positive, pregnant
LH	16 mU/mL	*Female:*
		Prepubertal: <5 mU/mL
		Pre- or postovulatory: 3–35 mU/mL
		Ovulatory surge: 40–150 mU/mL
		Postmenopausal: >30 mU/mL
FSH	3.4 mU/mL	*Female:*
		Prepubertal: <5 mU/mL
		Pre- or postovulatory: 5–20 mU/mL
		Ovulatory surge: 12–40 mU/mL
		Postmenopausal: >30 mU/mL
Prolactin	24 ng/mL	5–25 ng/mL
Testosterone, total	84 ng/dL	Female: 20–90 ng/dL
Testosterone, free	1.8 ng/dL	Female: 0.1–1.3 ng/dL
DHEA-sulfate	642 μg/dL	Female: 80–443 μg/dL
Glucose, fasting	118 mg/dL	70–110 mg/dL, fasting

Amenorrhea in a sexually active woman in this age group should prompt a pregnancy test. Although many aspects of Ms. Jackson's history suggest that she is not pregnant, it is important to do this simple, inexpensive test to be sure that pregnancy is not the reason for her amenorrhea. Ms. Jackson has oligoamenorrhea in a pattern that is consistent with anovulation and is associated, in her case, with evidence of relative androgen excess. The initial evaluation has ruled out pregnancy and premature menopause. The gonadotropin levels are similar to those seen in other patients with chronic anovulation and androgen excess. The LH concentration is more than 2.5 times the FSH value.

There are a number of conditions that should be considered in the evaluation of relative androgen excess and chronic anovulation. Adrenal and ovarian tumors can secrete large amounts of androgens and could be the etiology in this case. The androgen excess caused by such tumors, however, typically exhibits a rapid onset of symptoms and very high levels of androgens. Because these tumors may be relatively small, ultrasound studies and CT scans may not always provide anatomic evidence.

Cushing's syndrome is another condition that can cause androgen excess and chronic anovulation. Ms. Jackson does not have the physical stigmata of Cushing's syndrome, but either an overnight dexamethasone suppression test or a 24-hour urine test for free cortisol would be appropriate in her evaluation.

Late-onset forms of congenital adrenal hyperplasia with enzyme deficiencies in the adrenal steroid biosynthetic pathway also can result in relative androgen excess and chronic anovulation. For many women, obesity leads to changes in steroid hormone economy, with increases in both androgen and estrogen levels that can lead to chronic anovulation.

Ms. Jackson underwent some additional diagnostic tests:

Test	Florence Jackson	Normal
Urinary 17-ketosteroid excretion	14.1 mg/d	Female (adult): 3.0–15.0 mg/d
Urinary free cortisol excretion	42 μg/d	20–70 μg/d

Pelvic ultrasound: **Slightly enlarged ovaries with multiple small cysts**

These data suggest that Ms. Jackson does not have Cushing's syndrome or an adrenal tumor. She does have mild increases in both DHEA-sulfate, a weak adrenal androgen, and free testosterone. Because androgen excess results in a decrease in SHBG, some patients have elevated free testosterone levels even though their total testosterone level is normal.

Ms. Jackson has the clinical, biochemical, and anatomic features of polycystic ovary syndrome (PCO). Originally described as chronic anovulation associated with hyperandrogenism, this syndrome also can be described in biochemical and anatomic terms. Almost all patients with the clinical combination of oligomenorrhea and evidence of increased androgens exhibit cystic ovaries on an ultrasound study. The biochemical finding typically involves, as in Ms. Jackson's case, an LH concentration that is more than 2.5 times the FSH level.

The pathophysiology of PCO is not well defined, but a number of factors have been elucidated. One finding is that the theca cells of the ovary produce increased amounts of androgens in response to LH. Interestingly, insulin also may be involved in this process. Women with PCO have elevated insulin levels, without necessarily having abnormal glucose levels, and peripheral resistance to the effects of insulin has been demonstrated. Obesity is a frequent, but not consistent, finding in patients with PCO, and appears to play a role in resistance to insulin and in the abnormal production of androgens. High levels of insulin act in synergy with LH to increase ovarian androgen production. Within the ovary, the high androgen levels result in inhibition of normal maturation of follicular cysts and lack of progression to ovulation. High levels of androgens from other sources, either adrenal or endogenous, can cause a similar ovarian morphology and a clinical syndrome identical to PCO.

The treatment of patients with PCO involves a number of factors. One goal is to protect the endometrium from unopposed estrogen, because endometrial hyperplasia and even endometrial carcinoma can result when progesterone is not present to counterbalance the endometrial effects of estrogen. The patient also may desire treatment of the symptoms of androgen excess, hirsuitism and acne. A discussion of contraception and fertility, and the associated metabolic issues, specifically the potential for glucose intolerance or diabetes, is very important.

Periodic treatment with a progestational agent such as medroxyprogesterone acetate, daily for 10 to 14 days, three or four times a year, should induce withdrawal bleeding and protect the endometrium from hyperplasia and carcinoma secondary to the effects of unopposed estrogen. Oral contraceptives are another convenient way of providing endometrial protection.

The problems of androgen excess can be dealt with by local measures, such as depilatories and waxing for unwanted hair. In addition, spironolactone, an androgen receptor–blocking agent, can be helpful for some women with this syndrome.

Contraception is another important issue. The irregular bleeding pattern makes the detection of pregnancy, should it occur, difficult. Barrier methods of contraception usually are recommended for women who are not already using oral contraceptives for endometrial protection. Although patients with PCO tend to be relatively infertile, it is important that the condition not be relied upon as a form of contraception.

When conception is desired, on the other hand, a number of possibilities are available. Clomiphene citrate is an antiestrogenic agent that blocks the negative feedback effect of endogenous estrogens and androgens on gonadotropin secretion, resulting in increases in both LH and FSH secretion, and triggers ovulation for approximately 70% to 80% of patients. The conception rate following such treatments is approximately 40%. The complications of clomiphene include multiple gestation—primarily twins. In addition, on rare occasions, ovarian hyperstimulation can lead to marked ovarian enlargement. Gonadotropins and pulsatile GnRH also can be used to induce fertility. In the past, ovarian wedge resection, surgically opening the hardened capsule of the ovary, had a moderate degree of success in inducing an ovulatory state. Clomiphene therapy has decreased the need for surgical treatment. Finally, assisted reproductive technologies are available and may be helpful for patients with PCO.

For those women with this syndrome who are overweight, weight loss can lead to the return of menstrual cycles and improvement in fertility. Medications such as metformin and troglidizone, which increase insulin sensitivity, also are being tried for this syndrome, with encouraging results.

Two days after completing a 10-day course on medroxyprogesterone acetate, Ms. Jackson had her first menstrual period in over 6 months. She decided to start oral contraceptives, both for contraception and for regulation of menstrual bleeding. In addition, she joined a health club and signed up for nutrition classes. She has decided to make a major effort to control her weight now that it has begun to affect her health.

Six weeks later, she returned for a follow-up examination. She had had one period since beginning the birth control pills and had lost about 10 pounds.

Physical Examination
   Weight: **199 pounds**
   Blood pressure: **120/72**

The facial hair growth is still a problem, but she hopes that, with more weight loss, her hormonal status will improve and the unwanted hair will be more manageable.

CASE PRESENTATION: CASE 7

Secondary amenorrhea in a 21-year-old woman who runs 5 miles per day

Erica Long is 21 years old and has not had a menstrual period in 9 months. Ms. Long had the onset of menses at age 11 and, after 6 months or so of irregular spotty bleeding, began to have regular periods until age 16. At age 16, she became actively involved with the cross-country team at her high school. She began running between 3 and 8 miles a day. Shortly after she began running regularly, she stopped having menstrual periods, except during the winter, when she didn't run as frequently. Each spring, when she started running again, she would stop having menstrual periods.

Since finishing high school, Ms. Long has been working as a bank teller. She runs at least 5 or 6 miles every day. Ms. Long describes eating at least two meals a day and denies inducing vomiting or being concerned about her weight.

Ms. Long's past medical history and a detailed review of systems are unremarkable. She has never been pregnant and is not sexually active.

Physical Examination

General:	A thin, healthy-appearing woman
Height:	66″
Weight:	104 pounds
Vital signs:	Blood pressure 110/70; pulse, 48, regular
HEENT:	Normal, teeth in good repair without enamel abnormalities
Neck:	Normal
Chest:	Normal
Heart:	Normal
Breasts:	Normal, no galactorrhea
Abdomen:	Normal
Pelvic exam:	Normal external genitalia
	Healthy-appearing vagina and cervix (Pap smear and vaginal smear for cytology obtained)
	Bimanual examination: Normal uterus, ovaries not palpable
Extremities:	Normal

Laboratory Studies

Test	Erica Long	Normal
hCG—beta subunit	Negative	Negative, not pregnant Positive, pregnant
Prolactin	15 ng/mL	5–25 ng/mL

LH	2.4 mU/mL	*Female:*
		    Prepubertal: <5 mU/mL
		    Pre- or postovulatory: 3–35 mU/mL
		    Ovulatory surge: 40–150 mU/mL
		    Postmenopausal: >30 mU/mL

FSH	3.0 mU/mL	*Female:*
		    Prepubertal: <5 mU/mL
		    Pre- or postovulatory: 5–20 mU/mL
		    Ovulatory surge: 12–40 mU/mL
		    Postmenopausal: >30 mU/mL

Vaginal cytology	Low estrogen effect	Depends on phase of menstrual cycle
TSH	0.8 mU/L	0.3–5.0 mU/L
8 a.m. cortisol	24 μg/dL	15–25 μg/dL

Ms. Long has *secondary amenorrhea*—she has lost menstrual function after having an established menstrual pattern. Her menstrual function does seem to be correlated with her activity level. Her laboratory studies show low levels of gonadotropin and low estrogen effect. These findings would be normal if she were 7 years old, but at age 21, they are abnormal. The hypogonadotropic hypogonadism seen in Ms. Long could have a pituitary or hypothalamic basis. Because other functions of the anterior pituitary appear to be normal, it is unlikely that a pituitary lesion accounts for her condition. The clinical setting of increased activity, low body weight, and oligoamenorrhea in a woman who has developed normally suggests hypothalamic amenorrhea. In this condition there is a return of hormone patterns to a prepubertal level, with low gonadotropin and estrogen levels. The relative levels of gonadotropins and estrogen at various stages of life are shown in Figure 9-13.

Because estrogen levels are low, endometrial protection is not a major concern. The low levels of estrogen, however, may have significant effects. One important issue is the effect of low estrogen levels on bone density. Although Ms. Long has stopped growing, her bones are still increasing in density, a process that requires the presence of estrogen. Insufficient amounts of estrogen at this point in her development can lead to a significant reduction in bone density and to the premature development of osteoporosis.

Estrogen replacement therapy would be one way of dealing with Ms. Long's condition. Birth control pills would provide both estrogen and endometrial protection. Another approach would be to encourage Ms. Long

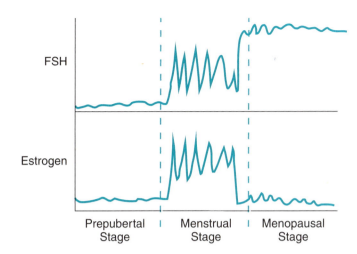

Figure 9-13. Pattern of estrogen and gonadotropin (FSH) secretion during different stages of life in women. Before puberty, both FSH and estrogen levels are low. During puberty and during the menstrual stage, FSH stimulates estrogen production in a cyclic fashion. After menopause, when ovarian function and significant estrogen production cease, FSH levels rise and remain elevated.

to gain weight and lower her level of exercise. The amenorrhea that is seen in athletes is a function of both body weight and exercise level. For many women, there is a critical body weight below which menstruation does not occur and above which menses are much more likely to occur on a regular basis.

For some patients, gaining weight may be difficult. Eating disorders, which can result in loss of significant amounts of body fat, are commonly associated with oligomenorrhea, and with gonadotropin and estrogen levels similar to those seen in athletes. Eating disorders may be difficult to detect clinically. Many patients are reluctant to be frank about their eating pattern, the induction of vomiting, or the abuse of laxatives or diuretics. Etching of dental enamel that can result from frequent vomiting may be a sign that an eating disorder is present. Although oral contraceptives can be of use, attaining a more normal weight, if possible, is the most helpful therapeutic maneuver.

After discussing the test results, Ms. Long has decided to start oral contraceptives. In addition, she plans to make an effort to increase her intake of calcium and vitamin D. She'll also try to increase her weight by at least 10 pounds, though she is not sure she wants to cut back on running.

CASE PRESENTATION: CASE 8

Erectile impotence in a 57-year-old man with diabetes

Paul Davis is 57 years old. For the past 32 years, he has had insulin-dependent diabetes. Recently, he has been taking three or four injections of insulin each day, and he does frequent finger-stick blood sugar measurements. He has had some mild background retinopathy, which has required laser therapy, but renal function has been normal.

Over the last several years, he has developed a painful nocturnal burning in his feet that is most painful when he goes to bed at night. He has recently tried some topical capsaicin cream, which has provided some relief.

For the last 3 years, Mr. Davis has had increasing difficulty both having and maintaining erections. He no longer has erections on awakening in the morning. He and his wife have been married for 32 years and have four children. Gloria Davis is healthy and does not have any gynecologic problems. Mr. Davis does not have any other sexual partners.

Mr. Davis does not use alcohol or smoke cigarettes and is on no medications other than insulin.

Physical Examination

General:	A healthy-appearing man
Vital signs:	Blood pressure 140/84; pulse 78, regular
HEENT:	Background retinopathy and laser scars
Neck:	Normal
Chest:	Normal
Heart:	Normal
Abdomen:	Normal
Genitals:	Normal penis, testes normal consistency, 4 × 3 × 3 cm bilaterally
Neurologic:	Decreased peripheral sensation in both lower extremities, up to mid-calf
	Absent ankle-jerk reflexes

Laboratory Studies

Test	Paul Davis	Normal
Testosterone	564 ng/dL	*Male:* Prepubertal: <100 ng/dL Adult: 300–1000 ng/dL
LH	16.8 mU/mL	*Male:* Prepubertal: <5 mU/mL Adult: 3–18 mU/mL
Prolactin	18 ng/mL	5–25 ng/mL

Mr. Davis' hormonal levels are normal, indicating that his impotence does not have a hormonal basis. After years of diabetes, many men develop erectile impotence. The mechanism is probably related to a combination of neuropathy and vasculopathy with decreased inflow.

An erection is an hydraulic event that is the result of a number of vascular, neurologic, and endocrine events. During an erection, the vascular channels of the corpora cavernosa, normally empty in the flaccid penis, become filled with blood at pressures near systemic arterial pressure. Arteriolar and sinusoidal smooth muscles of the corpora relax, allowing the inflow of blood. Venous return is impaired by an increase in venous resistance and by the mechanical pressure of the blood-filled sinusoids, which compress the sinusoidal draining venules against the minimally distensible tunica albuginea, which surrounds the shaft of the penis. To have an erection, vascular inflow must be adequate. In addition, local neurologic function must be adequate to decrease arteriolar resistance and decrease venous return. Appropriate central nervous system input or lack of inhibition also must be present for erection to occur.

Erectile dysfunction is a common complication of diabetes mellitus and usually is seen, as in Mr. Davis' case, in combination with other signs of neuropathy. A number of medications—including antihypertensives, psychotropics, and CNS depressants such as alcohol and narcotics—can interfere with erectile performance. In many instances, erectile failure has a psychogenic basis. Men with psychogenic impotence often are capable of having erections in some situations, e.g., on arising in the morning with a full bladder, with masturbation, or with a different partner.

When no correctable cause of erectile dysfunction is found, several options are available. Rigid condoms can be helpful for some men. External vacuum devices that pull increased blood volume into the penis can be used. The penile engorgement induced by the vacuum is then maintained by an appropriately sized tourniquet-like band placed at the base of the penis, which impedes venous return. This provides an erection adequate for penetration for some men with erectile impotence. Injection of the vasoactive substances papaverine or prostaglandin E1 (alprostadil) into the corpora cavernosa of the penis results in an erection in many men. A urethral suppository of alprostadil also is available and usually is effective. A firm erection induced in this fashion or with penile injection indicates that an adequate vascular supply is available for erection, providing evidence that atherosclerotic restriction of blood inflow is not the primary cause of the impotence. Surgical implantation of a rigid prosthesis is another way some men choose to deal with erectile dysfunction.

Sildenafil citrate is an orally administered medication that enhances erectile function. The drug inhibits a phosphodiesterase and thereby allows higher levels of cyclic guanosine monophosphate (cGMP) to be maintained in the corpus cavernosum. cGMP relaxes vascular smooth muscle, allowing engorgement and enhancing the development of an erection.

After reviewing the options, Mr. Davis and his wife decided that they would like to try sildenafil. They had watched the videotapes provided by the manufacturers of the various medication and devices on the market.

Sildenafil significantly improved Mr. Davis' erectile function without any apparent side effects.

KEY POINTS AND CONCEPTS

- The reproductive axis is a four-tiered system involving the (1) hypothalamus, (2) anterior pituitary, (3) gonad, and (4) tissues that respond to the effects of sex steroid hormones.
- The hypothalamic hormone (GnRH), the pituitary hormones (LH and FSH), and the sex steroid hormones (androgens, estrogens, and

progesterone) are precisely the same molecules in both males and females. The relative amounts of the steroid hormones differ significantly between the sexes, as do the patterns of feedback control that regulate gonadal function.

- Female internal and external genital tract development is the default process and does not require hormonal stimulation.
- Male reproductive duct development requires the presence of a testicle that can make testosterone and mullerian inhibitory substance (MIS).
- Between infancy and puberty there is essentially no activity of the reproductive axis.
- At puberty, the reproductive axis awakens with hormonal changes that result in the development of secondary sexual characteristics.
- In the adult female, the menstrual cycle is the result of a complex set of events. The first half of the cycle, the follicular phase, occurs in response to ovarian stimulation by LH and FSH and involves the development of a dominant follicle and increasing levels of estrogen. At ovulation, which is induced by a mid-cycle surge of LH, the hormonal secretion of the ovary changes to include progesterone in addition to estrogen.
- When a pregnancy is established, placental hCG stimulates continued ovarian steroid hormone secretion. If no pregnancy occurs, the corpus luteum becomes less responsive to the gonadotropins, steroid hormone levels fall, and menstruation occurs.
- When the ovary is depleted of follicles, it ceases to function, menstruation stops, and menopause begins. High levels of gonadotropins are seen in the postmenopausal woman.
- Male reproductive axis function is under tonic, negative feedback control by products of testicular function. LH stimulates and also is controlled by testosterone production. FSH stimulates sperm production and is controlled by a by-product of sperm production, inhibin.
- Disorders of reproductive function usually involve hypofunction and may be either primary—failure of the system to develop and function normally as a result of genetic, anatomic, or acquired abnormalities—or secondary—failure of function after the establishment of normal function as a result of autoimmune, inflammatory, or infectious processes.
- Treatment of reproductive axis dysfunction can, depending on the pathology and the needs of the individual patient, be focused at any of the four tiers of reproductive endocrine function.

SUGGESTED READING

Bagatell CJ, Bremner WJ. Androgens in men—uses and abuses. N Engl J Med 334: 707–714, 1996.

Braunstein G. Gynecomastia. N Engl J Med 328:490–495, 1993.

Franks S. Polycystic ovary syndrome. N Engl J Med 333:853–861, 1995.

Griffin JE. Androgen resistance—the clinical and molecular spectrum. N Engl J Med 326:611–618, 1992.

Marshall LA. Clinical evaluation of amenorrhea in active and athletic women. Clin Sports Med 13:371–387, 1994.

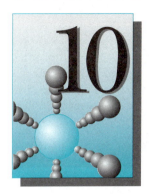

Endocrine Aspects of Blood Pressure Regulation

Arterial blood pressure is controlled and supported by several endocrine mechanisms. Low blood pressure stimulates neural and hormonal systems that influence blood volume, venous capacitance, vascular resistance, and heart rate and contractility. Simply getting up in the morning—going from lying to standing—calls on a number of mechanisms that preserve blood pressure and the flow of blood to vital organs.

As in other aspects of endocrinology, the effects of the hormones involved in the regulation of blood pressure are most apparent in the presence of hormonal excess or deficiency. Although these extremes of hormonal excess and deficiency are relatively uncommon, understanding the role of hormones in the regulation of blood pressure can be very helpful in the evaluation and treatment of blood pressure disorders of any cause.

Although rare, excess production of adrenocortical steroids and catecholamines are important causes of arterial hypertension. Renovascular disease and other conditions that result in increased renin production also can result in hypertension. Moderate hypertension can occur in states of growth hormone excess, hyper- and hypothyroidism, hyperparathyroidism, and conditions associated with excess insulin; while hypotension is seen in Addison's disease and autonomic neuropathy resulting from diabetes or other causes.

The term *essential hypertension* is used to describe the condition in most patients with hypertension, because there is no clearly definable cause. Most hypertensive patients have no symptoms and have normal laboratory studies. Evaluation usually shows only hypertension and, for some patients, its consequences—heart disease, renal dysfunction, and cerebrovascular disease. Early detection and effective treatment are the top priorities in managing hypertension. In many patients, elevation of blood pressure is clearly related to genetic and lifestyle factors. Stress, excessive alcohol intake, obesity, and high salt intake are all correlated with hypertension. In such cases, lifestyle modification is the foundation of therapy. Medications are added when lifestyle modifications do not work or when the hypertension is severe. When essential hypertension is difficult to control or is associated with hypokalemia, an endocrine cause should be considered.

ADRENAL CORTEX

Excess levels of glucocorticoid, and especially mineralocorticoid hormones, can result in significant hypertension. Table 10-1 presents some of the mechanisms related to the renin-angiotensin system or the adrenal cortex that can cause hypertension. Adrenal insufficiency is associated with hypotension, especially postural hypotension and hypotension at times of volume depletion and significant stress. The mechanism of the hypotension caused by adrenal insufficiency is related in part to volume depletion caused by the lack of aldosterone. In addition, the lack of cortisol affects vascular smooth muscle reactivity and contributes to hypotension.

MINERALOCORTICOIDS

The production and release of aldosterone by the glomerulosa cells of the adrenal cortex normally is stimulated by potassium and angiotensin. ACTH stimulation plays a relatively small role in non-stress situations (see Fig. 5-7 in Chapter 5). Mineralocorticoids cause increased sodium resorption in the distal nephron. When they are present in excess or in uncontrolled amounts, the resultant increase in total body sodium leads to volume expansion. The increased blood volume that follows can result in increased blood pressure. Edema usually is not present because of a compensating, escape phenomenon—an increased glomerular filtration rate (GFR) and decreased proximal sodium reabsorption result in some reduction of the excess volume. There is, however, little or no escape from the hypokalemia and alkalosis associated with mineralocorticoid excess.

Excess mineralocorticoid production can result from increased renin secretion or angiotensin production. Overproduction of mineralocorticoids also can occur as an autonomous process, independent of stimulation by angiotensin. Such uncontrolled secretion of aldosterone can be seen with an adrenal cortical adenoma and diffuse or nodular hyperplasia, or when a significant abnormality in the control of secretion occurs, as in *glucocorticoid remediable hypertension*. A mechanism for apparent mineralocorticoid excess in the absence of truly elevated hormone levels also has been identified.

Cortisol and aldosterone have equal affinity for and effectiveness in stimulating the mineralocorticoid receptor (see Chapter 5). The fact that cortisol is present in much larger molar concentrations than is aldosterone presents an interesting control system problem. In those tissues where aldosterone has its principle effect (e.g., renal collecting duct, parotid gland, colon), the enzyme 11β-hydroxysteroid dehydrogenase is present. This enzyme inactivates cortisol by converting the OH group at the 11 position to a ketone, thereby creating cortisone, an inactive hormone that has a very low affinity for the mineralocorticoid receptor. This process eliminates cortisol as a competitor and allows aldosterone access to the receptor (see Fig. 5-6 in Chapter 5). A deficiency or inhibition of 11β-hydroxy-

TABLE 10-1. *HYPERTENSION SYNDROMES INVOLVING THE RENIN-ANGIOTENSIN SYSTEM AND THE ADRENAL CORTEX*

CONDITION	COMMENTS
Renin/Angiotensin Excess	
Coarctation of the aorta	Decreased renal blood flow stimulates renin secretion—hypertension above the coarctation, normo- or hypotension below.
Renal artery stenosis	Renovascular hypertension—narrowing of the renal artery from atherosclerosis or fibromuscular hyperplasia—results in increased renin secretion.
Renin-secreting tumor	Rare; hemangiopericytomas contain elements of juxtaglomerular cells and secrete renin in an unregulated fashion.
Estrogen-induced (pregnancy, oral contraceptives, estrogen replacement therapy)	Renin substrate production is increased.
Malignant hypertension	In severe hypertension of any cause, renin levels are increased.
Aldosterone or Mineralocorticoid Excess	
Cushing's syndrome	Increased concentrations of glucocorticoid hormones result in increased mineralocorticoid effect.
Solitary aldosterone-secreting adenoma	Autonomous overproduction of aldosterone—also known as Conn's syndrome.
Bilateral nodular adrenal hyperplasia	Idiopathic overproduction of aldosterone by multiple adenomata—surgery does not correct hypertension, but does correct hypokalemia.
Adrenal cortical enzyme deficiencies (11 and 17 OH-ing)	In an effort to make adequate amounts of cortisol, precursor compounds above the enzymatic block are released in excess and, although "weak" mineralocorticoids, the excessive levels result in mineralocorticoid hypertension.
Glucocorticoid remedial hypertension	A genetic lesion in which the gene for aldosterone synthetase is fused with the regulatory region of 11b-hydroxylase, an ACTH-dependent enzyme—ACTH in physiologic amounts stimulates production of excess amounts of aldosterone.
Apparent Aldosterone or Mineralocorticoid Excess	
Licorice ingestion	Inhibition of 11-β hydroxysteroid dehydrogenase.
11-β hydroxysteroid dehydrogenase deficiency	Absence of the enzyme that inactivates cortisol at the mineralocorticoid receptor.

ACTH, adrenocorticotrophic hormone.

steroid dehydrogenase would allow the larger quantities of cortisol usually present to have a significant mineralocorticoid effect.

GLUCOCORTICOIDS

The mechanism of glucocorticoid-induced hypertension is not clearly understood, but it is thought to involve the presence of some mineralocorticoid effects in the setting of high levels of glucocorticoids, levels that may overwhelm the 11-β hydroxysteroid dehydrogenase enzyme system in mineralocorticoid-sensitive cells. In some cases, adrenal cortical overactivity results in the production of glucocorticoid precursors that have significant mineralocorticoid effects. In addition, direct effects of glucocorticoids on smooth muscle increase peripheral vascular resistance. Glucocorticoid hormones raise insulin levels, which, in turn, may raise blood pressure as a result of an effect of insulin on vascular smooth muscle. Both endogenous and exogenous glucocorticoids can elevate blood pressure.

ADRENAL MEDULLA

The adrenal medulla is both an endocrine organ and a highly specialized part of the sympathetic nervous system. In contrast to most of the autonomic nervous system, the adrenal medulla is not involved in the minute-to-minute regulation of physiologic processes. It is a stress-responding organ that becomes active when marked deviations from normal homeostasis occur. The catecholamine hormones that are released from the adrenal medulla have multiple effects on cardiovascular and metabolic function, effects that enable the delivery of blood and nutrients at times of significant stress.

ANATOMY

The adrenal medulla is derived from neural crest tissue, which migrates to join the developing adrenal cortex. In many species, the tissues that correspond to the adrenal medulla and adrenal cortex are separate, but in humans and most mammalian species, they are united into one structure, with cortical tissue surrounding the medullary component of the gland. With three separate arterial inputs, the rich vascular supply of the adrenal gland supplies both the cortex and the medulla. There is, in addition, a limited portal system within the adrenal gland. Blood that has perfused the cortex also may perfuse a capillary bed of the medulla, allowing the delivery of a high concentration of glucocorticoids to the adrenal medulla. The presence of high levels of glucocorticoids can effect adrenal medullary function. Venous drainage is into the single adrenal vein that serves each adrenal gland (see Fig. 5-1 in Chapter 5).

The adrenal medulla is made up of chromaffin cells, also referred to as pheochromocytes because of their histologic staining characteristics. The cells of the adrenal medulla are arranged in nests or cords and are in close contact with capillaries and vascular sinusoids. Preganglionic fibers of the sympathetic nervous system innervate the cells of the adrenal medulla. These fibers release acetylcholine, which, in turn, results in the secretion of catecholamines into the vascular system.

CHEMISTRY

The adrenal medulla produces several catecholamines, each of which is a modification of the tyrosine molecule. The principal catecholamines and the biosynthetic pathway are shown in Figure 10-1. The tyrosine that serves as the precursor can be derived from dietary sources, or can be synthesized in the liver from phenylalanine. In addition to being produced by the adrenal medulla, dopamine is found in many tissues throughout the body, where it serves as a neurotransmitter. Norepinephrine is found in other tissues as well, including the brain and peripheral sympathetic nerves. Epinephrine is essentially found only in the adrenal medulla. Phenylethanolamine-N-methyltransferase (PNMT), the enzyme that cat-

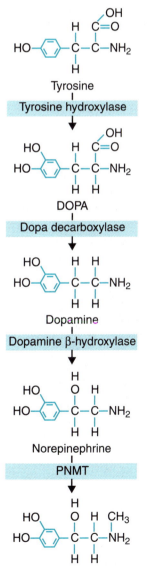

Figure 10-1. Biosynthesis of catecholamines. Starting with tyrosine, the principle catecholamines—dopamine, norepinephrine, and epinephrine—are synthesized in a series of enzymatic reactions. PNMT, phenylethanolamine-N-methyltransferase.

TABLE 10-2. ADRENERGIC RESPONSES OF SELECTED TISSUES		
ORGAN OR TISSUE	**RECEPTOR**	**EFFECT**
Heart	β_1	Increased contractility Increased heart rate
Blood vessels	α_1 β_2	Vasoconstriction Vasodilation
Bronchioles	β_2	Dilation
Kidney	β_1	Increased renin secretion
Liver	α, β_2	Increased glycogenolysis Increased gluconeogenesis
Pancreatic islet cells	α_2 β_2	Decreased insulin release Increased insulin release
Adipose tissue	α, β_2	Increased lipolysis
Skin	α	Increased sweating

alyzes the conversion of norepinephrine to epinephrine, is induced by the high levels of glucocorticoids that are delivered from the adrenal cortex to the medulla by the portal system described earlier.

Catecholamines are stored in granules and are released by exocytosis when the gland is stimulated by input from the sympathetic nervous system. Once released, the catecholamines of the adrenal medulla are weakly bound to circulating plasma proteins. The effects of circulating catecholamines are relatively short-lived. In addition to direct excretion by the kidney, circulating catecholamines are taken up by sympathetic nerve endings and metabolized to inactive forms, especially in the liver and in the kidneys.

Catecholamines initiate their regulatory physiologic effects by binding to receptors on the cell surface. These adrenergic receptors are transmembrane proteins that are part of the G-protein superfamily of cell surface receptors. Other members of the same family include the receptors for vasopressin, glucagon, luteinizing hormone (LH), and thyroid-stimulating hormone (TSH). A large number of different adrenergic receptors have been identified. Starting with physiologic observations, it was clear that there are at least two types of adrenergic receptors, termed *alpha* and *beta*. Subsequent physiologic and pharmacologic studies and, more recently, molecular biology techniques, have identified at least nine subtypes—five alpha and four beta—of adrenergic receptors. The precise function of each of these receptors has not yet been identified. Table 10-2 presents the adrenergic receptor–mediated effects on selected tissues.

DISORDERS OF ADRENAL MEDULLARY FUNCTION

Hypofunction of the adrenal medulla has surprisingly few effects. Individuals who have Addison's disease or who have undergone bilateral adrenalectomy do not need replacement of adrenal medullary hormones. They may, however, especially if they also have diabetes, be more susceptible to hypoglycemia. Adrenal medullary hypofunction probably is involved in the postural hypotension that is seen in patients with autonomic insufficiency of various etiologies. Diabetic autonomic neuropathy is the most common form, followed by the autonomic insufficiency associated with Parkinson's disease.

Adrenal medullary hyperfunction, on the other hand, usually is dramatic and life-threatening, but it is curable if diagnosed and treated appropriately. Both familial and sporadic forms of pheochromocytoma, the functional tumor of the adrenal medulla, have been described. They can be solitary, bilateral, or even extra-adrenal in location. In some patients, pheochromocytoma is associated with other endocrine tumors (e.g., MEN 2—see Chapter 11).

THE PHYSIOLOGIC BASIS OF CLINICAL TESTS TO EVALUATE THE ENDOCRINE ASPECTS OF ABNORMAL BLOOD PRESSURE

Blood Pressure Measurement. Blood pressure should be measured in both arms and both in the supine position and after standing for 2 minutes with an appropriately sized cuff. A rise in diastolic pressure on standing often is seen in normotensive individuals and in patients with essential hypertension. In hypertensive patients, a drop in blood pressure while standing suggests the presence of a secondary form of hypertension. The systolic blood pressure can be measured in one leg and the result correlated with blood pressure measured in the patient's arm to look for the possible presence of a coarctation of the aorta.

For patients with hypotension, the blood pressure and pulse rate responses to standing (if such testing can be done safely) provide useful information. A rise in heart rate suggests volume depletion. When heart rate does not increase in the presence of postural hypotension, neuropathy, the effects of a medication, or heart disease should be suspected.

Electrolytes. When renal function and diet are normal, and in the absence of vomiting, diarrhea, or medications the serum potassium level gives a good estimate of the level of mineralocorticoid activity. A potassium concentration lower than normal indicates increased mineralocorticoid function, whereas a high value points to possible mineralocorticoid deficiency. Because mineralocorticoids also promote the excretion of hydrogen ions, mineralocorticoid excess results in an alkalosis that leads to an increase in the measured bicarbonate concentration. The mild acidosis of mineralocorticoid deficiency, conversely, leads to a fall in the serum bicarbonate concentration. The serum sodium concentration usually is unchanged, because it is largely a function of water balance rather than sodium balance. Sodium concentrations lower than normal are seen in cortisol deficiency and in states of ADH excess.

Plasma Renin Activity. The level of renin activity can be measured in plasma and can be used to help define the mechanism of a patient's hypertension. The value is highly dependent on sodium intake and position, and can be affected by a number of medications. Coexisting illnesses, such as diabetes, heart failure, or hepatic cirrhosis, also can influence the result. Higher values are seen in states of volume depletion (either effective or real), diuretic therapy, catecholamine excess, and severe hypertension. Elevations of plasma renin activity also are seen in conditions that cause renal artery stenosis, or its functional equivalent, coarctation of the aorta above the renal arteries. High sodium intake, volume expansion, and adrenergic blocking agents are associated with low plasma renin activity levels. Elevated glucocorticoid and mineralocorticoid levels lower renin activity.

Renin levels are especially valuable in interpreting aldosterone levels. When both aldosterone and renin activity are elevated, renovascular disease or malignant hypertension should be suspected. When both are low, hyporeninemic hypoaldosteronism, a condition that presents as hyperkalemia and usually is seen in diabetic patients, is present. A low renin level and an elevated aldosterone level are seen in conditions of autonomous or abnormally controlled aldosterone production.

In patients with essential hypertension, assessment of renin activity can, on occasion, be helpful in designing a drug regimen. Patients with high renin levels may respond well to angiotensin-converting enzyme (ACE) inhibitors and adrenergic blocking agents, medications that decrease renin effectiveness or block its secretion. Diuretics and calcium channel blockers might be better initial options when treating essential hypertension in patients with low renin levels.

Plasma Aldosterone. Like renin levels, aldosterone concentrations can span a wide range and are significantly influenced by sodium intake, the patient's position, and associated medical conditions. The serum potassium level also has a profound influence on aldosterone levels. Hyperkalemia is a potent stimulus for aldosterone secretion. When hypokalemia that cannot be attributed to diuretic therapy is seen in hypertensive patients, aldosterone should be measured. A high aldosterone level indicates either autonomous overproduction or secretion stimulated by high levels of renin or ACTH. Simultaneous renin activity and aldosterone levels can be very helpful in evaluating patients with hypertension and potassium abnormalities.

Tests of Catecholamine Secretion. Catecholamines are metabolized into several related compounds. Although the life of the actual catecholamines in the circulation is very short, their metabolites are present for longer periods, and the measurement of these compounds may be an effective way to capture evidence of excess catecholamine production. Figure 10-2 presents the major metabolites of the catecholamines. Metanephrines are measurable in both plasma and urine. Traditional testing for the possible presence of a pheochromocytoma has been based on the urinary excretion of the catecholamines themselves or of their metabolites, measured over a 24-hour period. A recent study supports the use of plasma metanephrine levels in the diagnosis of pheochromocytoma.

Other Tests. Evaluation of patients with blood pressure abnormalities also should include testing that is directed by the patient's personal and family history and physical examination. When cortisol or growth hormone excess is suspected, appropriate studies should be ordered. The extremes of thyroid hyper- and hypofunction also can be associated with hypertension. Adrenal insufficiency and autonomic neuropathy should be considered in patients with postural hypotension.

Patients with hypertension should be evaluated to assess organ damage and associated correctable cardiovascular risk factors. In addition to a careful physical examination, it usually is appropriate to perform an electrocardiogram, a chest X-ray, and blood tests of renal function. Testing for diabetes and lipid abnormalities also are part of a thorough evaluation of a patient with hypertension.

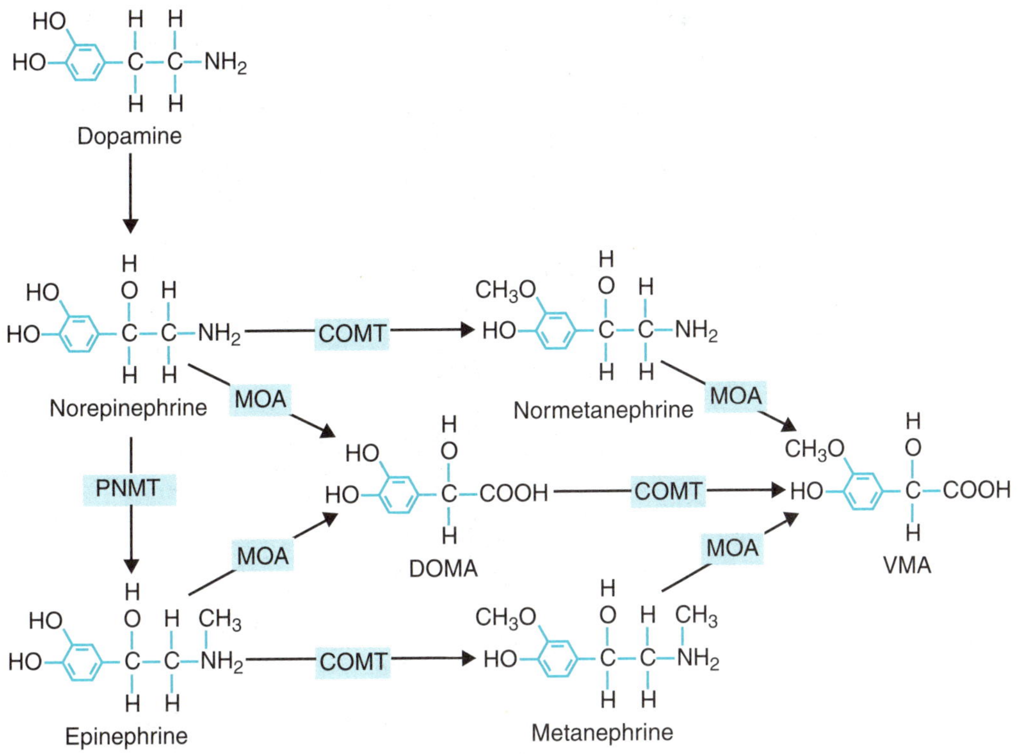

Figure 10-2. Metabolites of catecholamines. Through a series of reactions, catecholamines are broken down into metanephrines and vanillylmandelic acid (VMA). COMT, catechol-O-methyltransferase; MAO, monoamine oxidase; PNMT, phenylethanolamine-N-methyltransferase.

When the evaluation of hypertension points to a possible adrenal or reno-vascular cause, further testing often includes imaging studies. Magnetic resonance imaging (MRI) and computed tomographic (CT) scans can provide valuable information, especially when combined with an assessment of the clinical presentation and the biochemical data.

CASE PRESENTATION: CASE 1

Headaches, palpitations, and drenching sweats in a 35-year-old man

Headaches, other than occasional, clearly stress-related ones, had never been a problem for Larry Budman. Mr. Budman was 35 when he began to have daily, pounding headaches—"all over my head." Aspirin helped somewhat, but never completely relieved the pain. In addition, he had episodes of palpitations and drenching sweats that were very embarrassing. These spells were interfering with his work. Mr Budman owns and operates a small delicatessen that does a brisk breakfast and lunch business. When he has one of these spells, he has to stop slicing meat or making sandwiches because the sweat really pours off his forehead.

Mr. Budman's past medical history is unremarkable. He is on no medications and does not smoke. He has 4 to 5 cups of coffee each day and drinks about 6 cans of beer a week.

His parents are in their late 60s, and both are healthy; neither has hypertension. Mr. Budman's three siblings and his two children are healthy.

A detailed review of systems is negative.

Physical Examination
    General: A healthy-appearing man

Vital Signs:

Position	BP	Pulse
Lying (15 minutes)	180/120 (right arm)	90
	178/— (left leg by palpation)	
Sitting	160/110	110
Standing	150/100	110

HEENT:	**Normal**
Neck:	**Normal, thyroid not enlarged**
Chest:	**Normal**
Heart:	**Rapid, normal heart sounds**
Abdomen:	**Soft, normal bowel sound, no bruits, no masses or organomegaly**
Genitals:	**Normal**
Extremities:	**Normal**

Laboratory Studies

Test	Larry Budman	Normal
HCT	54%	42%–52% (male)
Sodium	144 mEq/L	135–145 mEq/L
Potassium	4.1 mEq/L	3.5–5.0 mEq/L
BUN	26 mg/dL	8–22 mg/dL
Creatinine	0.9 mg/dL	0.3–1.5 mg/dL
Glucose, fasting	138 mg/dL	70–110 mg/dL, fasting

While waiting for additional test results, Mr. Budman is started on the beta-blocker, atenolol, 50 mg per day.

Mr. Budman presents with severe hypertension and a history of spells of palpitations and excessive diaphoresis. His examination reveals that his blood pressure is elevated in both the upper and the lower extremities, making a coarctation of the aorta unlikely. In addition to hypertension, Mr. Budman has evidence of functional volume depletion. Although he is still hypertensive when standing, his blood pressure falls significantly. The elevated hematocrit and the fact that his BUN is elevated in the presence of a normal serum creatinine level suggest that he has some degree of intravascular volume depletion. Catecholamine excess could account for all of these findings.

Although rare (<0.1% of hypertensive patients), pheochromocytoma is both life-threatening and potentially curable. More than 90% of patients with pheochromocytoma have hypertension, and over half have sustained elevations of blood pressure. Headache, sweating, and palpitations are so common that the lack of all three would virtually exclude the diagnosis of pheochromocytoma. Postural hypotension and hypotension following surgery or trauma are explained by volume depletion, which is the result of chronic alpha-adrenergic–induced vasoconstriction. Dampened baroreflex function also is a factor. In most patients, pheochromocytoma is a sporadic occurrence, but it can be both familial and associated with other endocrine tumors, such as medullary carcinoma of the thyroid and parathyroid hyperplasia. Once clinically suspected, by symptoms, signs, or an adrenal mass, the diagnosis is supported by biochemical data—elevated urinary excretion or plasma levels of catecholamines or their metabolites. In patients with paroxysmal symptoms, a 24-hour urine collection starting at the time of an episode can improve diagnostic yield. Provocative and suppressive testing are indicated only in isolated, unusual cases.

After 1 week on the beta-blocker, Mr. Budman still has significant headaches and some sweating, but the palpitations are less severe.

Physical Examination
   Blood pressure: 180/130

Laboratory Studies

Test	Larry Budman	Normal
24-hour urinary catecholamine excretion:		
Epinephrine	188 μg/d	1.7–22.4 μg/d
Norepinephrine	205 μg/d	12.1–85.5 μg/d
Total	393 μg/d	<100 μg/d
24-hour urinary metanephrines	18.6 mg/d	<1.2 mg/d

Mr. Budman was admitted to the hospital and started on a nitroprusside drip to lower his blood pressure. The atenolol was discontinued, and the next morning his blood pressure was 150/90. Phenoxybenzamine was started, and the nitroprusside drip was tapered. During the next 2 weeks, Mr. Budman's blood pressure was controlled with phenoxybenzamine, and after several days of alpha blockade, atenolol was restarted to control tachycardia.

MR imaging revealed a 4-cm right adrenal mass.

Beta-adrenergic blockade alone in patients with pheochromocytoma can result in even higher blood pressure levels. Beta-mediated vasodilatation is blocked, and unrestrained alpha-adrenergic activity can exacerbate both the blood pressure and the clinical situation. Beta-blockers should be used with great caution in patients who have a history of, or physical examination suggestive of, a pheochromocytoma.

When clinical and biochemical data suggest a pheochromocytoma, noninvasive imaging studies—e.g., CT scanning, MR imaging, ultrasound, radiolabeled octreotide scanning, and MIBG (^{131}I-meta-iodobenzylguanidine) scanning—usually can localize the lesion and help identify bilateral and extra-adrenal pheochromocytomas (80% are unilateral, 10% bilateral, and 10% extra-adrenal).

Surgery after adequate preoperative preparation is the treatment of choice. Alpha-adrenergic blockade with phenoxybenzamine usually controls the hypertension; volume repletion reduces postural hypotension. Once alpha-blockade has been established, beta-blockers may be added to control tachycardia and arrhythmias. Preoperative therapy should proceed for at least 2 weeks before surgery to allow for volume repletion and the return of normal baroreflex function. For inoperable cases, alpha-blockade can be combined with other antihypertensives, such as ACE inhibitors and calcium channel blockers.

After 3 weeks of therapy with both an alpha-blocker, phenoxybenzamine, and a beta-blocker, atenolol, Mr. Budman feels well. He is free of headaches and is no longer having palpitations or episodes of sweating.

During surgery to remove the right adrenal mass, Mr. Budman's blood pressure fluctuated widely. Initially, with manipulation of the adrenal mass, his blood pressure rose to 200/140, and short-acting alpha- and beta-blockers were administered. After the adrenal vein was tied off and the adrenal mass was removed, Mr. Budman became hypotensive, requiring a dopamine drip and transfusion of one unit of blood and 1 L of saline.

Postoperatively, Mr. Budman's blood pressure has been normal off all medications and he fells well. He is back to slicing meat and making sandwiches without interruption.

Manipulation of the pheochromocytoma during surgery increases the release of preformed catecholamines and can have major effects on blood pressure and circulation. Once the tumor is removed, catecholamine levels fall, and the residual effects of adrenergic blocking agents can lead to significant hypotension.

Because pheochromocytomas can be multiple and can recur, Mr. Budman will need careful follow-up care to monitor his blood pressure and to watch for the return of catecholamine excess. In addition, his family members should be carefully evaluated.

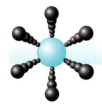

CASE PRESENTATION: CASE 2

Leg cramps, weakness, and hypokalemia in a 48-year-old man

Martin Carteras was 48 when painful leg cramps began to interrupt his sleep. He tried an over-the-counter quinine preparation, but it did not help. He also noted that he had to urinate more frequently, that he was drinking

more water, and that his muscles were weaker than usual. Because these symptoms were similar to those that his cousin Anthony had had when he was diagnosed with diabetes, Martin thought that he too had diabetes. He checked his blood sugar using Anthony's finger-stick glucose meter. The value was 108 mg/dL about 2 hours after breakfast.

Mr. Carteras works as an office manager in a large insurance company and lives with his wife and three teenage children. His past medical history is unremarkable. He is on no medications. A detailed review of systems is negative.

Physical Examination
 General: A healthy-appearing man

Vital Signs:

Position	Blood Pressure	Pulse
Lying (15 minutes)	170/100	90
Sitting	168/102	94
Standing (2 minutes)	170/98	90

HEENT:	Normal
Neck:	Normal, no thyroid enlargement
Chest:	Normal
Heart:	Normal
Abdomen:	Normal
Extremities:	Normal, no edema
Neurologic:	Normal

Laboratory Studies

Test	Martin Carteras	Normal
Glucose (fasting)	92 mg/dL	70–110 mg/dL, fasting
Sodium	144 mEq/L	135–145 mEq/L
Potassium	2.1 mEq/L	3.5–5.0 mEq/L
Chloride	100 mEq/L	98–106 mEq/L
Bicarbonate	34 mEq/L	21–30 mEq/L
BUN	16 mg/dL	8–22 mg/dL
Creatinine	1.0 mg/dL	0.3–1.5 mg/dL

While waiting for some additional lab studies, Mr. Carteras was started on potassium supplements and atenolol, 25 mg per day, to control his blood pressure.

In addition to significant hypertension, Mr. Carteras has profound hypokalemia. Hypokalemia can cause muscle weakness and irritability, which would explain some of his presenting symptoms. Significant hypokalemia has effects on renal function that lead to a mild nephrogenic diabetes insipidus. This acquired defect in renal concentrating ability does not respond to antidiuretic hormone (see Chapter 3) and may account for Mr. Carteras' polyuria and polydipsia.

The cause of this profound hypokalemia is not obvious from his history. He is not on any medications, and he does not have a history of either vomiting or diarrhea. His dietary intake has been normal, and he does not show evidence of conditions that might shift potassium into cells, such as alcohol withdrawal, catecholamine excess, or acidosis. Because he does not have evidence of extrarenal potassium loss or shifts, renal potassium loss is the most likely explanation.

The hypokalemia seen in Mr. Carteras is associated with an alkalosis, as indicated by the elevated bicarbonate concentration. The effect of aldosterone on the distal nephron is to induce sodium reabsorption in exchange for potassium and hydrogen ions. Increased aldosterone secretion or effectiveness can cause hypertension with hypokalemia and metabolic alkalosis. The mechanism of the possible excess aldosterone effect is unclear. It could be secondary to volume depletion, which triggers the renin-angiotensin system to stimulate aldosterone secretion, but there is no clinical evidence of volume depletion. Hyperkalemia, the other major stimulus for aldosterone secretion, clearly is not a factor, because Mr. Carteras is significantly hypokalemic. Excess ACTH seems unlikely, because he does not appear to be cushingoid, and his blood sugar is normal. He is not taking any medications that have a mineralocorticoid effect. Another possibility is consumption of licorice: when eaten in large amounts, it can inhibit the effect of the 11-β hydroxysteroid dehydrogenase enzyme in mineralocorticoid-sensitive cells and can cause hypertension and hypokalemic alkalosis.

After 7 days on atenolol and potassium supplementation, Mr. Carteras has noted no significant change in his symptoms. Additional history reveals that he is not eating licorice. His blood pressure is 150/96, and his pulse is 80.

Additional Laboratory Studies

Test	Martin Carteras	Normal
Potassium	2.4 mEq/L	3.5–5.0 mEq/L
Aldosterone	42 ng/dL	2–5 ng/dL supine 7–20 ng/dL standing
Plasma renin activity	<0.3 μg/L per hour	Normal diet: 0.3–1.9 μg/L per hour supine 0.3–3.6 μg/L per hour standing

Based on these results and the failure of potassium supplements to correct his hypokalemia, spironolactone was started at a dose of 50 mg twice a day. The atenolol was stopped and an MR image of the adrenal was scheduled.

The laboratory findings confirm the clinical suspicion of excess aldosterone. They also suggest that there is autonomous overproduction of aldosterone, because the plasma renin activity (PRA) is low. If the PRA were elevated, a renovascular lesion, diuretic use, or a renin-secreting tumor could be the explanation. Autonomous overproduction of aldosterone, or *primary aldosteronism,* can occur via several different mechanisms. A single adenoma, multiple adenomata, primary hyperplasia, and adrenal cortical carcinoma can all produce excessive amounts of aldosterone. Each of these conditions should be visible with CT scanning or MR imaging of the adrenal gland. When the adrenal glands appear anatomically normal, essential overproduction of aldosterone, i.e., *idiopathic* or *primary* hyperaldosteronism, usually is the explanation, but an ectopic source, such as an ovarian tumor that makes aldosterone or a condition referred to as *glucocorticoid remedial hypertension,* is another possibility.

In glucocorticoid remedial hypertension, the curious, serendipitous finding that physiologic replacement doses of glucocorticoids corrected both the hypertension and the hypokalemia in some familial forms of hyperaldosteronism elucidated a unique mechanism of aldosteronism. In this particular type of aldosteronism, which is autosomal dominant, the form of the 11β-hydroxylase enzyme that is present in the glomerulosa (P450$_{aldo}$) of the adrenal cortex becomes activated by ACTH. This phenomenon results in an increase of 11β-hydroxylase activity, which, in turn, leads to increased aldosterone production. Aldosterone production in this condition is controlled primarily by ACTH secretion, not by the renin-angiotensin system or the serum potassium concentration. By decreasing ACTH secretion, exogenous glucocorticoids decrease aldosterone secretion and correct the hypertension and hypokalemia.

Glucocorticoid remedial hypertension and other forms of aldosteronism that involve both adrenal glands usually are treated pharmacologically, because unilateral adrenalectomy is unlikely to correct the condition. For some patients with evidence of bilateral hyperfunction, even bilateral adrenalectomy, although it corrects the hypokalemia, may not correct the hypertension. The evaluation of aldosteronism is directed not only at finding the source of the excess aldosterone, but also at predicting the success of surgery in correcting the hypertension and hypokalemia.

The next steps in the evaluation of Mr. Carteras for aldosterone excess are anatomic and pharmacologic. The goal is to determine the mechanism of the elevated aldosterone level and to use that information to plan the most effective form of therapy. The CT scan should be able to define the anatomy of the adrenal glands and might indicate whether the process is bilateral or unilateral. Further anatomic and functional information can be obtained with adrenal vein catheterization. Catheters are threaded into each of the adrenal veins through a transcutaneous route, and samples are simultaneously obtained from each adrenal gland and from the inferior vena cava below the adrenal glands. A step up in the concentration of aldosterone on one side helps lateralize the pathology and can be valuable in planning surgery.

The pharmacologic evaluation is performed to see if the administration of an aldosterone receptor–blocking agent, such as spironolactone, can correct both the hypertension and the hypokalemia. Failure of spironolactone to correct the hypertension usually means that surgery will not correct the hypertension either.

Over the next 3 weeks, the dose of spironolactone was gradually increased to a total of 400 mg per day. On this regimen Mr. Carteras felt well. He no longer had the weakness, cramps, and polyuria that he had had before.

Physical Examination
    Blood pressure: 130/80

Laboratory Studies

Test	Martin Carteras	Normal
Potassium	3.8 mEq/L	3.5–5.0 mEq/L

MR images: See Figure 10-3
               12-mm adenoma of the right adrenal cortex

To verify the functionality of the lesion seen on MRI, adrenal venous sampling was performed:

Vein	Aldosterone (ng/dL)	Cortisol (μg/dL)	Aldosterone-to-Cortisol Ratio
Right adrenal	2804	423	6.6
Left adrenal	190	518	0.4
Inferior vena cava	56	28	2.0

Based on this information, Mr. Carteras decided to proceed with surgery. He had laparoscopic removal of the right adrenal gland. The pathology report revealed a benign 11-mm adenoma. Postoperatively, Mr. Carteras became normotensive and normokalemic without any medications.

Although the adrenal vein sampling may not have been absolutely necessary in this evaluation, it did help reassure the patient and his doctors that surgery would have a high likelihood of correcting both the hypertension and the hypokalemia. The aldosterone levels measured in the right adrenal vein were markedly elevated. Expressing the levels as a ratio with cortisol as the denominator allows a more accurate comparison of the adrenal vein effluent values. Because Mr. Carteras' other adrenal gland is intact, he did not and will not need corticosteroid coverage.

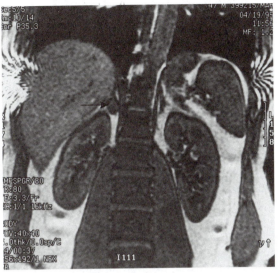
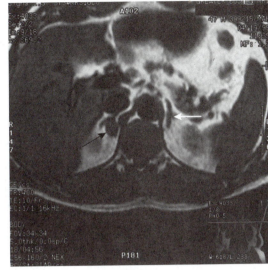
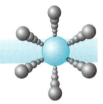

A   **B**

Figure 10-3. Abdominal MRI images of Martin Carteras. (**A**) Coronal view of the abdomen. A nodule (*arrow*) is seen above the right kidney, medial to the liver. (**B**) Axial view of the abdomen. A normal, triangle-shaped, left adrenal gland is present (*white arrow*). A nodule (*black arrow*), distorts the normal triangular shape of the right adrenal gland.

CASE PRESENTATION: CASE 3

Postural hypotension in a 48-year-old woman with diabetes

Getting up quickly had become a significant problem for Heather Henson. If she didn't slowly go from lying to standing, Ms. Henson would become very light-headed and, on a couple of occasions, she actually fainted. The problem really started several months ago, but has worsened over the past month. The symptoms are especially prominent when she gets up in the morning or when she stands up after eating a large meal.

Heather Henson is 48 years old and has had diabetes mellitus for the past 34 years. Although there were times when her diabetic control was less than ideal, for the last 20 years she has made a major effort to control her glucose levels. She is now on three shots per day of insulin, and she does finger-stick blood glucose determinations three or four times a day. She has an occasional mild hypoglycemic episode, and at times her sugars are very high. The memory module in her glucose meter indicates an average blood sugar of 138 mg/dL over the past month.

Mild retinopathy has led to laser therapy in each eye, but her vision has been quite good. A painful burning discomfort in her feet, which is especially prominent when she goes to bed, has been the most difficult complication of her diabetes. About 2 years ago Ms. Henson began to have nocturnal diarrhea that was unpleasant and difficult to control, until she started on an antibiotic regimen.

Physical Examination
    General: A healthy-appearing woman

Vital Signs:

Position	BP	Pulse
Lying (15 minutes)	140/92	84
Sitting	122/80	82
Standing (2 minutes)	80/56	88

HEENT:	Diabetic retinopathy with multiple laser scars, both eyes
Neck:	Normal, no thyromegaly
Chest:	Clear, excellent air movement
Heart:	No murmurs, normal heart sounds
Abdomen:	Soft, normal bowel sounds, no organomegaly
Extremities:	No edema, mild dependent rubor
Neuro:	**Mental status: Normal**
	Cranial nerves: Intact
	Motor: Normal
	Sensory: Decreased light touch, both lower extremities, in a stocking distribution up to the mid-calf
	Reflexes: Absent ankle-jerk reflexes

Ms. Henson has significant postural hypotension. The drop in blood pressure that occurs when she stands up is occurring in the setting of borderline supine hypertension and is not associated with the expected increase in heart rate. In the absence of cardiac conducting system disease or medications that might affect heart rate, the lack of a reflex tachycardia suggests that Ms. Henson has autonomic neuropathy. She clearly has evidence of a distal, symmetrical, peripheral sensory neuropathy in a pattern that is commonly seen in patients with diabetes. In addition, her nocturnal diarrhea is likely due to autonomic neuropathy affecting her colon. The bacterial overgrowth that sometimes occurs with decreased colonic motility can, for some patients, be counteracted with antibiotics. The several neuropathies that are associated with diabetes (see Chapter 7) often are present together in various combinations in the same patient.

Further evaluation of patients with postural hypotension should involve a thorough evaluation of the pumping, volume, and vascular components of the cardiovascular system that help maintain blood pressure when position is changed. Heart disease could be a factor. In patients with diabetes and autonomic neuropathy, significant ischemic heart disease can be present without the usual symptoms of pain that are associated with ischemia. Depending on the clinical situation, a stress test or an electrophysiologic study may be appropriate in the evaluation of patients with postural hypotension.

Additional evaluation revealed a normal electrocardiogram and normal electrolytes. 8 a.m. cortisol and thyroid function tests also were normal. An

exercise tolerance test failed to show evidence of ischemia, but Ms. Henson had difficulty reaching her target heart rate.

Adding some salt to her diet and raising the head of her bed by about 8 inches did improve her symptoms, although she still had to be very careful getting up. When her evaluation was completed, Ms. Henson started taking fludrocortisone. After about 4 weeks the dose was increased to 0.3 mg each day, a dose that is about three times the physiologic replacement dose of this aldosterone-like medication.

With fludrocortisone added, Ms. Henson had much less difficulty with postural symptoms.

Physical Examination

Vital Signs:

Position	BP	Pulse
Lying (15 minutes)	160/100	84
Sitting	140/96	82
Standing (2 minutes)	110/64	88

Laboratory Studies

Test	Heather Henson	Normal
Potassium	2.8 mEq/L	3.5–5.0 mEq/L

Although Ms. Henson's symptoms are somewhat better, she now has very significant supine hypertension and marked hypokalemia, two potentially dangerous conditions. The presence of hypertension increases her risk for cardiovascular complications and is especially worrisome with regard to her renal function. The combination of hypertension and diabetes increases the risk of chronic renal failure. The hypokalemia can be associated with weakness, muscle cramps, and an increased risk of cardiac arrhythmias.

In addition to fludrocortisone, elevating the head of the bed, and increasing salt intake, constrictive garments that prevent pooling of blood in the lower extremities can help patients manage postural hypotension. Erythropoietin administration can increase blood volume and has been used in patients with postural hypotension. Midodrine, a selective alpha$_1$-adrenergic agonist, is available, but, like fludrocortisone and erythropoietin, it can cause supine hypertension.

Because of the patient's supine hypertension, the dose of fludrocortisone is reduced to 0.15 mg each day. Ms. Henson still has some postural dizziness, but she is learning to cope with the symptoms. On the lower dose, her supine pressure is 138/84 and her potassium is in the normal range at 3.6 mEq/L.

KEY POINTS AND CONCEPTS

Hypertension

- Essential hypertension is the most common form of hypertension.
- A postural fall in blood pressure suggests a possible endocrine pathogenesis.
- When hypokalemia is present, mineralocorticoid or glucocorticoid excess should be considered.
- When headache, palpitations, and diaphoresis are associated with hypertension, a pheochromocytoma should be considered.

Hypotension

- Postural hypotension may be caused by any of several mechanisms:
  - Volume depletion.
  - Medications that block cardiovascular reflexes.
  - Mineralocorticoid or glucocorticoid deficiency.
  - Cardiac disease—rhythm or pump disturbances.
  - Autonomic neuropathy.

SUGGESTED READING

Blumenfeld JD, Sealy JE, Schussel Y, et al. Diagnosis and treatment of primary hyperaldosteronism. Ann Intern Med 121:877–885, 1994.

Cryer PE. Pheochromocytoma. West J Med 156:399–407, 1992.

Insel PA. Adrenergic receptors—evolving concepts and clinical implications. N Engl J Med 334:580–585, 1996.

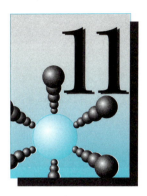

Integrative Endocrinology

POLYGLANDULAR SYNDROMES AND ENDOCRINE ASPECTS OF VARIOUS MEDICAL CONDITIONS

The cases discussed in this chapter involve variations and combinations of clinical concepts discussed earlier. The basic pathophysiology, and the basis for clinically useful tests of function and anatomy, are found in the preceding chapters.

POLYGLANDULAR SYNDROMES

Syndromes of both hypofunction and hyperfunction involving multiple glands have been described. The pathophysiologic basis for these curious combinations of malfunction of more than one gland has become better understood in the past several years.

Autoimmune induced impairment of endocrine gland function is the most common cause of glandular failure syndromes. Lymphocyte- and antibody-mediated destruction of gland architecture or impairment of gland function results in hypofunction. For some patients, the autoimmune process also includes other glands and nonendocrine target tissues.

Most diseases that involve hormonal overproduction are associated with cellular proliferation within the affected gland. In some cases, the stimulus for hyperplasia is an external one. Graves' disease, for example, is caused by an antibody that mimics TSH. In other cases, hyperplasia and hormonal overproduction appear to be triggered by internal or intracellular phenomena, usually a mutation that disrupts the cell's mechanism for controlling its growth, hormone production, and hormone release. It is this latter mechanism, in one form or another, that accounts for most syndromes of polyglandular hormonal excess.

Diabetes, Addison's disease, hypothyroidism, and vitiligo in a 19-year-old woman

At the age of 12, shortly after the onset of menstruation, Bertha Coombs suddenly began to experience polyuria and polydipsia and lost approximately 10 pounds in 4 days. Nausea and vomiting developed and became so severe that her parents brought her to the emergency room, where the following laboratory data were generated:

Test	Bertha Coombs	Normal
Glucose	396 mg/dL	70–110 mg/dL, fasting
Serum ketones	Strongly positive	Negative

Therapy with intravenous fluids and insulin was begun, and 2 days later Bertha was home, reconstituted and back to her usual self. She quickly mastered the use of insulin and finger-stick blood glucose determinations. Her usual insulin dose was 20 units of NPH insulin and 4 units of regular insulin in the morning, followed by 8 units of NPH insulin and 6 units of regular insulin at supper. On this basic regimen, Bertha did well, having infrequent mild episodes of hypoglycemia and keeping her glycohemoglobin within a good range.

At age 16, Bertha began to have frequent insulin reactions. The palpitations, sweatiness, irritability, and feelings of hunger usually meant that her blood sugar was very low. She documented the low sugars with her finger-stick meter and made appropriate adjustments in her diet, activity plans, and insulin dose. Her total daily insulin dose decreased to 20 units per day, down from the original 38 units.

One day at school, an unfortunately scheduled mid-term exam forced Bertha to deviate from her usual routine. She had intended to eat a late lunch after her mid-term, but she had a major motor seizure during the test. In the ambulance on the way to the hospital, she had a finger-stick blood glucose of 19 mg/dL. She was given 50 mL of 50% glucose in water. She promptly regained consciousness, but could not remember any details of what had transpired. On arrival at the Emergency Room, the following additional information was generated:

Physical Examination
  Blood pressure: 90/60 supine
                  60/? sitting
  Pulse: 100 supine
            124 sitting

Skin:	**Bronze tan with pigmentation of palmar creases and areolae**
HEENT:	**Normal**
Chest:	**Clear**
Heart:	**Normal**
Abdomen:	**Normal**
Extremities:	**Normal**

Intravenous saline was started at 200 mL/hour.

Laboratory Studies

Test	Bertha Coombs	Normal
Glucose—20 minutes after 50% glucose	452 mg/dL	70–110 mg/dL, fasting
Sodium	123 mEq/L	135–145 mEq/L
Potassium	6.2 mEq/L	3.5–5.0 mEq/L
BUN	34 mg/dL	8–22 mg/dL
Creatinine	0.9 mg/dL	0.3–1.5 mg/dL

There are a number of different conditions that can cause a type 1 diabetic to exhibit reduced insulin requirements. Declining renal function and counterregulatory hormone deficiencies are the most important mechanisms to consider. Although for many patients, a change in activity level or food intake may account for an alteration in insulin needs, hypoglycemic episodes that are not readily explained require further evaluation. Evaluation of Bertha's declining insulin requirements was prompted by a seizure, a severe manifestation of hypoglycemia. Luckily, she was treated quickly, thereby lowering the risk of permanent CNS damage.

Bertha's declining insulin requirements, her hyperpigmentation, her postural hypotension, and her serum electrolytes all point to the diagnosis of adrenocortical insufficiency. A lack of the glucocorticoid hormone, cortisol, has significant effects on glucose metabolism (see Chapter 5). Without the presence of cortisol, insulin is more effective in lowering glucose levels. In addition, the counterregulatory effects of cortisol are important in maintaining a normal blood sugar and preventing hypoglycemia. The lack of both cortisol and aldosterone could account for Bertha's hypotension and clinical volume depletion. Her hyperkalemia could be caused by a lack of mineralocorticoid function. Although her BUN is elevated, the normal creatinine concentration suggests that she is volume depleted and that she probably does not have parenchymal renal disease.

When the question of adrenal insufficiency was raised, an ACTH level was drawn, followed by a cosyntropin stimulation test. After receiving 2 L of saline, Bertha began to feel much better, and her blood pressure no longer dropped significantly when she sat up. After the cosyntropin test was completed, Bertha received 100 mg of hydrocortisone intravenously.

Cosyntropin Stimulation Test

	Bertha Coombs	
Time (min)	Cortisol (μg/dL)	Aldosterone (ng/dL)
0	4	6
30	3	6
60	5	7

ACTH Level

Test	Bertha Coombs	Normal
ACTH	652 pg/mL	8 a.m., fasting <80 pg/mL

Bertha was started on hydrocortisone and fludrocortisone and was discharged from the hospital the following day. At home she planned to readjust her insulin dose and schedule a make-up exam. After 5 days, Bertha was back to a total daily insulin dose of 38 units. She did well on the make-up exam and quickly resumed her normal activities.

Bertha has developed adrenocortical insufficiency. She now has two major endocrine deficiency conditions. Two separate polyglandular failure syndromes have been described. The two types overlap significantly in two areas, although there are important differences (Table 11-1). Type 1 usually presents in childhood and almost always is associated with mucocutaneous candidiasis. It is familial, as well, and transmitted as an autosomal recessive trait. Adult onset of symptoms and low likelihood of hypoparathyroidism characterize type 2 polyglandular failure syndrome. Although type 2 clearly has characteristic HLA associations, other factors, possibly environmental, must play a role, because identical twins may not be similarly affected.

Although the role of organ-specific autoantibodies in the pathogenesis of organ hypofunction is unclear, these autoantibodies usually are measurable before hypofunction develops. Antibody measurements can be used to assess the likelihood of subsequent disease, but they do not predict when glandular failure will occur. Histologic examination of the target gland usually reveals lymphocytic infiltration and inflammation and, later, fibrosis.

The treatment of each hypofunctioning system is the same for patients with polyglandular failure syndromes as for patients with single system failures. Bertha Coombs' history demonstrates that there can be important interactions between affected glandular systems.

Three years later, during her sophomore year in college, Bertha began to gain weight, and her menstrual periods, which had previously been regular, became more frequent—every 10 days, on average—and very heavy. Bertha initially attributed these changes to the stress of a heavy academic load

TABLE 11-1. CLINICAL FEATURES OF AUTOIMMUNE POLYGLANDULAR SYNDROMES		
CONDITION OR CHARACTERISTIC	**TYPE 1**	**TYPE 2**
Age of onset	Childhood	Adult
Inheritance	Autosomal recessive	HLA association
Mucocutaneous candidiasis	Common	Not seen
Adrenal cortical failure (Addison's disease)	Common	Common
Thyroid disease	Rare	Common
Hypoparathyroidism	Common	Rare
Primary hypogonadism	Common	Occurs
Type 1 diabetes	Occurs	Common
Pituitary failure	Occurs	Occurs
Autoimmune hepatitis	Occurs	Not seen
Pernicious anemia	Occurs	Occurs
Vitiligo	Occurs	Occurs
Alopecia	Common	Occurs
Myasthenia gravis	Not seen	Occurs

and a busy social life, but when her weight gain reached 15 pounds, she decided to seek medical attention.

Physical Examination

Height:	5'6"
Weight:	159 pounds
Vital signs:	Blood pressure 140/84; pulse 62
Skin:	Hypopigmented areas of forearms, dorsum of hands, and left thigh
HEENT:	Mild, puffy, periorbital edema
Neck:	Easily visible and palpable thyroid, about 2 times normal size
Chest:	Clear
Heart:	Normal
Abdomen:	Normal
Pelvic examination:	Normal
Extremities:	Normal
Neuro:	Cranial nerves: Normal
	Motor: Normal
	Sensory: Normal
	Cerebellar: Normal
	Reflexes: Delayed relaxation of Achilles and biceps tendon reflexes

Laboratory Studies

Test	Bertha Coombs	Normal
TSH	98 mU/L	0.3–5.0 mU/L
T$_4$	2.0 μg/dL	5–12 μg/dL

Based on these results, thyroid hormone therapy was begun. After about 12 weeks on 0.125 mg of thyroxine (T$_4$) each day, Bertha was feeling very well and her menstrual periods have returned to normal. Taking a single thyroid hormone pill each day was, Bertha noted, the easiest part of her medical regimen.

The vitiligo—the hypopigmented patches on her hands, arms, and thigh—is a problem. Bertha understands that the condition sometimes is progressive. She has found a cosmetic lotion that hides it well, but she hates to add yet another chore to her daily personal care.

Bertha often wonders what medical problem will appear next. She would like to avoid developing another full-blown hormone deficiency syndrome. She is especially worried about the possibility of premature ovarian failure, and asks what can be done to prevent it.

Laboratory Studies

Test	Bertha Coombs	Normal
Anti-ovarian antibodies	Negative	Negative

Bertha has developed both vitiligo and primary hypothyroidism, adding two more autoimmune conditions to her list of diagnoses. Vitiligo develops when the autoimmune process involves melanocytes, resulting in patchy areas of depigmentation. Although neither of these new conditions is life threatening, such an accumulation of medical problems can be very depressing for patients with these syndromes. Bertha's worries about hypogonadism are quite reasonable. Hypogonadism is one of the most difficult autoimmune conditions to manage. In both sexes, replacing end-organ sex steroid hormones is relatively easy and free of complications, but replacing reproductive potential is very difficult. Although Bertha's antibody titer is negative, she still is at risk for autoimmune oophoritis and premature ovarian failure. Unfortunately, there currently is no method of preventing glandular failure in patients with this syndrome. Careful follow-up care, periodically looking for preclinical manifestations of other associated conditions, is clearly indicated.

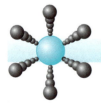

CASE PRESENTATION: CASE 2

Pheochromocytoma, medullary carcinoma of the thyroid, and hyperparathyroidism in a 35-year-old man

Gary Sadler was 35 years old when he began to experience severe, exertion-related headaches and palpitations. His job as a railroad maintenance engineer often involved moving railroad ties and pounding spikes.

Nearly every time he had to help lift a tie he would develop a severe head-ache, palpitations, and diaphoresis and would have to sit down for 25 to 30 minutes.

Mr. Sadler's foreman was both fed up and worried, and sent him to the local hospital. On arrival at the outpatient clinic Mr. Sadler's blood pressure was measured at 200/160, and he was admitted for evaluation and management.

Past Medical History

Illnesses:	No diabetes, TB, or hepatitis
Surgery:	Tonsillectomy at age 7
Medications:	None
Habits:	Alcohol: 2 drinks per day
	Cigarettes: 1 pack per day
	Coffee: 6 cups per day
OTC medications:	Acetaminophen for headaches, up to 10 per day
Allergies:	None

Family History

Father:	Died at age 29 of heat stroke
Mother:	Died at age 62 of pneumonia
No siblings	
3 children:	Andrew, 3, alive and well
	Martin, 5, alive and well
	Amy, 8, alive and well

Physical Examination

Thin, well-developed man in some discomfort

Vital Signs	Supine	Standing (10 minutes)
Blood pressure:	190/150	160/120
Pulse:	90	110

HEENT:	Arteriolar narrowing, scattered retinal hemorrhages, both eyes
Neck:	1.5-cm firm nodule right thyroid lobe, near isthmus, no adenopathy
Chest:	Clear
Heart:	Rapid, normal
Abdomen:	No palpable masses or organomegaly. Palpation of the abdomen was immediately followed by a paroxysm of severe hypertension
Genitals:	Normal
Extremities:	Normal
Neuro:	Normal

Laboratory Studies

Test	Gary Sadler	Normal
Calcium	12.2 mg/dL	8.5–10.5 mg/dL
Phosphorus	1.8 mg/dL	3–4.5 mg/dL
T_4	9.9 μg/dL	5–12 μg/dL
TSH	1.2 mU/L	0.3–5.0 mU/L
24-hour urinary VMA	52 mg/d	2–7 mg/d
24-hour catecholamine excretion:		
Epinephrine	204 μg/d	1.7–22.4 μg/day
Norepinephrine	230 μg/d	12.1–85.5 μg/day
Total	434 μg/d	<100 μg/day

X-rays:
 Chest: Normal
 Abdomen: **Shifting of renal axis by suprarenal masses bilaterally**

Clearly, the most important of Mr. Sadler's presenting problems is his severe hypertension. His clinical history of severe hypertension with exertion-related paroxysms of headache and palpitations should raise the possibility of a pheochromocytoma. In addition, he has both anatomic evidence of adrenal masses (shifting of the renal axes on abdominal X-rays) and biochemical evidence of excessive catecholamine production. The death of Mr. Sadler's father at age 30 of "heat stroke" raises the possibility that Mr. Sadler is part of a kindred of familial pheochromocytoma.

The diagnosis of pheochromocytoma alone, however, does not explain all of Mr. Sadler's clinical findings. The thyroid nodule clearly needs further evaluation, even in the face of normal thyroid function tests. In addition, Mr. Sadler has evidence of hyperparathyroidism. His serum calcium level is significantly elevated, with a very low serum phosphate level—another problem needing further evaluation. Exploratory neck surgery will be an efficient way of dealing with both the nodule and the hyperparathyroidism, but the pheochromocytoma must be dealt with first.

In preparation for surgery to remove the pheochromocytomas, Mr. Sadler was started on alpha-adrenergic blocking agents, with a beta-blocking agent added to control tachycardia. After 3 weeks, his blood pressure was 140/84 and he no longer had a significant postural drop in blood pressure.

During these 3 weeks of preparation some additional studies were completed:

 MR image of the abdomen: Bilateral adrenal masses, consistent with bilateral pheochromocytomas
 Thyroid scan: Uptake 28% (normal 10%–25%)
         Cold nodule, 1.5 cm, right lobe near isthmus

Laboratory Studies

Test	Gary Sadler	Normal
Calcium	12.1 mg/dL	8.5–10.5 mg/dL
PTH (intact molecule)	235 pg/mL	10–65 pg/mL
Calcitonin	327 pg/mL	Male: 0–14 pg/mL Female: 0–28 pg/mL

The PTH level is markedly elevated in the face of an elevated calcium concentration, a combination diagnostic of hyperparathyroidism (see Chapter 6). Calcitonin, a protein hormone product of the parafollicular, or C cells, of the thyroid is a marker for medullary carcinoma of the thyroid. This malignancy of the thyroid originates in the parafollicular cells and usually is more aggressive than papillary or follicular thyroid cancer.

Each of Mr. Sadler's three conditions—pheochromocytoma, hyperparathyroidism, and medullary carcinoma of the thyroid—can be hereditary or sporadic. Inherited syndromes of endocrine neoplasia involving multiple glands have been described and are referred to as multiple endocrine neoplasia (MEN) (Table 11-2). Studies of kindreds that exhibit these syndromes have broadened our understanding of endocrine neoplasia.

Most endocrine tumors appear to develop as monoclonal expansions. Elegant genetic studies based on the fact that one X chromosome is inactivated early in the embryonic development of somatic cells in females have supported this conclusion. If tumor cells from a woman contain only one type of X chromosome in the active state, clonal expansion of a single cell or small group of similar cells is likely. A tumor containing both active forms

TABLE 11-2. *CLINICAL FEATURES OF MULTIPLE ENDOCRINE NEOPLASIA SYNDROMES*

MEN type 1
  Hyperparathyroidism
  Anterior pituitary tumors
  Pancreatic tumors

MEN type 2a
  Hyperparathyroidism
  Medullary thyroid carcinoma
  Pheochromocytoma

MEN type 2b
  Medullary thyroid carcinoma
  Pheochromocytoma
  Mucosal neuromas

MEN, multiple endocrine neoplasia.

of the X chromosome suggests that monoclonal expansion did not occur, because the tumor contains a mixture of cells of different origins. This has been well studied in tumors that cause hyperparathyroidism. Adenomas, the most common cause of primary hyperparathyroidism (see Chapter 6), are the product of monoclonal expansion. Parathyroid hyperplasia, on the other hand, is a polyclonal process involving all four glands.

The mechanism of monoclonal expansion that results in the formation of an adenoma appears to reside in genetic mutations. Two different types of mutations have been elucidated. Cell proliferation can be induced when a mutation results in the development of a stimulating oncogene. Another mechanism of cellular proliferation involves the mutation of a tumor suppressor gene, which allows cellular proliferation to proceed without the normal constraints. Both mechanisms appear to be involved in the etiology of the MEN syndromes.

Type 1 MEN develops when a combination of mutations, both inherited and somatic, occurs in a tumor suppressor gene located on chromosome 11. The abnormal gene that results does not suppress cell growth normally, and neoplasia develops. The mechanism of the MEN type 2 syndromes involves mutations of a proto-oncogene referred to as RET, located on chromosome 10. The RET gene encodes a member of the tyrosine protein kinase family of receptors located on the cell surface. Although the gene is not highly expressed in most adult tissues, it is expressed in medullary thyroid cancer and in pheochromocytoma cell lines. The two subtypes of the MEN 2 syndrome result from different mutations of the same RET gene. Changes in the extracellular portion of the receptor result in the MEN 2a syndrome, whereas mutations that affect the intracellular domain of the receptor protein are seen in the MEN-2b form of the syndrome.

At surgery, Mr. Sadler had bilateral pheochromocytomas removed. Although there were wide fluctuations in his blood pressure during the procedure, Mr. Sadler tolerated the surgery well. Because it is not possible to separate the adrenal cortex from the pheochromocytoma tissue, the surgery left Mr. Sadler with adrenocortical insufficiency. Stress-dose glucocorticoids were started at the time of surgery, and the dose was gradually tapered to a physiologic replacement level. By the 5th postoperative day, Mr. Sadler was able to walk without assistance, bowel function returned to normal, and he was discharged with a blood pressure of 134/82, without any postural change. His discharge medications included hydrocortisone, 20 mg each morning and 10 mg each afternoon along with fludrocortisone, 0.1 mg each day.

Six weeks after the bilateral adrenalectomy, Mr. Sadler was readmitted for neck exploration. At surgery, a total thyroidectomy was performed. The cold nodule in the right lobe and four of 16 lymph nodes removed from the anterior neck revealed medullary thyroid carcinoma. In addition, all four parathyroid glands were identified and appeared to be enlarged. A frozen section showed probable parathyroid hyperplasia—a diffuse increase in cellularity without an obvious rim of normal appearing parathyroid tissue. Based on this finding, Mr. Sadler underwent a subtotal parathyroidectomy, leaving $\frac{1}{2}$ of one gland. Postoperatively, after a transient period of hypocalcemia, Mr. Sadler's calcium returned to normal.

Case 2: Pheochromocytoma, Medullary Carcinoma of the Thyroid, and Hyperparathyroidism

Three months after the neck surgery Mr. Sadler returned for a follow-up visit. His neck incision had healed well. No adenopathy was found.

Bone scan: Negative
Liver scan: Normal liver and spleen

Laboratory Studies

Test	Gary Sadler	Normal
Calcium	9.3 mg/dL	8.5–10.5 mg/dL
Phosphate	3.8 mg/dL	3–4.5 mg/dL
Calcitonin	3.8 pg/mL	Male: 0–14 pg/mL Female: 0–28 pg/mL <10.0 post–total thyroidectomy

Individual	RET Proto-Oncogene
Andrew Sadler	Negative
Emily Sadler	Negative
Martin Sadler	Positive
Gary Sadler	Positive

It is vital to screen family members for the genes associated with MEN syndromes, especially for the MEN type 2 syndromes. Early detection of the syndrome permits the performance of a total thyroidectomy before medullary carcinoma, the most difficult of the MEN type 2 neoplasms to manage, develops. In the past, early detection was based on pentagastrin or calcium infusion to stimulate calcitonin secretion. When values exceeded guideline levels, C cell hyperplasia or early medullary thyroid carcinoma was suspected. Unfortunately, false-positive tests resulted in unnecessary thyroidectomies in a number of children suspected of having the gene. Current screening is based on DNA analysis that looks for the specific mutations associated with the MEN syndromes.

One of Mr. Sadler's children, Martin, carries the abnormal gene and will need a total thyroidectomy in the near future. He also will need to be screened periodically for the development of pheochromocytoma. Serum calcium levels should be checked periodically, but hyperparathyroidism appears to occur less often in patients who undergo total thyroidectomy at a young age.

Over time, Mr. Sadler will need to be followed carefully, with serial calcitonin levels to look for recurrent disease. In addition to the neck, the mediastinal lymph nodes, lung, liver, and bone can be the site of metastatic disease.

ENDOCRINE ASPECTS OF VARIOUS MEDICAL CONDITIONS

A number of medical conditions have important endocrine aspects. Hormones or hormone analogues are used in the treatment of several illnesses. The anti-inflammatory effects of glucocorticoids, for example, can dramatically reverse the pathophysiology of asthma or inflammatory bowel disease. Although the pharmacologic uses of glucocorticoids can be life saving and are vital in the management of patients with these and other conditions, there can be, and often are, important sequelae. Case 4 in Chapter 5 illustrates a number of the consequences of exogenous steroids—cushingoid appearance, adrenal insufficiency, and osteoporosis.

Malignancies of several tissues can be associated with the production of hormones or substances that act like hormones. Case 3 in the Chapter 3 describes a patient with a lung tumor that makes ADH, with significant effects on water balance. Another lung malignancy is the cause of Cushing's syndrome resulting from ectopic ACTH production, as presented in Case 2 in Chapter 5. Knowledge of the endocrine aspects of cases like these can lead to important therapeutic interventions. In addition, hormones or hormone analogues made by tumors can be markers that allow monitoring of the success of therapy.

Endocrine interventions also can be used to palliate or significantly alter the course of a number of malignancies. Inhibition or interference with estrogen production or the target tissue effects of estrogen can improve the course of breast cancer. Similarly, shutting off androgen production or blocking androgen receptors can slow the course of prostate cancer in some men.

Obesity is seen in several endocrine syndromes. Obesity also has significant effects on intermediary metabolism and is highly correlated with diabetes and hypertension. HIV infection and the opportunistic infections associated with it can also have significant effects on endocrine function.

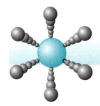

CASE PRESENTATION: CASE 3

Breast cancer in a 51-year-old woman

Sarah Schwartz was 44 years old when a routine mammogram showed a suspicious calcification. The biopsy revealed an invasive breast cancer. The decisions that had to be made were not easy, but Ms. Schwartz decided on a simple mastectomy, perhaps with reconstruction at a later date. This would avoid the radiation therapy that was recommended if she were to have a lumpectomy alone. At the time of the mastectomy, axillary lymph node sampling was performed. Three of ten axillary nodes were positive for cancer. The tumor was estrogen receptor–positive.

Soon after she had recovered from the surgery Sarah Schwartz had the first of six courses of CMF (cyclophosphamide, methotrexate, and fluorouracil) chemotherapy. During the chemotherapy she was very fatigued and lost almost all of her scalp hair. After the second cycle of chemotherapy, she also stopped menstruating and began to have hot flashes. Her hair grew

back, and the hot flashes gradually went away, but menstrual periods never returned. Although she was concerned about her family history of coronary artery disease and osteoporosis, Ms. Schwartz was convinced that estrogen replacement for her premature menopause was not safe.

Breast cancer is the most common malignancy in women in the United States and will develop in about 12% of women. Although the exact mechanisms that lead to breast cancer are not fully understood, a number of factors are known to be important. Genetic predisposition is clearly a factor. In addition, radiation exposure to the breast area, especially at an early age, appears to play a role. Obesity, low parity, advanced age at first pregnancy, and alcohol consumption are each correlated with increased risk. Although oral contraceptives do not appear to increase the risk of breast cancer, there is some evidence that long-term use of postmenopausal estrogen may increase the risk of breast cancer. This makes the decision of whether to take postmenopausal estrogen especially difficult for many women. The benefits of estrogen replacement for prevention of osteoporosis and heart disease must be weighed against the small, but real, risk of breast cancer.

The facts that Ms. Schwartz was premenopausal when she developed her cancer and that the tumor was estrogen receptor–positive suggest that there may be potentially important hormonal contributions to her treatment. Breast tumors that are rich in the cytoplasmic protein that binds estrogen and carries it to the nucleus, the site of estrogen effect, are considered to be estrogen receptor–positive (ER+), and are more likely to respond to hormonal manipulation. The available hormonal treatments may be additive or ablative.

Medical or surgical induction of ovarian failure often can have a significant positive effect on the course of breast cancer. Ms. Schwartz's chemotherapy did, as it does with many patients, induce ovarian failure and premature menopause. For Sarah Schwartz, estrogen replacement therapy clearly would be very risky because of the potential stimulation of any remaining breast cancer tissue. If ovarian function remains after adjuvant chemotherapy, oophorectomy can be considered, or it may be reserved for the future should the tumor recur. Long-acting gonadotropin-releasing hormone (GnRH) analogues suppress gonadotropin secretion and thereby reduce ovarian steroid hormone production. The resulting medical oophorectomy can be effective in increasing disease-free survival.

For the next 3 years, Sarah Schwartz had no evidence of breast cancer. She had a mammogram of her remaining breast every year, and every 6 months had a careful examination of the mastectomy site and axilla. Shortly before the 4th anniversary of her mastectomy, Ms. Schwartz noted a crust developing on the mastectomy scar with a small nodule adjacent to the crusting. The biopsy revealed breast cancer, histologically similar to her primary tumor. A bone scan and chest X-ray were both negative.

Although Ms. Schwartz had hoped that any further surgery would be for reconstruction of her missing breast, she underwent resection of the recurrent lesion, followed by 6 weeks of radiation therapy. After completing the radiation therapy she started on tamoxifen.

Tamoxifen is an example of an additive form of hormonal therapy. It is both an estrogen agonist and antagonist. In some areas—bone and endometrium—it has estrogen-like effects, while at the same time having an antiestrogen effect on breast tissue. The estrogen-like effect of tamoxifen on the endometrium brings with it an increased risk of endometrial carcinoma, a fact that has tempered the early enthusiasm that hailed tamoxifen as an effective and safe agent for preventing breast cancer. For patients like Sarah Schwartz, the palliative effects on breast cancer clearly are worth the risk of endometrial cancer, a process that should be curable if detected at an early stage.

For the next 3 years, Ms. Schwartz continued on tamoxifen and was clinically free of disease. Just after her 51st birthday, Ms. Schwartz began to have some pain in her left hip. X-rays showed a questionable lesion, and a bone scan showed multiple areas of metastatic disease—in both femurs, in the skull, and in several ribs (Fig. 11-1).

Because tamoxifen appeared to have provided some benefit, Ms. Schwartz continued the tamoxifen, and aminoglutethimide was added, together with hydrocortisone. The bone pain responded to a short course of

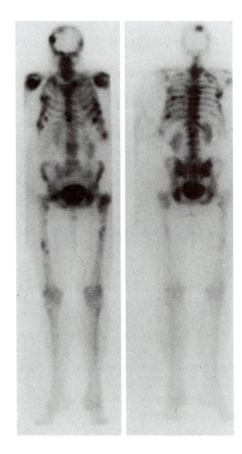

Figure 11-1. Bone scan: Sarah Schwartz. Both the anterior view on the left and the posterior view on the right show multiple areas of increased isotope uptake in bone. The patchy, widespread uptake seen in the ribs, skull, and femurs exhibits a pattern that is seen in metastatic disease.

local radiation therapy to the hip area, and Sarah Schwartz was able to resume all her normal activities.

Because Ms. Schwartz seemed to have responded favorably to hormonal manipulations—chemotherapy-induced early menopause followed by tamoxifen, it seemed that another attempt at decreasing steroid hormone levels might be effective. Aminoglutethimide inhibits cholesterol side-chain cleavage in steroid hormone–producing tissues and is so effective that hydrocortisone is added to replace the adrenocortical insufficiency that results. The decrease in steroid molecule production leads to a decreased availability of precursor molecules for aromatization to estrogen in body fat and other tissues. This regimen and other pharmacologic approaches to decreasing estrogen levels have largely replaced surgical adrenalectomy, a procedure done in the past to palliate the course of breast and other steroid-responsive cancers. Like other patients with bony metastases, Sarah Schwartz is at risk for hypercalcemia (see Case 3 in Chapter 6).

It is hoped that Sarah Schwartz will have a long remission with the latest interventions. Unfortunately, these interventions are usually palliative rather than curative. They are important tools in the management of breast cancer, however.

CASE PRESENTATION: CASE 4

Prostate cancer in a 71-year-old man

Getting up to urinate two or three times a night really interfered with Samuel Phillips' sleep. He had always been a light sleeper, experiencing difficulty getting back to sleep if awakened. This was Mr. Phillips' only complaint. He is 71 years old, his past medical history is unremarkable, and he takes no medications.

A physical examination was unremarkable except for an enlarged (+3 out of 4) prostate and a very firm nodule of the right lobe of the prostate noted on rectal examination.

Laboratory Studies

Test	Samuel Phillips	Normal
Prostate-specific antigen	18.6 μg/mL	0–4 μg/mL

Under ultrasound guidance, several transrectal biopsies of the nodule were taken.

Biopsy results: **4 of 6 biopsy specimens revealed Gleason grade 5 adenocarcinoma of the prostate**

Bone scan: **No evidence of metastatic disease, osteoarthritis of both knees**

**Pelvic CT scan: Probable metastases to pelvic lymph nodes and
seminal vesicles**

Mr. Phillips has prostate cancer that has spread beyond the capsule of
the prostate gland. The finding of disease outside the prostate indicates that
the condition is not curable and that radical surgery is not appropriate. Radical surgery brings with it a high likelihood of urinary incontinence and
erectile dysfunction. Because androgens are cofactors in the growth of prostate cancer, hormonal therapy offers the hope of stemming the course of
the disease process. There are several ways in which androgen levels can be
lowered, and when different modalities are combined, very low androgen
levels can be achieved.

Figure 11-2 illustrates the sites of action of various androgen-lowering
therapies. Estrogen and GnRH analogues block gonadotropin secretion. Ke-

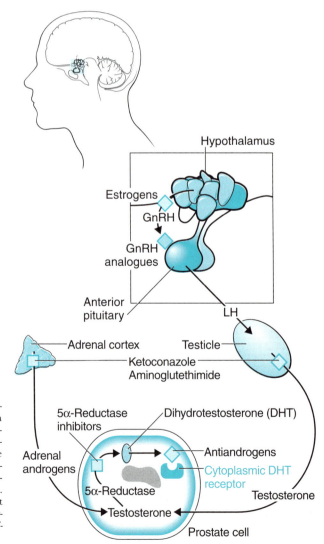

Figure 11-2. Sites of action of androgen-lowering therapies. Androgens can be lowered by a
number of medications. Gonadotropin secretion can be blocked by GnRH analogues. Adrenal and testicular steroid production can be
blocked by several drugs, including ketoconazole and aminoglutethimide. 5α-reductase inhibitors and antiandrogens also can be used.
Combinations of drugs, with effects at different
points in the axis, can be very effective in lowering androgen levels and in reducing the effects of androgens.

toconazole and aminoglutethimide inhibit the production of steroid hormones at both the adrenocortical and gonadal levels. The antiandrogens cyproterone and flutamide block the binding of dihydrotestosterone to the cytoplasmic receptor.

After considering the options, Mr. Phillips decided to have radiation therapy together with hormonal therapy. Other than some diarrhea and rectal urgency, Mr. Phillips tolerated the radiation treatments well.

He also started on monthly injections of goserelin acetate, a synthetic decapeptide analogue of GnRH. For several days after the first injection, he had some hot flashes, but these have stopped completely. Since starting the radiation treatments and the GnRH analogue, Mr. Phillips has been unable to have an erection that is adequate for intercourse. He is not able to ejaculate, and no longer has erections on awakening in the morning. Although fertility is no longer an issue, Mr. Phillips and his wife would like to be able to have intercourse on occasion.

Two months after Mr. Phillips started the goserelin, the following laboratory studies were obtained:

Test	Samuel Phillips	Normal
PSA	1.2 μg/L	0–4 μg/L
Testosterone, total	22 ng/dL	*Male:* Prepubertal: <100 ng/dL Adult: 300–1000 ng/dL

Goserelin is a synthetic analogue of GnRH. After initially stimulating the hypothalamic–pituitary–gonadal axis, this agent is a potent inhibitor of the axis. Prolonged stimulation of the gonadotropin-secreting cells of the anterior pituitary results in down-regulation and a marked decrease in the secretion of LH and FSH. As a result of the initial brief stimulation of the axis, some patients who are symptomatic may have worsening of bone pain or other symptoms, which is then followed by significant improvement. After 2 months of therapy, Mr. Phillips' testosterone level is very low, indicating successful suppression of the axis.

The problems of sexual performance that most men face in the course of treatment of prostate cancer are multifactorial in origin. The low testosterone levels that are desired to stem tumor growth may result in loss of both libido and erectile function. In addition, both radiation therapy and surgery in the region of the prostate can interfere with nerve function that is vital to normal erectile performance. An erection results when the flow of blood out of the corpora cavernosa of the penis is restricted and the inflow of blood is maintained or increased. Neural mechanisms control the inflows and outflows that can result in an erection.

For men with impotence, several options for improving erectile performance are available. The easiest is a semirigid condom that can be worn over the penis and may allow adequate vaginal penetration for intercourse.

External vacuum devices work by encasing the penis with a vacuum, which fills the corpora with blood. This penile engorgement is maintained by the placement of a properly-sized tourniquet band at the base of the penis. Surgically implanted rigid or inflatable devices also are available. Prostaglandins, either injected into the corpora or placed in the urethra, induce an erection in many impotent men. Each of these erectile assistance modalities, except the rigid condom and the implanted devices, requires adequate inflow of blood to achieve an erection and may not work for men whose impotence is based on vascular insufficiency.

After viewing the videotape, Mr. Phillips and his wife have decided that they would like to try the vacuum system. After a couple of practice sessions, they were able to have some sexual activity. Although it was different than it had been 20 years earlier, they were both pleased that they were able to resume some sexual activity.

Mr. Phillips will continue the goserelin injections. It is hoped that his cancer will stay in remission.

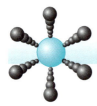

CASE PRESENTATION: CASE 5

Pneumonia in a 37-year-old man with HIV

Stephen Jenkins began using heroin shortly after he dropped out of medical school. In addition to working as a casual laborer, he supported himself and his drug usage by shoplifting and occasional opportunistic car theft. One bungled car theft resulted in a prison term of 6 months, and an opportunity to become drug-free. Shortly after his release from prison, however, he was back to using heroin and stealing cars. In prison, he learned that he had had hepatitis B at some point and also that he was HIV-positive. He was started on antiretroviral therapy, but because he felt well and the clinic visits and medication regimen were a hassle, he stopped them.

For the past 2 years, Mr. Jenkins has been homeless. Possessions that do not fit in the supermarket cart that he pushes around the city are stored under a bridge abutment near a railroad station. Once or twice a week he stays in a homeless shelter for the night, but most of the time he sleeps in a park or under a bridge. Now, at age 37, Stephen Jenkins is no longer using heroin. He buys food and cigarettes with money he gets from returning the bottles and cans that he picks up in the street and in the parks.

Cough, fever, shortness of breath, and marked weakness brought Mr. Jenkins to the emergency room.

Physical Examination

A disheveled, thin man with yellow stains on the second and third fingers of his right hand

Height:	**5′11″**
Weight:	**137 pounds**

Vital signs:

Blood Pressure	Pulse	Respirations	Temperature
Supine: 100/60	110, regular	22/min	101.2°F
Sitting: 80/50	130, regular		

HEENT:	**Poor oral hygiene, otherwise unremarkable**
Neck:	**Normal, no thyromegaly**
Chest:	**Fair air movement, clear**
Heart:	**Rapid, normal heart sounds**
Abdomen:	**Normal**
Genitals:	**Normal**
Extremities:	**Needle track marks in both antecubital fossae**
O$_2$ saturation on room air:	**78% (normal: >90%)**
Chest X-ray:	**Multiple healed rib fractures**
	Normal heart
	Prominent hila with ground-glass appearance of lung parenchyma

Laboratory Studies

Test	Stephen Jenkins	Normal
WBC	2900/mm^3	4300–10,800/mm^3
HCT	40.5%	42%–52%
Sodium	122 mEq/L	135–145 mEq/L
Potassium	5.9 mEq/L	3.5–5.0 mEq/L
Glucose	125 mg/dL	70–110 mg/dL, fasting

Based on these results, therapy with oxygen and intravenous fluids was begun. A cosyntropin test was performed, and while waiting for the results, Mr. Jenkins was started on hydrocortisone, 100 mg every 8 hours, intravenously.

Patients with advanced HIV disease occasionally display findings suggestive of adrenal insufficiency. Postural hypotension, hyponatremia, and hyperkalemia in any patient should raise the suspicion of adrenal insufficiency (see Chapter 5). Definitive testing for this possibility and treatment of the suspected adrenal insufficiency is, therefore, very appropriate. Adrenalitis resulting from cytomegalovirus (CMV) is seen in a significant proportion of HIV patients with CMV infection. Complete destruction of the adrenal cortex, however, is a very rare and very late complication of HIV. CMV and other opportunistic infections also can affect the anatomy and function of the hypothalamus and pituitary, leading to significant defects in anterior pituitary function.

Many medications used in the treatment of patients with HIV infection have an impact on the function of the adrenal cortex. Ketoconazole inhibits the p-450 side-chain cleavage and 11-hydroxylase enzymes and thereby decreases adrenocortical hormone production. Rifampin, phenytoin, and opiates are known to shorten the half-life of cortisol.

Some patients with HIV disease may exhibit high levels of cortisol without clinical evidence of cortisol excess. For some of these patients, the elevated cortisol levels are a reaction to the stress of the clinical situation, with cytokines stimulating the release of corticotropin-releasing hormone (CRH). For others, the elevated cortisol is caused by changes in cortisol-binding globulin. In addition, some patients develop an apparent acquired resistance to glucocorticoids. These patients have weakness and hyperpigmentation and have preservation of a diurnal ACTH rhythm, but at levels higher than normal. A change in glucocorticoid receptor affinity is a possible explanation for these findings.

Factors other than adrenal insufficiency could account for Mr. Jenkins' hyponatremia and hyperkalemia. Volume depletion and SIADH (see Chapter 3) from various causes, including pneumonia, can cause hyponatremia. Similarly, hyperkalemia can be the result of factors unrelated to adrenocortical function, induced by drugs or resulting from HIV-related nephropathy.

Later on the day of admission, an induced sputum showed *Pneumocystis* pneumonia, and intravenous trimethoprim-sulfamethoxazole was started. High-dose glucocorticoids also were started in the form of prednisone, 80 mg per day, and the hydrocortisone was discontinued.

Twenty-four hours after admission the results of the cosyntropin test became available, and the sodium and potassium levels were repeated:

Time (min)	Cortisol (μg/dL)
0	22
30	32
60	29

Test	Stephen Jenkins	Normal
Sodium	132 mEq/L	135–145 mEq/L
Potassium	4.5 mEq/L	3.5–5.0 mEq/L

Although Mr. Jenkins had several features consistent with adrenal insufficiency, his baseline cortisol level and the response to the ACTH stimulation were normal. The high-dose steroids were started to decrease that inflammatory reaction that the *Pneumocystis* organism generates in the lung parenchyma. The dose will be tapered over a 20-day period, and Mr. Jenkins should be able to stop all steroids at the end of that taper. There will be some suppression of hypothalamic–pituitary–adrenal axis function, but he should be able to recover from this quickly.

His electrolytes have improved. The hyponatremia probably was the result of a combination of volume depletion and some inappropriate ADH secretion triggered by the lung infection. The mechanism of the hyperkalemia is unclear, but it may have involved a transient change in renal function, related to volume status.

Several other endocrine abnormalities have been described in patients with HIV infection. Some patients develop hypocalcemia as a result of malnutrition or malabsorption. Some of the drugs used in the treatment of AIDS affect vitamin D activity, whereas others result in magnesium wasting, compromising parathyroid hormone function. The thyroid axis also can be affected during the course of HIV disease. Thyroid-binding globulin increases as CD4 counts decrease, altering thyroid function test results. Thyroid function usually is well maintained, however, except in the very rare cases when an opportunistic infection such as *Pneumocystis* causes a painful thyroiditis.

Gonadal function may be affected at several levels in patients with HIV disease. Oligoamenorrhea often is seen in women with HIV. In men, low levels of testosterone are common. Hypogonadotropic hypogonadism can be the result of the stress of severe illness, malnutrition, or infiltration of the hypothalamus or pituitary with CMV or toxoplasmosis. End-organ gonadal dysfunction as a result of opportunistic infections also is possible. Drugs used in the treatment of HIV-related illnesses also may affect the gonadal axis. For female patients, the use of oral contraceptives is an easy way to replenish sex hormones. For men, testosterone replacement may improve lean body mass, muscle strength, feelings of well-being, and sexual function.

After 10 days in the hospital and feeling very much better, Mr. Jenkins was discharged to a halfway house set up for individuals with HIV disease. He has started on a complicated retroviral regimen and will have some help managing his medications at the halfway house. He has a part-time job lined up at the homeless shelter where he used to stay on occasion. He hopes that he can start over and has promised to give it a try.

CASE PRESENTATION: CASE 6

Morbid obesity in a 34-year-old man

Robert McLaughlin has struggled with his weight since he was a teenager. He weighed 242 pounds and was 5'9" tall when he graduated from high school. After basic training in the Army, Mr. McLaughlin was the trimmest he had ever been, at 190 pounds. Following his discharge from the Army, and his return to a less active life as a computer repair technician, the weight just seemed to pour back on. He quickly surpassed his high school graduation weight and now, at age 34, he weighs about 325 pounds.

Mr. McLaughlin's life is significantly limited by his weight. His sleep is characterized by loud snoring and frequent episodes of apnea. During the day he can fall asleep very easily. Although he has not fallen asleep while driving, he keeps the radio turned up loud and the windows open. He is no longer able to climb more than one flight of stairs because of shortness of breath and knee pain.

Physical Examination

Height:	5′9″
Weight:	347 pounds
Body mass index (BMI):	51.5
Blood pressure (large cuff):	160/100, right arm, sitting
Pulse:	88, regular
Respiratory rate:	18/minute
HEENT:	Normal
Chest:	Clear
Heart:	Normal
Abdomen:	Obese, nonpigmented stretch marks, no organomegaly
Genitals:	Normal penis and testicles
Extemities:	Venous stasis changes of both lower extremities

Laboratory Studies

Test	Robert McLaughlin	Normal
Glucose, fasting	110 mg/dL	70–110 mg/dL, fasting
Cholesterol, fasting	283 mg/dL	<200 mg/dL (ideal)
TSH	1.2 mU/L	0.3–5.0 mU/L
24-hour urinary free cortisol	38 μg/24 hrs	20–70 μg/24 hrs

Although some endocrinopathies (e.g., hypothyroidism and Cushing's syndrome) are associated with weight gain, massive obesity is not often caused by an endocrine condition. Severe obesity does, however, have significant effects on the several aspects of endocrine function. Obesity results in insulin resistance and leads to hyperinsulinemia. If pancreatic B-cell function is limited or impaired, overt hyperglycemia and diabetes can result. In addition, for many patients with severe obesity, plasma lipid values become significantly elevated, bringing with them the risks of premature vascular disease. Hypertension and osteoarthritis also are often seen in patients with severe obesity. Sleep apnea, with symptoms similar to those of Mr. Mc-Laughlin, is much more common in massively obese patients.

Obesity is the most prevalent nutrition-related problem in industrialized societies. One third of adults in the United States are obese, a disproportionate number of whom are African American and Hispanic women. About 20% of children in the United States are obese. Obesity can be assessed by calculating the body mass index (BMI)—dividing the patient's weight in kilograms by the square of the height in meters:

$$BMI = kg/m^2$$

BMI correlates with body fat and with risks for heart disease, diabetes, hypertension, degenerative joint disease, dyslipidemias, and certain types of cancer. These risks increase significantly with a BMI of 25 or higher. The distribution of body fat plays an important role in the medical risks associated with obesity. The risk of associated morbidity and mortality is related to how much fat is located in the abdominal region, both intraabdominal and subcutaneous. Upper body, or android, obesity ("apple-shaped" obesity) often is accompanied by hyperinsulinemia, glucose intolerance, and hypertriglyceridemia, whereas lower body, or gynecoid, obesity ("pear-shaped" obesity) usually is benign.

Studies of twins, adoptees, and families indicate that as much as 80% of the variance in BMI can be attributed to genetic factors. The level of physical activity, the resting metabolic rate, and the various aspects of feeding behavior account for a smaller percentage of that variance. Obesity that develops early in life appears to be more likely to have a genetic component than does obesity that develops during adulthood. The inverse relationship between obesity and social class, however, is strong evidence of potent environmental influences.

The gene or genes that influence our eating patterns, basal metabolism, and physical activity remain a mystery, as does the way in which these genes exert their control over these functions. Geneticists have identified a number of such genes in several species of rodents, including the ob/ob mouse, which lacks the gene that encodes the blueprint for leptin, a hormone produced by adipose tissue. Without leptin, these mice have voracious appetites, are hypometabolic and hypothermic, and grow to three times normal weight. When these mice are given leptin, their appetites diminish, they lose weight, and their O_2 consumption and body temperature normalize. Leptin is thought to act as an afferent satiety signal in a feedback loop that affects the appetite and satiety centers in the hypothalamus. Humans possess an ob gene on chromosome 7q32.1, and its expression is increased in humans who are obese, but the relationship between leptin and human obesity remains unclear. A strong correlation exists between serum leptin concentrations and the percentage of body fat. The paradox of a high concentration of leptin, a hormone that suppresses appetite, in the face of obesity suggests that obese humans are insensitive to the actions of leptin. Whether this insensitivity reflects defects in the leptin receptor, postreceptor abnormalities in signal transmission, or other flaws in hypothalamic function remains an enigma. Leptin appears to be merely one of several factors in the dysregulated system linking the brain, food intake sensors, and adipose tissue mass. Additional factors that may contribute to the dysfunction that eventuates in obesity include neuropeptides that induce hyperphagia, deficiency of anorexigenic neuropeptides, and increased secretion of insulin or glucocorticoids.

Weight reduction by the mobilization of body fat stores can be achieved by creating an energy deficit. This goal is most easily achieved by expending more energy through activity than is taken in through eating. Restricting energy intake may necessitate merely choosing healthier foods or may include intentional caloric restriction. Experienced counselors advise that to increase long-term success and avoid severe caloric deficits, modest energy deficits (in the range of 500 kcal/day) should be recommended. Although very-low-calorie diets (<800 kcal/day) produce more immediate results, the chance of long-term success is low, and the possibility of mineral and vitamin deficits is high.

The primary method of increasing energy expenditure is increasing physical activity. Any energy-using activity that is appealing and feasible for the individual is beneficial. Persons who do not engage in regular activity should begin by incorporating a few minutes of increased activity during the day. Those who are already somewhat active often benefit from a plan to increase that activity or initiate a formal exercise routine. For obese individuals who have difficulty performing traditional exercises, dancing, floor exercises, water aerobics, and swimming are recommended.

Pharmacologic agents may be a useful adjunct to, but are never a substitute for, the necessary changes in eating patterns and physical activity. The effectiveness of pharmacologic agents depends on their use with appropriate dietary intervention as well as increased physical activity and alterations in lifestyle. Available over-the-counter medications include bulk-producing products that fill the stomach and suppress appetite. Agents that selectively interfere with fat absorption or increase energy expenditure are being developed. The anorexic agents that are currently available by prescription act on neurotransmitters in the brain to partially suppress appetite and reduce caloric intake. Coexisting conditions that contraindicate pharmacotherapy always must be considered. These include pregnancy, lactation, severe cardiovascular disease, and a number of concurrent medications. The effectiveness of anorexic medication should be evaluated early, because not all patients respond, and individuals who are not responsive after 3 to 6 weeks are unlikely to have any benefit.

Surgical treatment for obesity contributes to the establishment of an energy deficit by restricting caloric intake and by affecting absorption of nutrients. A surgical approach is considered only in people whose BMI is greater than 35 and who have comorbidities or other risk factors. The Roux-en-Y gastric bypass and the vertical banded gastroplasty are the procedures most commonly performed. Modifications of the gastric bypass that increase the malabsorptive component of the procedure with biliopancreatic diversion do increase weight loss, but they cause substantial increases in nutritional and metabolic complications. Surgical procedures require lifetime follow-up and should be performed only by experienced surgeons in collaboration with a knowledgeable healthcare team.

Three days before his scheduled follow-up visit, Mr. McLaughlin fell asleep while driving and ran into a utility pole. Luckily, no one was injured, but the car was seriously damaged. Mr. McLaughlin also fell asleep in the waiting room while waiting to be seen for his follow-up appointment. His loud snoring disturbed several people in the waiting room. Mr. McLaughlin was embarrassed when awakened. Following the accident, he decided that he had to do something about his weight.

He remembered basic training in the Army—hours of strenuous phys-

ical activity each day—but he was not sure that his knees would take the stress. Armed with some information about meal planning and portion size and with a plan for a graded exercise program, Mr. McLaughlin is embarking on a program that he hopes will allow him to make a major and, most importantly, permanent change in his weight. He plans to join the Walking Club at his church and will return for a follow-up appointment in 1 month.

Although many patients are successful in losing weight for brief periods, permanent, significant weight loss is a goal that is very difficult to achieve. Unfortunately, the motivation to make a change often comes when a complication of obesity, such as sleep apnea, a myocardial infarction, or a pulmonary embolus, develops. In addition to motivation and education, support and encouragement from professionals, family, and friends are important components of a successful weight management program.

KEY POINTS AND CONCEPTS

- Failure of one glandular system as a result of autoimmune destruction increases the possibility of other glandular failure syndromes.
- There are three types of multiple endocrine neoplasia (MEN):
  - MEN 1: pituitary, pancreas, parathyroid.
  - MEN 2a: medullary thyroid carcinoma, pheochromocytoma, hyperparathyroidism.
  - MEN 2b: medullary thyroid carcinoma, pheochromocytoma, mucosal neuromas.
- DNA screening of family members of patients with MEN syndromes is vitally important.
- Hormonal therapy may palliate the course of several malignancies. Hormonal therapy may be ablative or additive.
- Obesity has significant effects on intermediary metabolism, causing insulin resistance and hyperinsulinemia.
- HIV and related diseases may have an important impact on glandular systems, occasionally resulting in hypofunction.

SUGGESTED READING

Ahonen P, Myllamiemi S, Sipila I, et al. Clinical variation of autoimmune polyendocrinopathy-candidiasis-ectodermal dystrophy (APECED) in a series of 68 patients. N Engl J Med 322:1829–1836, 1990.

Colditz GA, Hankinson SE, Hunter DJ, et al. The use of estrogens and progestins and the risk of breast cancer in postmenopausal women. N Engl J Med 332:1589–1593, 1995.

Garnick MB, Fair WR. Prostate cancer: emerging concepts. Parts I and II. Ann Intern Med 125:118–125, 205–212, 1996.

Grinspoon SK, Bilezikian JB. HIV disease and the endocrine system. N Engl J Med 327:1360–1365, 1992.

Lips CJM, Landsvater RM, Hoppener JWM, et al. Clinical screening as compared with DNA analysis in families with multiple endocrine neoplasia type 2A. N Engl J Med 331:828–835, 1994.

Ravussin E, Swinburn BA. Energy expenditure and obesity. Diabetes Reviews 4:403–422, 1996.

Table of Normal Values

CHEMISTRY (BLOOD, PLASMA, AND SERUM)

ANALYTE	NORMAL RANGE	UNITS
Albumin	3.5–5.5	g/dL
Alkaline phosphatase	30–120	U/L
Amylase	60–180	U/L
Bicarbonate	21–30	mEq/L
BUN (blood urea nitrogen)	8–22	mg/dL
Calcium	8.5–10.5	mg/dL
Chloride	98–106	mEq/L
Cholesterol, total	<200 (ideal)	mg/dL
Cholesterol, HDL	>60 (ideal)	mg/dL
Cholesterol, LDL	<130 (primary prevention)	mg/dL
	<100 (secondary prevention)	mg/dL
Creatinine	0.3–1.5	mg/dL
Electrolytes		
Sodium	135–145	mEq/L
Potassium	3.5–5.0	mEq/L
Chloride	98–106	mEq/L
Bicarbonate	21–30	mEq/L
Gases, arterial blood		
P_{O_2}	80–100	mmHg
P_{CO_2}	35–45	mmHg
pH	7.38–7.44	
Glucose, fasting	70–110	mg/dL
Ketones (serum or plasma)	Negative	
Lipid profile, fasting		
Total cholesterol	<200 (ideal)	mg/dL
HDL cholesterol	>60 (ideal)	mg/dL
Triglycerides	<160 (ideal)	mg/dL
LDL cholesterol	<130 (primary prevention)	mg/dL
	<100 (secondary prevention)	mg/dL

CHEMISTRY (BLOOD, PLASMA, AND SERUM)
(Continued)

ANALYTE	NORMAL RANGE	UNITS
Magnesium	1.5–2.4	mg/dL
Osmolality	285–295	mOsm/kg
Phosphatase, alkaline	30–120	U/L
Phosphorus (phosphate)	3.0–4.5	mg/dL
Potassium	3.5–5.0	mEq/L
Prostate-specific antigen (PSA)	0.0–4.0	μg/L
Sodium	135–145	mEq/L
Triglycerides, fasting	<160	mg/dL
Urea nitrogen (BUN)	8–22	mg/dL

HEMATOLOGY

ANALYTE	NORMAL RANGE	UNITS
CBC (complete blood count)		
Hematocrit		
Female	37–48	%
Male	42–52	%
Hemoglobin		
Female	11.2–15.3	g/dL
Male	13.6–17.2	g/dL
White blood cell count	4300–10,800	cells/mm^3
Platelet count	140,000–430,000	cells/mm^3
Erythrocyte sedimentation rate (Westergren)		
Female	0–20	mm/hr
Male	0–15	mm/hr

ENDOCRINE CHEMISTRY (BLOOD, PLASMA, AND SERUM)

ANALYTE	NORMAL RANGE	UNITS
ACTH, 8 a.m.	<80	pg/mL
Aldosterone (normal sodium intake)		
Supine	2–5	ng/dL
Standing	7–20	ng/dL
Calcitonin		
Female	0–14	pg/mL
Male	0–28	pg/mL
Post–total thyroidectomy	<10	pg/mL
Chorionic gonadotropin (hCG, beta subunit), qualitative		
Pregnant	Positive	
Not pregnant	Negative	
Cortisol		
8 a.m.	5–25	μg/dL
5 p.m.	3–12	μg/dL
1 hour after cosyntropin	>18	μg/dL
Overnight dexamethasone suppression at 8 a.m.	<5	μg/dL
Dehydroepiandrosterone sulfate (DHEA-S)		
Male, adult	155–446	μg/dL
Female, adult	80–443	μg/dL
Follicle-stimulating hormone (FSH)		
Female		
Prepubertal	<5	mU/mL
Pre- or postovulatory	5–20	mU/mL
Ovulatory surge	12–40	mU/mL
Postmenopausal	>30	mU/mL
Male		
Prepubertal	<5	mU/mL
Adult	3–18	mU/mL
Growth hormone		
Fasting	2–6	ng/mL
After glucose load	<2	ng/mL
After stimulation	>7	ng/mL
Hemoglobin A_{1c} (HGB A_{1c})	3.5–5.6	%
17-hydroxyprogesterone (17-OH-progesterone)		
Female		
Follicular phase	0.1–1.0	μg/L
Luteal phase	0.5–3.5	μg/L

ENDOCRINE CHEMISTRY (BLOOD, PLASMA, AND SERUM) *(Continued)*

ANALYTE	NORMAL RANGE	UNITS
IGF-1 (insulin-like growth factor-1)		
Female (adult)	140–400	ng/mL
Male (adult)	54–325	ng/mL
Luteinizing hormone (LH)		
Female		
Prepubertal	<5	mU/mL
Pre- or postovulatory	3–35	mU/mL
Ovulatory surge	40–150	mU/mL
Postmenopausal	>30	mU/mL
Male		
Prepubertal	<5	mU/mL
Adult	3–18	mU/mL
Parathyroid hormone	10–65	pg/mL
Prolactin		
Female	5–25	ng/mL
Male	5–20	ng/mL
Renin activity (plasma)		
Normal diet		
Supine	0.3–1.9	μg/L per hr
Standing	0.3–3.6	μg/L per hr
Testosterone, total		
Female (adult)	20–90	ng/dL
Male		
Prepubertal	<15	ng/dL
Adult	300–1000	ng/dL
Testosterone, free		
Female (adult)	0.1–1.3	ng/dL
Male (adult)	3–24	ng/dL
Thyroid function tests		
T_4	5–12	μg/dL
T_3	80–200	ng/dL
T_3 resin uptake	25–35	%
TSH	0.3–5.0	mU/L
Vitamin D (25-dihydroxy, serum)		
Summer	15–80	ng/mL
Winter	14–42	ng/mL

URINE TESTS

ANALYTE	NORMAL RANGE	UNITS
Chorionic gonadotropin (hCG, beta subunit), qualitative		
Pregnant	Positive	
Not pregnant	Negative	
Microalbumin	<30	μg/mg creatinine
Osmolality (depends on volume status)	50–1200	mOsm/kg
Sodium		
Volume depleted	<25	mEq/L
Volume overloaded	>70	mEq/L
Urinalysis		
Color	Yellow, clear	
Specific gravity	1.001–1.020	
Protein	Negative	
Blood	Negative	
Glucose	Negative	
Ketones	Negative	
Protein	Negative	
Nitrite	Negative	
Leukocytes	<4/high-power field	
Red blood cells	<4/high-power field	

URINE TESTS: TIMED COLLECTIONS

ANALYTE	NORMAL RANGE	UNITS
Cortisol (urinary free cortisol)—24 hr	20–70	μg/24 hr
17-hydroxysteroid excretion (17-OH steroids)—24 hr		
Female	2.0–6.0	mg/24 hr
Male	3.0–10.0	mg/24 hr
17-ketosteroid excretion—24 hr		
Female (adult)	3.0–15.0	mg/24 hr
Male (adult)	9.0–22.0	mg/24 hr
Microalbumin		
Normal	<30	mg/24 hr
Microalbuminuria	30–300	mg/24 hr
Albuminuria	>300	mg/24 hr

OTHER TESTS

TEST	NORMAL RANGE	UNITS
Barr bodies		
Female	>50	%
Male	<20	%
Karyotype		
Female	46,XX	
Male	46,XY	
Radioactive iodine uptake, 24 hr	10–25	%
Semen analysis		
Volume	2–6 mL	mL
Count	>20	$\times 10^6$/mL
Motility	>60	% motile
Morphology	>60	% normal

Case Study Index

POSTERIOR PITUITARY (CHAPTER 3)

CASE	DIAGNOSIS	DESCRIPTION	NAME
1	Diabetes insipidus	Polyuria and polydipsia in a 24-year-old woman	Myra Wilson
2	Inappropriate secretion of ADH and diabetes insipidus	Wide fluctuations in water balance following pituitary surgery in a 58-year-old man	Charles McHenry
3	Inappropriate secretion of ADH as a result of a lung tumor	Hyponatremia in a 65-year-old man with a lung mass	Donald Granger

THYROID (CHAPTER 4)

CASE	DIAGNOSIS	DESCRIPTION	NAME
1	Graves' disease	Hyperthyroxinemia in a woman with a diffusely enlarged thyroid	Jane Jones
2	Toxic adenoma	Hyperthyroxinemia and a "hot" nodule in a 52-year-old man with coronary artery disease	James Richardson
3	Toxic multinodular goiter	Hyperthyroxinemia in an elderly woman with a multinodular goiter	Joan Stark
4	Increased thyroid-binding protein	Hyperthyroxinemia in a 25-year-old woman on oral contraceptives	Alice Avery
5	Subacute thyroiditis	Hyperthyroxinemia in a 30-year-old woman with a sore neck	Marian Masters
6	Excess exogenous thyroid hormone	Toxic effects of exogenous thyroid hormone in a 38-year-old man	Walter "Tiny" Griswald
7	Primary hypothyroidism	Hypothyroxinemia in a 32-year-old woman with menorrhagia and an enlarged thyroid gland	Susan Gilman
8	"Cold" nodule—papillary carcinoma of the thyroid	Thyroid nodule found during a routine physical examination in a 32-year-old man	Mark Cohen

ADRENAL CORTEX (CHAPTER 5)

CASE	DIAGNOSIS	DESCRIPTION	NAME
1	Cushing's disease	Truncal obesity, striae, hypertension, and glucose intolerance in a 39-year-old man	Charles Denney
2	Ectopic production of ACTH	Fatigue, hypokalemia, and a lung mass in a 65-year-old man	William Atkinson
3	Addison's disease	Fatigue, hyperpigmentation, and hyperkalemia in a 38-year-old woman	Anne Darlington
4	Cushing's syndrome caused by exogenous steroids	The problems of exogenous steroids in a 48-year-old woman	Marjorie Young
5	Congenital adrenal hyperplasia	Hirsutism and menstrual irregularity in a 21-year-old woman	Alison Rossiter

CALCIUM METABOLISM (CHAPTER 6)

CASE	DIAGNOSIS	DESCRIPTION	NAME
1	Hyperparathyroidism	Urolithiasis and hypercalcemia in a 54-year-old woman	Agnes Allen
2	Hypervitaminosis D	Coma and hypercalcemia in an older man	Clarence Hamilton
3	Hypercalcemia caused by metastatic disease	Lethargy and hypercalcemia in a 68-year-old woman with metastatic breast cancer	Emma Watson
4	Vitamin D deficiency	Hypocalcemia and bone pain in a 50-year-old woman	Maria Renaldi
5	Osteoporosis	Loss of height and back pain in a 70-year-old woman	Wilma Larson

GLUCOSE METABOLISM (CHAPTER 7)

CASE	DIAGNOSIS	DESCRIPTION	NAME
1	Type 1 diabetes mellitus	Polyuria, polydipsia, and weight loss in a 13-year-old girl	Robin Tyler
2	Type 2 diabetes mellitus	Fatigue and hypertension in a 53-year-old man	James Howard
3	Nonketotic hyperosmolar coma	Lethargy and marked hyperglycemia in a 72-year-old woman	Dorothy Lauer

LIPID METABOLISM (CHAPTER 8)

CASE	DIAGNOSIS	DESCRIPTION	NAME
1	Hypertriglyceridemia	Abdominal pain and lactescent serum in a 33-year-old man	William Leonard
2	Hypercholesterolemia	Hypercholesterolemia in a 39-year-old man with a strong family history of heart disease	Walter Anderson

REPRODUCTIVE DISORDERS (CHAPTER 9)

CASE	DIAGNOSIS	DESCRIPTION	NAME
1	Premature ovarian failure	Amenorrhea and dyspareunia in a 34-year-old woman	Eleanor O'Reardon
2	Testicular feminization	Primary amenorrhea in an 18-year-old woman	Theresa Fleming
3	Kleinfelter's syndrome	A 17-year-old male who has not yet gone through puberty	Charles Goddard
4	Exogenous androgen use	Steroid use in a 27-year-old body builder	J. J. Edmunds
5	Kallman's syndrome	Hypogonadism and anosmia in a 24-year-old man	Jason Fernandez
6	Polycystic ovary syndrome	Amenorrhea and hirsutism in a 27-year-old woman	Florence Jackson
7	Jogger's amenorrhea	Secondary amenorrhea in a 21-year-old woman who runs 5 miles per day	Erica Long
8	Erectile impotence	Erectile impotence in a 57-year-old man with diabetes	Paul Davis

A *t* following a page number indicates a table and an *f* following a page number indicates a figure. Drugs are listed under their generic names. When a drug trade name is listed, the reader is referred to the generic name.